RADIOLOGY

CASE REVIEW SERIES | Interventional Radiology

Notice

Medicine is an ever-changing science. As new research and clinical experience broaden our knowledge, changes in treatment and drug therapy are required. The authors and the publisher of this work have checked with sources believed to be reliable in their efforts to provide information that is complete and generally in accord with the standards accepted at the time of publication. However, in view of the possibility of human error or changes in medical sciences, neither the authors nor the publisher nor any other party who has been involved in the preparation or publication of this work warrants that the information contained herein is in every respect accurate or complete, and they disclaim all responsibility for any errors or omissions or for the results obtained from use of the information contained in this work. Readers are encouraged to confirm the information contained herein with other sources. For example and in particular, readers are advised to check the product information sheet included in the package of each drug they plan to administer to be certain that the information contained in this work is accurate and that changes have not been made in the recommended dose or in the contraindications for administration. This recommendation is of particular importance in connection with new or infrequently used drugs.

RADIOLOGY

CASE REVIEW SERIES | Interventional Radiology

Matthew DBS Tam, MA(Oxon), MRCS, FRCR, MClinEd

Consultant Interventional Radiologist
Department of Radiology
Southend University Hospital NHS Foundation Trust
Westcliff on Sea, Essex, United Kingdom

Honorary Senior Clinical Lecturer
Postgraduate Medical Institute
Anglia Ruskin University
Rivermead Campus, Essex, United Kingdom

Weiping Wang, MD, FSIR

Staff Interventional Radiologist
Section of Interventional Radiology
Imaging Institute
Cleveland Clinic, Cleveland
Ohio, United States

SERIES EDITOR

Roland Talanow, MD, PhD

President
Department of Radiology Education
Radiolopolis, a subdivision of InnoMed, LLC
Stateline, Nevada

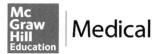

New York   Chicago   San Francisco   Athens   London
Madrid   Mexico City   Milan   New Delhi   Singapore
Sydney   Toronto

Radiology Case Review Series: Interventional Radiology

Copyright © 2014 by McGraw-Hill Education. All rights reserved. Printed in the U.S.A. Except as permitted under the United States Copyright Act of 1976, no part of this publication may be reproduced or distributed in any form or by any means, or stored in a data base or retrieval system, without the prior written permission of the publisher.

7 8 9 10 LKV 24 23 22 21

ISBN 978-0-07-176051-5
MHID 0-07-176051-2

This book was set in Times LT Std. by Thomson Digital.
The editors were Michael Weitz and Karen G. Edmonson.
The production supervisor was Richard C. Ruzycka.
Project management was provided by Shaminder Pal Singh, Thomson Digital.
The cover designer was Thomas De Pierro.
LSC Communications, was printer and binder.

This book is printed on acid-free paper.

CIP is on file with the publisher.

Dedicated to all radiology students who will find this text helpful in their studies.

Contents

Series Preface

Maybe I have an obsession for cases, but when I was a radiology resident I loved to learn especially from cases, not only because they are short, exciting, and fun—similar to a detective story in which the aim is to get to "the bottom" of the case—but also because, in the end, that's what radiologists are faced with during their daily work. Since medical school, I have been fascinated with learning, not only for my own benefit but also for the sake of teaching others, and I have enjoyed combining my IT skills with my growing knowledge to develop programs that help others in their learning process. Later, during my radiology residency, my passion for case-based learning grew to a level where the idea was born to create a case-based journal: integrating new concepts and technologies that aid in the traditional learning process. Only a few years later, the *Journal of Radiology Case Reports* became an internationally popular and PubMed indexed radiology journal—popular not only because of the interactive features but also because of the case-based approach. This led me to the next step: why not tackle something that I especially admired during my residency but that could be improved—creating a new interactive case-based review series. I imagined a book series that would take into account new developments in teaching and technology and changes in the examination process.

As did most other radiology residents, I loved the traditional case review books, especially for preparation for the boards. These books are quick and fun to read and focus in a condensed way on material that will be examined in the final boards. However, nothing is perfect and these traditional case review books had their own intrinsic flaws. The authors and I have tried to learn from our experience by putting the good things into this new book series but omitting the bad parts and exchanging them with innovative features.

What are the features that distinguish this series from traditional series of review books?

To save space, traditional review books provide two cases on one page. This requires the reader to turn the page to read the answer for the first case but could lead to unintentional "cheating" by seeing also the answer of the second case. Doesn't this defeat the purpose of a review book? From my own authoring experience on the *USMLE Help* book series, it was well appreciated that we avoided such accidental cheating by separating one case from the other. Taking the positive experience from that book series, we decided that each case in this series should consist of two pages: page 1

with images and questions and page 2 with the answers and explanations. This approach avoids unintentional peeking at the answers before deciding on the correct answers yourself. We keep it strict: one case per page! This way it remains up to your own knowledge to figure out the right answer.

Another example that residents (including me) did miss in traditional case review books is that these books did not highlight the pertinent findings on the images: sometimes, even looking at the images as a group of residents, we could not find the abnormality. This is not only frustrating but also time consuming. When you prepare for the boards, you want to use your time as efficiently as possible. Why not show annotated images? We tackled that challenge by providing, on the second page of each case, the same images with annotations or additional images that highlight the findings.

When you are preparing for the boards and managing your clinical duties, time is a luxury that becomes even more precious. Does the resident preparing for the boards truly need lengthy discussions as in a typical textbook? Or does the resident rather want a "rapid fire" mode in which he or she can "fly" through as many cases as possible in the shortest possible time? This is the reality when you start your work after the boards! Part of our concept with the new series is providing short "pearls" instead of lengthy discussions. The reader can easily read and memorize these "pearls."

Another challenge in traditional books is that questions are asked on the first page and no direct answer is provided, only a lengthy block of discussion. Again, this might become time consuming to find the right spot where the answer is located if you have doubts about one of several answer choices. Remember: time is money—and life! Therefore, we decided to provide explanations to *each* individual question, so that the reader knows exactly where to find the right answer to the right question. Questions are phrased in an intuitive way so that they fit not only the print version but also the multiple-choice questions for that particular case in our online version. This system enables you to move back and forth between the print version and the online version.

In addition, we have provided up to 3 references for each case. This case review is not intended to replace traditional textbooks. Instead, it is intended to reiterate and strengthen your already existing knowledge (from your training) and to fill potential gaps in your knowledge.

However, in a collaborative effort with the *Journal of Radiology Case Reports* and the international radiology community Radiolopolis, we have developed an online repository with more comprehensive information for each case, such as demographics, discussions, more image examples, interactive image stacks with scroll, a window/level feature, and other interactive features that almost resemble a workstation. In addition, we are planning ahead toward the new Radiology Boards format and are providing rapid fire online sessions and mock examinations that use the cases in the print version. Each case in the print version is crosslinked to the online version using a case ID. The case ID number appears to the right of the diagnosis heading at the top of the second page of each case. Each case can be accessed using the case ID number at the following web site: www.radiologycasereviews.com/case/ID, in which "ID" represents the case ID number. If you have any questions regarding this web site, please e-mail the series editor directly at roland@talanow.info.

I am particularly proud of such a symbiotic endeavor of print and interactive online education and I am grateful to McGraw-Hill for giving me and the authors the opportunity to provide such a unique and innovative method of radiology education, which, in my opinion, may be a trendsetter.

The primary audience of this book series is the radiology resident, particularly the resident in the final year who is preparing for the radiology boards. However, each book in

this series is structured on difficulty levels so that the series also becomes useful to an audience with limited experience in radiology (nonradiologist physicians or medical students) up to subspecialty-trained radiologists who are preparing for their CAQs or who just want to refresh their knowledge and use this series as a reference.

I am delighted to have such an excellent team of US and international educators as authors on this innovative book series. These authors have been thoroughly evaluated and selected based on their excellent contributions to the *Journal of Radiology Case Reports*, the Radiolopolis community, and other academic and scientific accomplishments.

It brings especially personal satisfaction to me that this project has enabled each author to be involved in the overall decision-making process and improvements regarding the print and online content. This makes each participant not only an author but also part of a great radiology product that will appeal to many readers.

Finally, I hope you will experience this case review book as it is intended to be: a quick, pertinent, "get to the point" radiology case review that provides essential information for the radiology boards in the shortest time available, which, in the end, is crucial for preparation for the boards.

Roland Talanow, MD, PhD

Preface

It is a pleasure and privilege to be an interventional radiologist. We are able to not only make diagnoses, but also treat a large variety of conditions all around the body using so many different techniques.

Interventional radiology skills are hard-earned and rely upon a broad medical training, diagnostic radiology skills, and an extensive and graduated exposure to all procedures rising in complexity through to fellowship.

Interventional radiology is what it is today, thanks to a wonderful faculty of extremely gifted and inspiring radiologists who have preceded us and continue to progress in the field with their research, innovation, and vision.

No book or educational endeavor can be comprehensive, but we hope that our case book can inspire and encourage future interventional radiologists and we are sure the second edition will have many new things

M.T.
W.W.

Matthew DBS Tam, MA(Oxon), MRCS, FRCR, MClinEd is a Consultant Interventional Radiologist at Southend University Hospital NHS Foundation Trust, and an Honorary Senior Clinical Lecturer at the Postgraduate Medical Institute, Anglia Ruskin University, United Kingdom.

Weiping Wang, MD, FSIR is a Staff Interventional Radiologist at Cleveland Clinic, Ohio, United States, and a Fellow of the Society of Interventional Radiology. Dr. Wang is the founder of CirClub, an online based cardiovascular and interventional radiology educational organization.

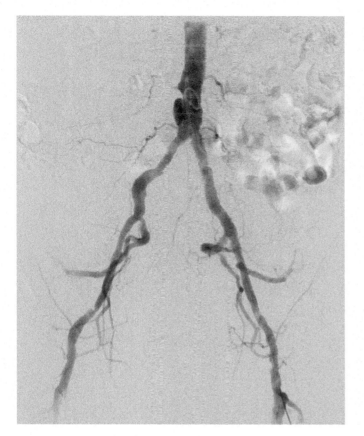 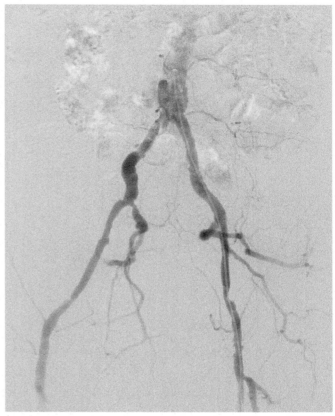

1. What are risk factors for aortoiliac disease?

2. Name some indications for angioplasty of iliac stenosis.

3. What is the most important safety consideration if you are undertaking iliac angioplasty?

4. What is the 3-year patency of iliac angioplasty?

5. Name some complications of iliac angioplasty.

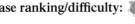 Case ranking/difficulty: 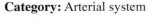 **Category:** Arterial system

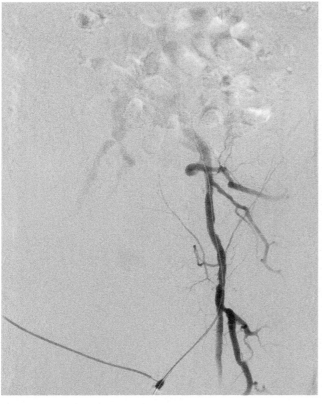

Left anterior oblique view, post angioplasty of left external iliac lesion.

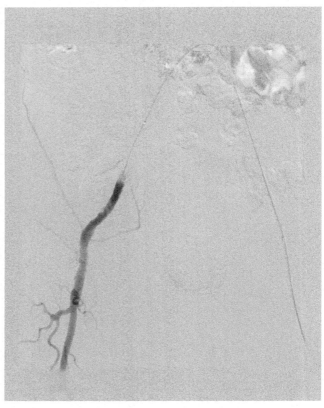

Post angioplasty of right external iliac lesion, treated from left side.

Answers

1. Smoking, hypertension, diabetes, and hypercholesterolemia are risk factors.

2. Iliac angioplasty is indicated for lifestyle-limiting claudication and critical ischemia. Asymptomatic lesions may be treated if this would facilitate EVAR, and high-grade contralateral lesions may become symptomatic after the ipsilateral lesion is treated (the patient may initially feel only limited by the left leg, but when this side is treated, previously masked symptoms become noticeable on the right side). Asymptomatic lesions found above grafts should also be treated.

3. Intravenous access, cardiopulmonary monitoring, and pre-procedural renal function and coagulation profiles are important but the storage of a covered stent in the suite is of critical importance as angioplasty can cause iliac rupture, and prompt placement of a covered stent may be life-saving.

4. This is reported to be around 70%.

5. Iliac artery rupture is a serious complication that is potentially life-threatening.

Pearls

- This case demonstrates bilateral external iliac stenotic disease. Note that multiple angiographic views are required in order to visualize the stenoses. Anteroposterior (AP) and both right anterior oblique (RAO) and LAO views are useful. The oblique will tend to open the contralateral iliac bifurcation, and as seen here, the LAO view demonstrates the right iliac bifurcation well. Note also how the left external iliac stenosis is not clearly seen on the AP but easily seen on the LAO view. Both lesions were successfully angioplastied.

Suggested Reading

Toshifumi Kudo, Fiona A Chandra, Samuel S Ahn. Long-term outcomes and predictors of iliac angioplasty with selective stenting. *J Vasc Surg.* 2005;42(3):466-475.

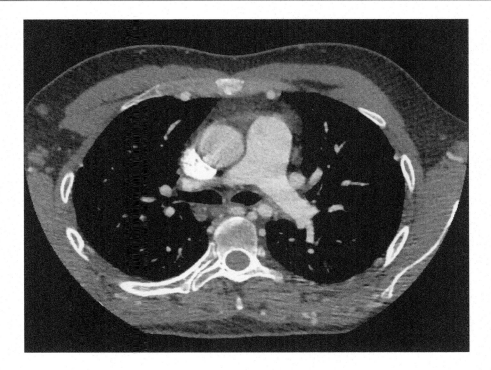

1. What is the diagnosis?

2. Which are the treatment options available?

3. Which investigation is most important after diagnosis?

4. What is the mean survival in this condition?

5. What are the complications of angioplasty in this condition?

Case ranking/difficulty: 🐾

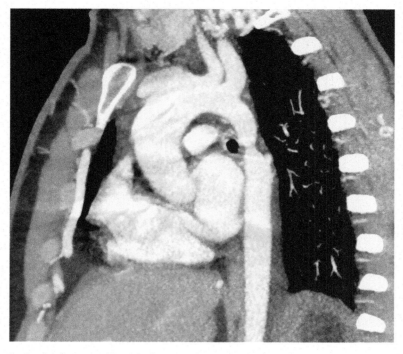

Sagittal reformatted image showing the site of coarctation.

Answers

1. This is postductal aortic coarctation.

2. Stenting, angioplasty, surgery, and conservative management are all options. Angioplasty has a largely palliative role as there is a higher rate of recurrence. Stent graft placement is evolving and may well have similar results to surgery.

3. Brain imaging is important, as 10% of those with coarctation have intracranial aneurysms.

4. Mean survival is 33 years; 90% of people with coarctation will die before reaching their sixth decade. About 20% of coarctations present in adulthood. With modern techniques, recoarctation rates are probably of the order of around 10%.

5. Angioplasty can lead to restenosis if under-sized, or aneurysm formation if over-sized. Patients, however, can outgrow stents and recoarctation can occur. Balloon size can be chosen by judging the size of the aorta at the diaphragmatic hiatus, and kissing balloon techniques allow the use of smaller sheath sizes in children.

Pearls

- Coarctation of the aorta accounts for 6% to 8% of congenital heart defects. It can affect any part of the descending thoracic, and also abdominal aorta.
- It can be classified into preductal, ductal, and postductal.
- It can present late in adolescence or early adulthood. Endovascular repair with stent graft or uncovered stents is safe and may be an alternative to surgery.
- Collateral vessels are responsible for the classical sign of rib notching.

Suggested Reading

Turner DR, Gaines PA. Endovascular management of coarctation of the aorta. *Semin Intervent Radiol.* 2007;24(2):153-166.

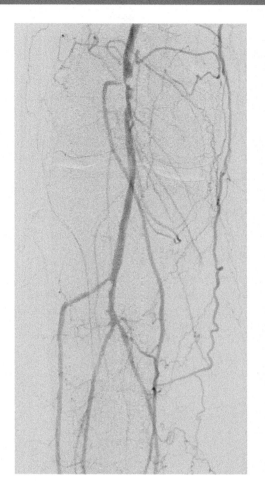 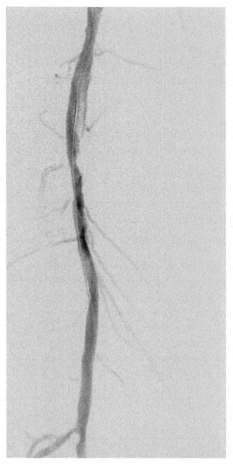

1. The popliteal artery always arises from the superficial femoral artery—true or false?

2. The popliteal artery always divides into the anterior tibial and tibioperoneal trunk—true or false?

3. List 4 pathologies, other than atherosclerosis, that can affect the popliteal artery.

4. What is the 1-year patency rate for popliteal angioplasty?

5. List some combinations of equipment that you would use to perform a popliteal angioplasty after obtaining arterial access.

Case ranking/difficulty: 🐢

Category: Arterial system

Answers

1. In one anatomic variant, this does not hold true. A persistent sciatic artery arises from the internal iliac artery, leaves the pelvis through the greater sciatic foramen, and continues in the posterior thigh, where it gives rise to the popliteal artery.

2. There are multiple variations in anatomy at this site, such as a high origin of the anterior tibial and a trifurcation.

3. Popliteal entrapment syndrome and cystic adventitial disease of the popliteal artery are important entities. Aneurysm formation and traumatic injury from a posterior knee dislocation also occur.

4. One-year patency is around 75%.

5. A 5 Fr sheath, 0.035" wire, and a 4 mm or 5 mm angioplasty balloon could be used. Similarly, low-profile 0.018" equipment can be used, which can be inserted through a 4 Fr sheath. Balloon-expandable stents are not recommended as they would be subject to external compression. Self-expanding stents may be used if there is elastic recoil or dissection but care should be taken with use of stents around the knee joint.

Pearls

- This is an image from an antegrade right leg angiogram. The image demonstrates stenotic disease in the popliteal artery. Note the collateral vessels. The anterior tibial artery, tibioperoneal trunk, common peroneal, and posterior tibial are patent but also have some mild stenotic disease. Postangioplasty images demonstrate improved patency and reduction in collaterals, with some residual irregularity that is acceptable and likely to remodel over time.

Suggested Reading

Adam DJ, Beard JD, Cleveland T, et al. Bypass versus angioplasty in severe ischaemia of the leg (BASIL): multicentre, randomised controlled trial. *Lancet.* 2005;366(9501):1925-1934.

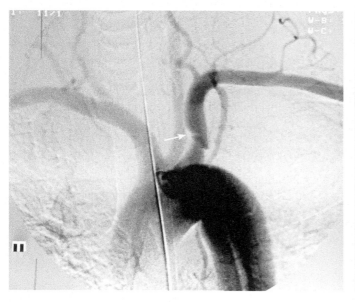 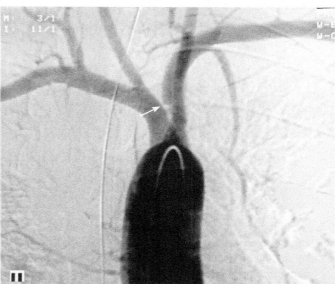

1. Which is the best projection for an arch aortogram?

2. What is the abnormality?

3. Which part of the left subclavian artery is more likely injured?

4. List 5 possible treatments for a subclavian artery trauma.

5. What other tests should be considered in this patient?

Case ranking/difficulty:

Category: Arterial system

Answers

1. Left anterior oblique view 30 to 40 degrees is usually the best projection.

2. There is irregularity of the left subclavian artery consistent with transection.

3. The origin of the left subclavian artery is most commonly injured as this is fixed to the aortic arch, whereas the distal artery is free and more mobile.

4. Surgical repair, ligation, or bypass are possible surgical options. Endovascular stent grafting can be performed. Conservative management is also possible as collaterals can develop.

5. Evaluation of the trauma patient will include CXR and CT. Esophagoscopy and bronchoscopy may also be indicated. There should always be a high index of suspicion for other injuries in major trauma.

Pearls

- Trauma to the subclavian artery is rare. It occurs more frequently as a result of blunt trauma or penetrating injury but those injured may not make it to a hospital setting. Endovascular approaches to repair are becoming more commonplace.

Suggested Reading

Shalhub S, Starnes BW, Hatsukami TS, Karmy-Jones R, Tran NT. Repair of blunt thoracic outlet arterial injuries: an evolution from open to endovascular approach. *J Trauma.* 2011;71(5):E114-E121.

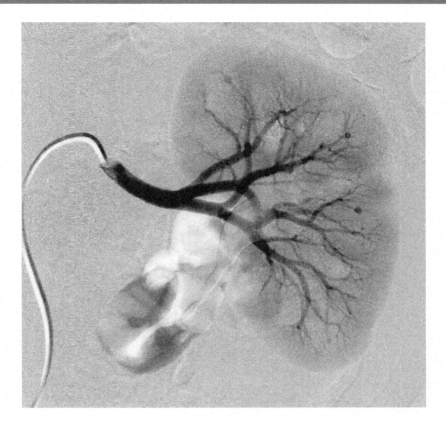

1. What is the diagnosis?

2. What are the key angiographic findings of this condition?

3. Which arterial territories may be affected?

4. What are recognized treatments for this condition?

5. What is the incidence?

Case ranking/difficulty:

Category: Arterial system

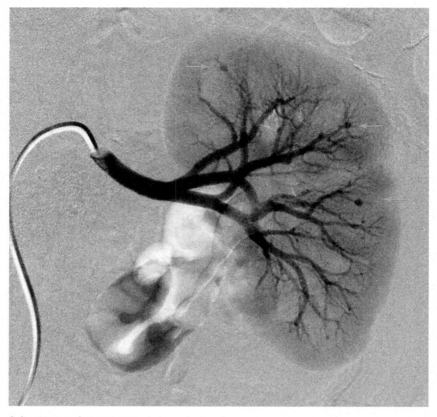

Selective renal angiogram.

Answers

1. Diagnostic catheter angiography shows polyarteritis nodosa (PAN).

2. Fusiform and saccular microaneurysm measuring 1 to 5 mm are diagnostic of PAN.

3. Renal, mesenteric, and hepatic branches are commonly affected.

4. Medical therapy includes corticosteroids and other immunosuppressive therapies.

5. A rare condition, with a reported incidence of 1.6 per 1,000,000 in European countries.

Pearls

- Polyarteritis nodosa is a vasculitis that affects small and medium-sized arteries.
- Multiple small microaneurysms (2- to 5-mm) are said to be pathognomic of this condition.

Suggested Reading

Jee KN, Ha HK, Lee IJ, et al. Radiologic findings of abdominal polyarteritis nodosa. *AJR Am J Roentgenol.* 2000;174(6):1675-1679.

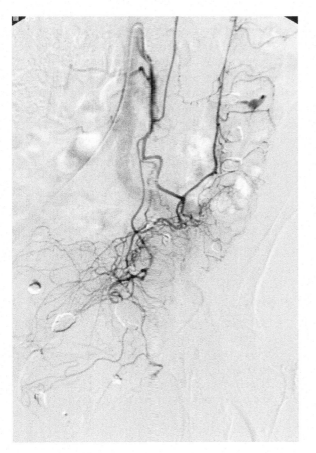
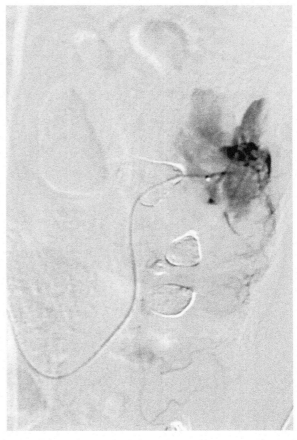

1. What is the cause of hemorrhage?

2. When would you perform angiography in GI bleeding?

3. What pharmaceutical agents may aid the detection of GI bleeding or its subsequent embolization?

4. Which is the embolic agent of choice in this case?

5. What is the risk of causing bowel infarction during an embolization procedure and what other factors can improve detection rates during angiography?

Case ranking/difficulty: 🌰

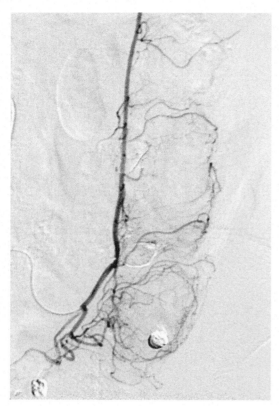

Angiogram after embolization showing cessation of contrast extravasation.

3. Buscopan and glucagon reduce bowel gas artifact. Glyceryl trinitrate reduces vasospasm. In the case of recurrent GI bleeds, "provocative mesenteric angiography" may be performed, where tissue plasminogen activator (tPA) and heparin are administered intraarterially in a controlled setting. Their use is not recommended in the acute setting. Methylene blue can also help localize bleeding if not seen at angiography; this can help at subsequent laparotomy.

4. Superselective embolization of the vasa recta is best achieved through the use of microcoils. Other agents would increase the risk of bowel ischemia.

5. Risk of bowel infarction after selective embolization is around 3%. Attention to technique in performing and framing angiograms can aid detection rates.

Pearls

- Left-sided diverticulosis is common in westernized nations.
- It is frequently a cause of massive lower GI tract bleeding.
- Selective inferior mesenteric artery (IMA) angiography and embolization is a therapeutic option.

Answers

1. The hemorrhage is from a bleeding diverticulum.

2. Hypotension, massive ongoing bleeding, and evidence of a positive site of bleeding on CT mean that angiography is more likely to show a target, and embolization likely to help.

Suggested Reading

Kuo WT, Lee DE, Saad WE, Patel N, Sahler LG, Waldman DL. Superselective microcoil embolization for the treatment of lower gastrointestinal hemorrhage. *J Vasc Interv Radiol.* 2003;14(12):1503-1509.

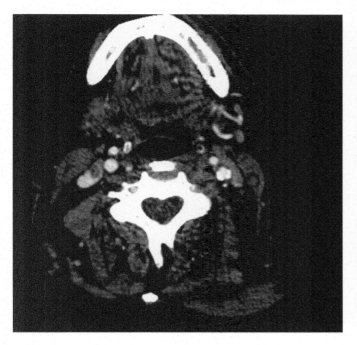 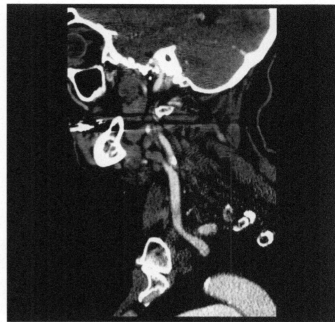

1. What are signs of a significant carotid stenosis?

2. What factors indicate a significant stenosis on ultrasound specifically?

3. How many branches does the internal carotid artery (ICA) have in the neck?

4. What unexpected findings might be seen on a carotid computed tomographic angiography?

5. What other features does the vascular surgeon want to know about?

Case ranking/difficulty: 🐢

Answers

1. A significant carotid stenosis is defined as being 70% to 99% stenosed. On computed tomography (CT), luminal narrowing can be assessed by comparing the lumen at the site of stenosis with the size of the artery above and below the lesion. Care must be taken to closely review the axial images and the multiplanar reformats. Maximum intensity projection (MIP) and volume rendering (VR) images should not be used to assess for stenosis.

2. An ICA of >230 cm/sec or an ICA–common carotid artery (CCA) ratio >4 indicates significant stenosis. If the ultrasonographic findings are equivocal or the ICA is hard to assess because of patient factors such as tortuosity, a short neck, and heavy calcification, CT can be used.

3. Zero.

4. Remember that the base of skull, intracranial vessels, arch, cervical spine, and lung apices are all well visualized on a CT carotid angiogram and must be reviewed and reported upon—the so-called nonvascular or incidental findings.

5. Knowing the level of the bifurcation, for example, relative to the angle of the mandible, is also particularly useful for the vascular surgeon.

Pearls

- Patients with symptomatic carotid artery stenosis present with stroke, transient ischemic attack, and amaurosis fugax. Data regarding significant stenotic disease is derived from the North American Symptomatic Carotid Endarterectomy Trial and the European Symptomatic Carotid Trial. Ultrasonography is the main diagnostic modality. Computed tomographic angiography is useful when ultrasonographic findings are uncertain because of heavy calcification. Carotid endarterectomy prevents strokes. Carotid stenting has similar results in terms of stroke prevention but may be associated with increased complications.

Suggested Reading

Schmidt KI, Papanagiotou P, Zimmer A, Schäfers HJ, Reith W. Carotid artery stenosis: current state of therapy [in German]. *Radiologe.* 2010;50(7):614-622.

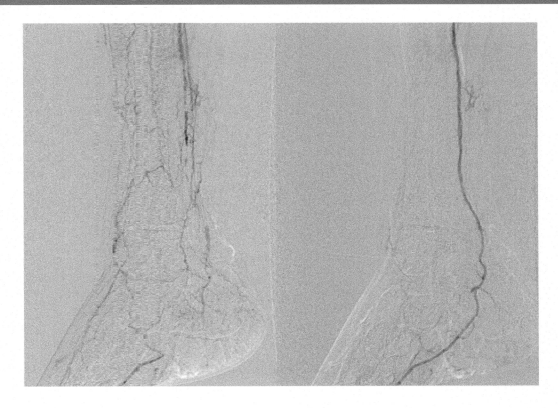

1. What is the definition of critical ischemia?

2. Do you know any classifications of peripheral arterial disease?

3. What is the main endpoint for infrapopliteal angioplasty?

4. If angioplasty was unsuccessful in this case, what would the next step be?

5. Which are useful intraprocedural medications?

Case ranking/difficulty:    Category: Arterial system

Answers

1. Rest pain, ulceration, and gangrene are features of critical limb ischemia.

2. Rutherford, Fontaine, and the Trans-Atlantic Inter-Society Consensus Document on the Management of Peripheral Arterial Disease (TASC II) are useful classifications. SAFARI (subintimal arterial flossing with antegrade-retrograde intervention) is a method of subintimal recanalization. ACT in these circles refers to activated clotting time, a method of monitoring heparinization.

3. The aim of infrapopliteal angioplasty is to promote wound healing. More than one vessel may be targeted. The most appropriate vascular territory is described by the "angiosome" concept.

4. Distal bypass using vein graft is the best alternative. Prosthetic grafts have worse results in this setting. However, the patient may not be fit for major surgery.

5. Use of sedoanalgesia, heparin, and arterial vasodilators is important.

Pearls

- Critical limb ischemia is defined as tissue loss or rest pain longer than 2 weeks with evidence of arterial disease. Typical presentations are those of rest pain, ulceration, and gangrene.
- Angioplasty distal to the popliteal artery should only be performed for critical ischemia, not for claudication. Patients are at risk of amputation without revascularization.
- Distal arterial disease is commonly seen in diabetics.

Suggested Reading

Markose G, Bolia A. Below the knee angioplasty among diabetic patients. *J Cardiovasc Surg (Torino)*. 2009;50(3):323-329.

55-year-old man with left thigh and buttock claudication

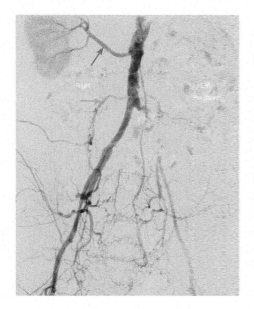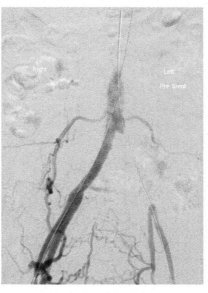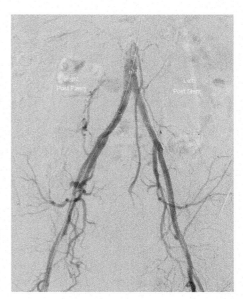

1. Name the vessel labelled with the red arrow.

2. Name the vessel labelled with the green arrow.

3. How would you deploy an iliac stent?

4. What special equipment might you use to perform subintimal recanalization of an iliac occlusion?

5. This case fits into which classification of TASC aortoiliac lesions?

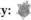

Category: Arterial system

Answers

1. This is an accessory right renal artery.

2. This is the fourth right lumbar artery.

3. Angiographic roadmaps or bony landmarks are helpful for stent positioning. Stents should be balloon angioplastied after deployment. Transient pain or discomfort often occurs. Pre-stent placement angioplasty increases the risk of distal embolization, but angioplasty with a small balloon may facilitate passage of the stent through a heavily calcified vessel. Self-expanding iliac stents are used.

4. Reentry catheters are designed to break back into the vessel lumen from the subintimal channel. A hydrophilic wire and torqueable catheter is commonly used. The back end of a wire, or a stiff wire, can facilitate the creation of a subintimal tract.

5. A long unilateral common iliac lesion is a TASC (TransAtlantic Inter-Society Consensus) type C lesion. The classification is a useful tool for research purposes.

Pearls

- Aortoiliac disease is common and can cause lifestyle limiting claudication or contribute to critical limb ischemia.
- Subintimal recanalization commonly requires the use of a directional catheter and hydrophilic guidewire. Occlusions can be crossed in an antegrade direction, or retrogradely using an "up and over" technique. Occasionally reentry catheters are required to reenter the lumen from a subintimal tract. Rarely, a through-and-through access (flossing) may be required to pass a catheter or stent across the occluded segment.

Suggested Reading

Norgren L, Hiatt WR, Dormandy JA, et al. Inter-Society Consensus for the Management of Peripheral Arterial Disease (TASC II). *J Vasc Surg*. 2007;45(suppl):S5-S67.

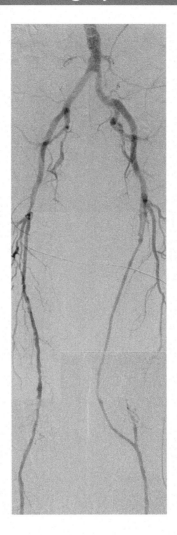

1. Review the angiogram. How is the left leg vascularized?

2. What is the ideal conduit for femoropopliteal bypass?

3. What is the 5-year patency of a vein bypass?

4. What is the 5-year patency of a synthetic graft?

5. What are the complications of bypass? And how would each be managed?

Case ranking/difficulty: 🐢

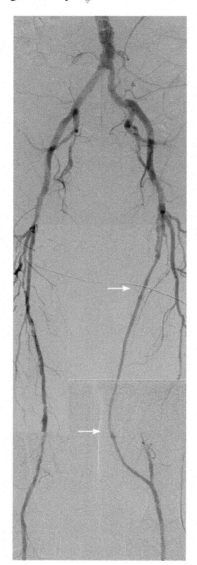

Angiogram of the lower limbs.

Answers

1. There is a left femoropopliteal vein graft.

2. Vein.

3. 70%.

4. 40%.

5. Early occlusion requires a return to the operation theater, for thrombectomy and revision. Late occlusion can be treated with lysis and angioplasty, or surgical revision. Infection would require graft excision and an alternate means for revascularization. Stenoses can be managed with angioplasty, and grafts should undergo ultrasonographic surveillance.

Pearls

- Ipsilateral great saphenous vein is the ideal bypass.
- Polytetrafluoroethylene (PTFE, Gore-Tex) or polyester (Dacron) synthetic grafts can also be used, but these have lower patency rates.
- Graft patency rates vary across studies but a recent review compared venous and PTFE bypass procedures reporting 5-year primary patency rates of 74% and 39%, respectively.
- Endovascular approaches to infrainguinal occlusive disease with angioplasty and stenting can be successful. Longer occlusions may be better treated with surgery. Graft complications include restenosis and occlusion, and so ultrasonographic surveillance of grafts can be useful. Graft infection can occur, and pseudoaneurysm formation can also occur at suture lines.

Suggested Reading

Klinkert P, Post PN, Breslau PJ, van Bockel JH. Saphenous vein versus PTFE for above-knee femoropopliteal bypass. A review of the literature. *Eur J Vasc Endovasc Surg.* 2004;27(4):357-362.

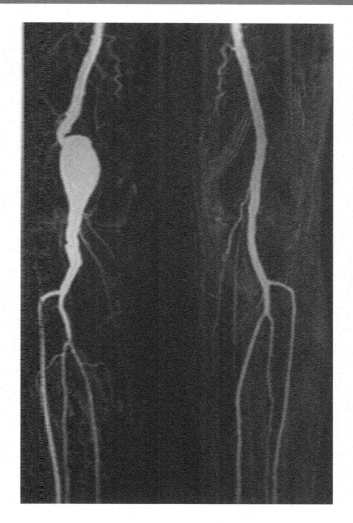

1. Popliteal aneurysms are the commonest peripheral aneurysm—true or false?

2. What percentage of popliteal aneurysms are bilateral?

3. What size of aneurysm should be treated in an asymptomatic patient?

4. List some treatment options for popliteal aneurysm.

5. Name 2 other important, but rare, pathologies of the popliteal artery.

Case ranking/difficulty: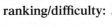

Category: Arterial system

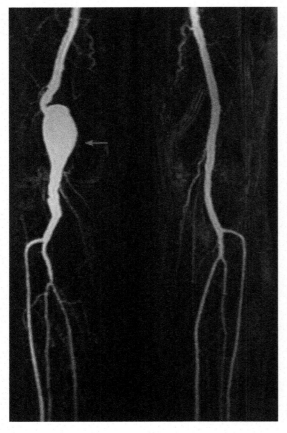

Right popliteal aneurysm.

Answers

1. The popliteal artery is the most common site of peripheral aneurysms.

2. About 50% to 70% have bilateral aneurysms.

3. The balance of risks and benefits and patient choice should always be considered in any management plan. Some operators think this should be when the aneurysm is >2 cm but complications can occur with any aneurysm.

4. Surgical bypass is performed, but endovascular stent graft placement is an alternative.

5. Popliteal entrapment syndrome and cystic adventitial disease of the popliteal artery are rare, but important, conditions.

Pearls

- Popliteal aneurysms are the commonest peripheral artery aneurysm and frequently occur in males. They are bilateral in 25% to 50% of cases and are associated with abdominal aortic aneurysms.
- Thrombosed popliteal aneurysm is best treated with surgical bypass grafting.

Suggested Reading

Foley WD, Stonely T. CT angiography of the lower extremities. *Radiol Clin North Am.* 2010;48(2):367-396, ix.

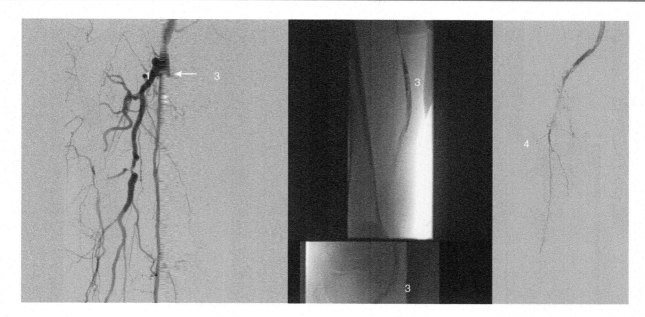

1. Review the pre-lysis images, label structures 1 through 4.

2. Name some contraindications to lysis.

3. What is alteplase?

4. What safety considerations are there during an infusional thrombolysis procedure?

5. What is the 5-year secondary patency rate after thrombolysis?

Case ranking/difficulty:

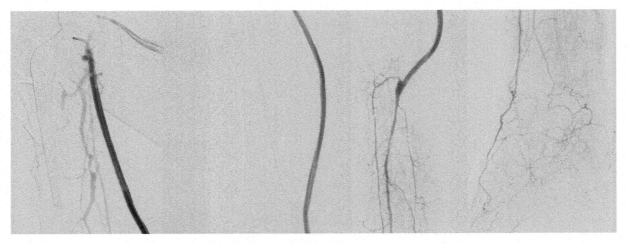

The patient cam to the interventional suite the following morning with a warm foot and post-thrombolysis angiogram shows patent graft and run off into the foot.

Answers

1. 1. Profunda femoris. 2. Native superficial femoral artery which is occluded in the lower thigh. 3. Occluded stump of the femoral graft. 4. Poor run-off.

2. Pregnancy, diabetic retinopathy, recent intra-cranial hemorrhage, active hemorrhage, and recent stroke are contraindications to thrombolysis. However, significant complications may be rare and need should be considered on a patient-to-patient basis.

3. Alteplase is well tolerated. It is a recombinant version of tissue plasminogen activator (rtPA). Previously available lytics such as streptokinase and urokinase were associated with anaphylactoid reactions.

4. Patients should be monitored in high-dependency units/ intensive care. Hemoglobin and fibrin levels should be monitored. Meticulous care of the sheaths and catheters and regular review of the access sites are required.

5. Five-year patency of a bypass after thrombolysis has been reported to be in the order of 23%.

Pearls

- Intraarterial lysis restores graft function. Technical success is reported to be in the order of 75%. There is often an underlying stenosis. Aspiration thrombectomy and thrombolysis with mechanical-rotational devices has also been reported.
- Complications of lysis include local and systemic hemorrhage (eg, intracranial, gastrointestinal, retroperitoneal). Alteplase (recombinant tissue plasminogen activator) is commonly used. Alteplase binds fibrin and then catalyzes the conversion of plasminogen into plasmin, which then itself causes the break-up of fibrin into degradation products.
- Alternatives to graft thrombosis include surgical thrombectomy and revision or a redo bypass.

Suggested Reading

Sandbaek G, Staxrud LE, Rosén L, et al. Outcome after catheter-directed thrombolysis of occluded prosthetic femoropopliteal bypasses. A prospective study. *Acta Radiol*. 2000;41(3):249-254.

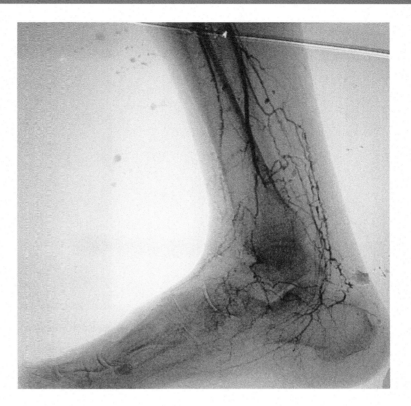

1. What is the diagnosis?

2. What is the most valuable laboratory test to definitively diagnose this condition?

3. What is the most effective treatment?

4. What arteriographic features are pathognomonic?

5. What are some complications of lower extremity amputation?

Case ranking/difficulty: 🔥

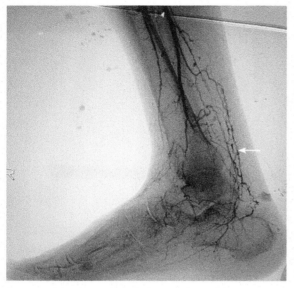

Digital subtraction angiography: abrupt occlusions with very tortuous collaterals.

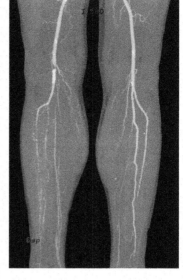

Coronal reformatted computed angiographic (CT) image of another patient.

Answers

1. This is thromboangiitis obliterans, also known as Buerger disease.

2. No specific laboratory test can be used to definitively diagnose Buerger disease. Erythrocyte sedimentation rate, C-reactive protein, antinuclear antibody, and other serological markers are normal.

3. There is no cure for Buerger disease. The most effective treatment is complete discontinuation of cigarette smoking or use of tobacco in any form.

4. Collaterals following the original arteries, corkscrew spiral collaterals, skip lesions, and tapering of the distal arteries are suggestive of, but not pathognomonic of, this condition.

5. Stump neuroma formation and phantom pain are particular complications of amputation.

Pearls

• In Buerger disease, suggestive angiographic findings include involvement of small vessels, preservation of proximal vessels with no evidence of atheroma, skip lesions, and spiral or "corkscrew" collaterals, which often follow the path of the main arteries. Outcome is best improved by encouraging the cessation of use of all tobacco products.

Suggested Reading

Kulkarni S, Kulkarni G, Shyam AK, Kulkarni M, Kulkarni R, Kulkarni V. Management of thromboangiitis obliterans using distraction osteogenesis: A retrospective study. *Indian J Orthop.* 2011;45(5):459-64.

67-year-old man presents for a procedure pre–endovascular aneurysm repair (EVAR)

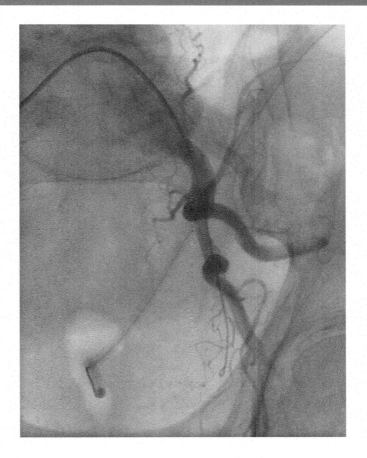

1. Where is the tip of the sheath?

2. What are the risks associated with bilateral internal iliac artery embolization?

3. What devices can be used to embolize the internal iliac artery?

4. What are the advantages of Amplatzer vascular plug (AVP) over coils?

5. What are the advantages of coils over AVP?

Case ranking/difficulty:

Category: Arterial system

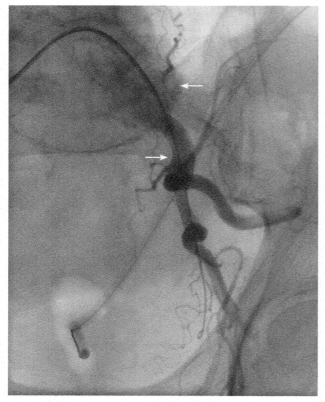

Preembolization. Angiogram via the sheath in the internal iliac artery. Note the reflux into the aneurysmal common iliac artery.

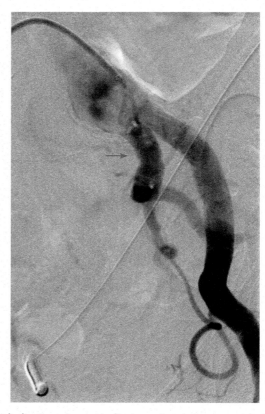

Postembolization. Arrows indicate an Amplatzer vascular plug (AVP) in the origin of the internal iliac artery and flow down the external iliac artery.

Answers

1. The tip of the sheath is in the left internal iliac artery. Note reflux into an aneurismal common iliac artery.

2. Spinal cord ischemia is rare but can occur. Other severe ischemic complications include buttock necrosis, bowel or bladder ischemia. Buttock or thigh claudication is common, at around 30%, and persists at 1 year in 10%. Sexual dysfunction may occur in 5%.

3. AVP and coils are commonly used.

4. AVP can be used as a single device, has a precise deployment mechanism, and the device can be released and recovered; also angiograms can be performed through the sheath to check position. It has also been reported to be cost-effective, with reduced procedure time and patient dose.

5. AVP may be limited by tortuosity due to its stiff wire, and so coils may be advantageous when there is severe tortuosity.

Pearls

- Internal iliac arteries can be embolized using AVPs or coils. The AVP appears to be more cost-effective. It may also reduce dose and treatment time, as a single plug is required, instead of multiple coils.
- This can be performed at the same sitting as EVAR, or as a staged procedure depending on local logistics.
- Branched iliac grafts preserve the internal iliac arteries but suitable anatomy must be present.

Suggested Reading

Pellerin O, Caruba T, Kandounakis Y, et al. Embolization of the internal iliac artery: cost-effectiveness of two different techniques. *Cardiovasc Intervent Radiol.* 2008;31(6):1088-1093.

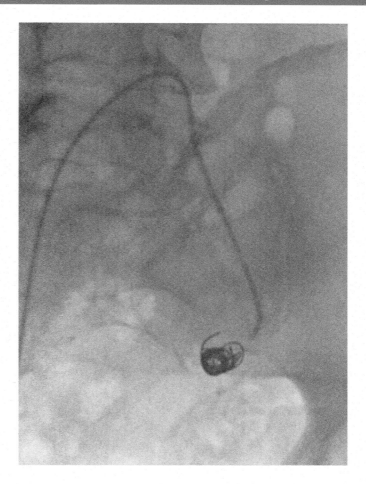

1. How can embolization coils be deployed?

2. What complications can occur during coil deployment?

3. How do coils cause vessel occlusion?

4. What sizes of coils are available?

5. What effects do coils have on computed tomography (CT) and magnetic resonance (MR) imaging?

Case ranking/difficulty: 🌑

Category: Arterial system

Answers

1. A wire or dedicated coil pusher can be used to push the coil out of the host catheter. Coils can also be flushed out with jets of saline. Detachable coils have manufacturer-specific deployment mechanisms, which can be mechanical, electrical, or laser based.

2. Coil migration and coil misplacement can occur. Correct sizing of coils and maintaining control of the host catheter are important.

3. Fibers attached to the coils lead to thrombosis and occlusion.

4. There is a wide range of sizes, from 0.018", to 0.035" to 0.052". Amplatzer vascular plugs have been shown to function effectively where otherwise large numbers of coils would be needed and are available in a range of designs and size.

5. Coils cause significant artifact on CT and so follow-up imaging of the embolized vascular structures can be difficult. Coils are MR compatible, but every device should be checked against the manufacturer instructions and MR safety databases.

Pearls

- Coils can be divided into macrocoils (>0.035") and microcoils (0.018"). The original Gianturco coils were 0.052" in size. In addition, 0.035"-coils are typically made from stainless steel, and 0.018"-microcoils from platinum. Coils can have simple cylindrical or complex shapes, can have a range of synthetic fibers to increase thrombogenicity, and can be detachable or expandable/hydrocoils.
- Standard coils can be delivered by flushing them out of the host catheter, or pushed out using either an end of a guidewire or a specifically designed coil pusher.
- Detachable coils can be deployed with various techniques, rotation, electrolysis, or laser technology.
- The thrombogenic effect occurs due to thrombosis induced by the fibers attached to the coil, not from mechanical occlusion of the coil itself.
- Coil migration and misplacement can occur. Misplaced coils can be retrieved with a snare or specific coil-retrieval devices.

Suggested Reading

Zhu X, Tam MD, Pierce G, et al. Utility of the Amplatzer vascular plug in splenic artery embolization: a comparison study with conventional coil technique. *Cardiovasc Intervent Radiol.* 2011;34(3):522-531.

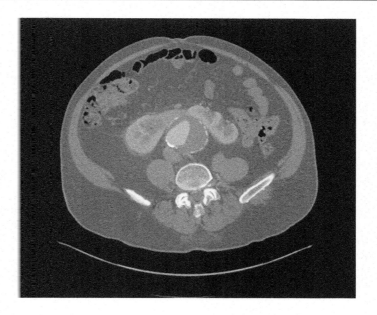

1. What is the diagnosis?

2. Where can its arteries arise from?

3. In aneurysm repair, all arteries should be preserved, true or false?

4. Endovascular repair is contraindicated—true or false?

5. Are there any special considerations for performing a nephrostomy here?

Case ranking/difficulty: 🦔

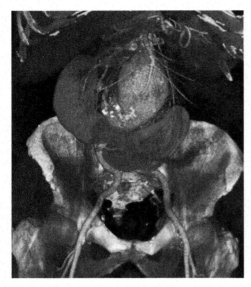

Volume rendered image from the CTA showing the aortic aneurysm and horseshoe kidney.

Answers

1. There is a horsehoe kidney and a triple A.

2. Horseshoe kidneys commonly take their supply from the aorta and common iliac arteries. The inferior mesenteric artery (IMA) can also supply the isthmus.

3. False. Small arteries up to 2 mm can be sacrificed.

4. Endovascular repair is possible and the aim is to spare as many renal arteries as possible. Open repair requires division of the isthmus.

5. The upper pole is usually more accessible.

Pearls

- Horseshoe kidneys have a variable blood supply. There can be multiple aortic branches, and accessory arteries can arise from the common and external iliac arteries.
- Endovascular aneurysm repair is possible in the presence of a horseshoe kidney. Special attention must be paid to the origin of any accessory arteries. Open repair involves surgical division of the isthmus.

Suggested Reading

Jackson RW, Fay DM, Wyatt MG, Rose JD. The renal impact of aortic stent-grafting in patients with a horseshoe kidney. *Cardiovasc Intervent Radiol.* 2004;27(6):632-636.

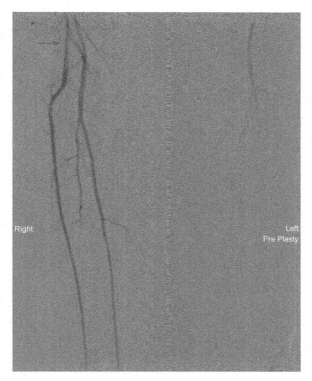

Lower limb angiogram.

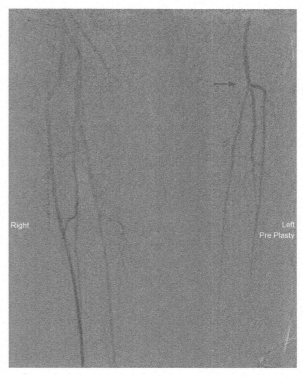

Lower limb angiogram.

1. What is the vessel labelled with an arrow on the left image?

2. The vessels on the left, in the figure on the right, are normal—true or false?

3. Name some recognized anatomic variations of the crural vessels.

4. Describe the embryologic development of the lower limb arteries.

5. What is the incidence of variant anatomy?

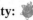
Answers

1. The image demonstrates a right-sided anterior tibial artery with high take-off.

2. In a later frame from the same angiogram, there is also variant anatomy on the left, a trifurcation.

3. There are multiple variations, which include absence of any of the 3 vessels, a long tibioperoneal trunk, a peroneal magna artery, and so-called island popliteal artery.

4. In the early developing limb bud, the sciatic artery (a branch of the internal iliac artery) is the main supply. Later, the femoral artery (a branch of the external iliac artery) anastomoses with the sciatic artery and the femoral artery becomes the main supply as the proximal primitive sciatic artery regresses.

   The middle and distal primitive sciatic arteries give rise to the popliteal and peroneal arteries.

   There is a superficial popliteal artery that gives rise to the definitive anterior tibial artery.

   Any failure of fusion or regression of the embryonal arteries can result in an anomaly, such as an island popliteal artery or persistent sciatic artery.

5. Normal pattern is seen in 90%. High anterior tibial artery is seen in around 5%, a trifurcation in 3%. Variation is not thought to increase the risk or severity of PVD. These findings are based on several published retrospective reviews of large series of lower limb angiograms.

Pearls

- Vascular variation is important, both diagnostically and therapeutically. Abnormal anatomy is important for the surgeon to know about—for distal bypass grafts and also for the harvesting of soft tissue flaps by plastic surgeon.

Suggested Reading

Kelly AM, Cronin P, Hussain HK, et al. Preoperative MR angiography in free fibula flap transfer for head and neck cancer: clinical application and influence on surgical decision making. *AJR Am J Roentgenol.* 2007;188(1):268-274.

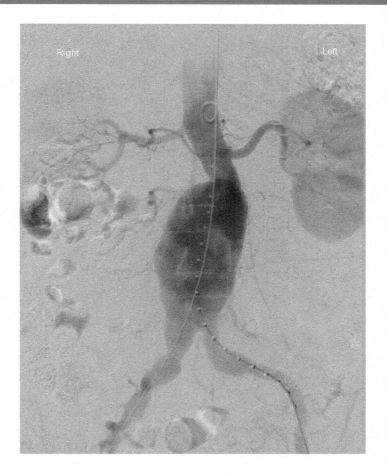

1. What nonpatient factors must be considered when planning an endovascular aneurysm repair?

2. What features of aortic anatomy must be considered?

3. Name some EVAR-related complications.

4. What are indications for EVAR?

5. What did the 'EVAR 2' trial find?

Case ranking/difficulty: 🌸

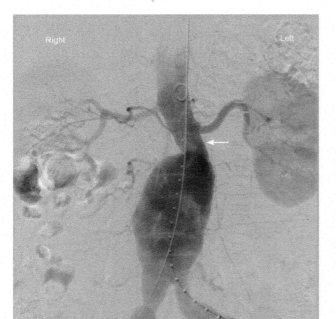

Aortogram. Arrow indicates the aneurysm neck.

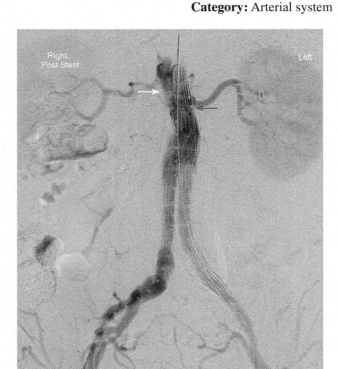

Aortogram. White arrow indicates uncovered "crown of thorns," and red arrow indicates the covered body just at the level of the lowest renal artery.

Answers

1. EVAR must be a well-coordinated activity and takes into account patient factors, aortic anatomy, knowledge of the device and appropriate components, and appropriately trained operators.

2. Aortoiliac angulation, diameters, lengths, tortuosity, as well as the location of visceral vessels are important parameters when planning EVAR and choosing a device.

3. Endoleaks, graft migration and thrombosis, renal impairment, infection, and groin and lower extremity complications can occur and delayed rupture is also reported. Post-EVAR surveillance is therefore required.

4. EVARS can be performed for ruptured aneurysms, suprarenal aneurysms (FEVAR, fenestrated EVAR), and thoracic aneurysms (TEVAR) and can incorporate and preserve internal iliacs (branched iliac grafts).

5. The EVAR 2 trial found no survival benefit of EVAR for patients deemed unfit for open repair. EVAR requires surveillance, and reintervention rates are quoted at around 15%.

Pearls

- EVAR is performed for patients who are suitably fit for open repair of infrarenal aneurysm repair.
- There are multiple devices available.
- The aneurysm morphology must be suitable to a particular device. This includes particular features of the aneurysm neck, visceral vessels, aneurysm sac, and iliac arteries and are commonly device specific.

Suggested Readings

EVAR trial participants. Endovascular aneurysm repair and outcome in patients unfit for open repair of abdominal aortic aneurysm (EVAR trial 2): randomised controlled trial. *Lancet.* 2005;365(9478):2187-2192.

EVAR trial participants. Endovascular aneurysm repair versus open repair in patients with abdominal aortic aneurysm (EVAR trial 1): randomised controlled trial. *Lancet.* 2005;365(9478):2179-2186.

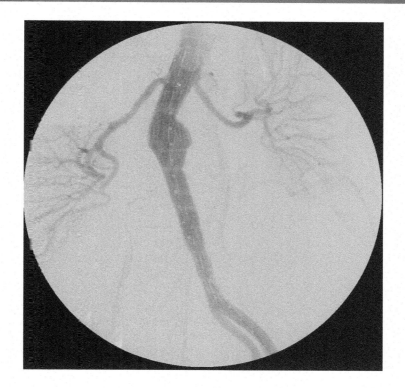

1. Review the image—what has been performed?

2. How is the right lower extremity vascularized?

3. What is done to the contralateral common iliac artery?

4. What conditions present in iliac arteries make an aorto-uni-iliac graft indicated?

5. What other non-iliac features might lead to aorto-uni-iliac graft?

Case ranking/difficulty: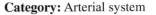

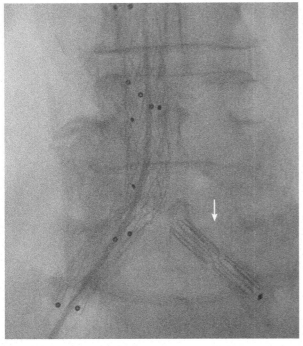

Occluder.

5. A narrow aortic bifurcation would preclude standard, bifurcated EVAR. An aortic bifurcation of more than 20mm is required to allow 2 limbs to sit unconstrained. Note AUI is an also option in rupture cases. Failure to cannulate the contralateral gate may also lead to conversion to an AUI.

Pearls

- Aorto-uni-iliac graft is an important tool in EVAR. It can be used in emergencies and also enables aneurysm to be treated when a standard bifurcation graft cannot be used.
- Advantages of aorto-uni-iliac grafts may include ability to achieve EVAR in the setting of iliac disease, stenosis, dissection or occlusion, and can also be performed in the acute setting.
- The contralateral common iliac artery is occluded with a specific graft component (an "occluder") or with other embolic devices (eg, an Amplatzer vascular plug [AVP]). The contralateral limb is then revascularized with a femoral-to-femoral cross-over graft.

Answers

1. An aorto-uni-iliac graft has been deployed.

2. Femoral-femoral cross-over graft is required.

3. If patent, the contralateral common iliac artery requires occluding, either with a specific occluding piece from the EVAR kit (a cuff is shown), or with an Amplatzer Vascular Plug. Otherwise, there is a risk of persistent retrograde sac perfusion and delayed rupture.

4. Iliac artery dissection, occlusion, stenosis, tortuosity, or circumferential calcification may be the reasons.

Suggested Readings

Heredero AF, Stefanov S, del Moral LR, et al. Long-term results of femoro-femoral crossover bypass after endovascular aortouniiliac repair of abdominal aortic and aortoiliac aneurysms. *Vasc Endovascular Surg.* 2008;42(5):420-426.

Hinchliffe RJ, Alric P, Wenham PW, Hopkinson BR. Durability of femorofemoral bypass grafting after aortouniiliac endovascular aneurysm repair. *J Vasc Surg.* 2003;38(3):498-503.

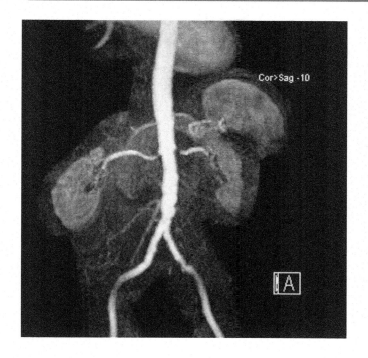

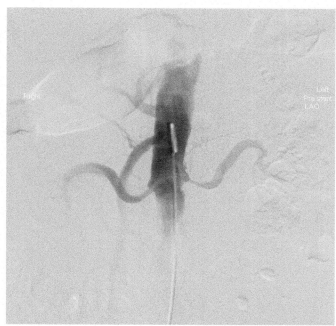

1. What is the role of ultrasound in diagnosing this condition?

2. What alternative contrast media are available to be used angiographically?

3. What is the incidence of variant renal artery anatomy?

4. What are the indications for treating renal artery stenosis?

5. Describe your technique for renal artery stenting. What are potential complications?

Case ranking/difficulty:

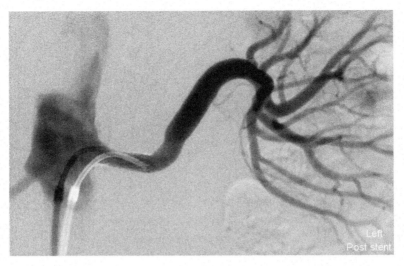

Poststent angiogram.

Answers

1. Renal artery velocity of more than 3.5 times that of the aorta and a peak systolic velocity of 180 cm/s are signs of stenosis. Renal size should be measured, as small kidneys respond poorly. A resistive index of <0.7 is associated with better outcomes.

2. Gadolinium can be used in patients with allergies to iodinated contrast media. Carbon dioxide can be used in patients with poor renal function. Hydration, bicarbonate infusions, and Mucomyst may reduce contrast nephropathy.

3. Around 70% of the population has accessory renal arteries.

4. Atherosclerotic renal artery stenosis is performed in patients with refractory hypertension, declining renal function, and in flash pulmonary edema.

5. Balloon-mounted stents are used. Stents should extend into the aortic lumen to reduce the risk of neointimal hyperplasia and recurrent renal artery stenosis. There is a risk for causing renal artery dissection and rupture, which can be managed with prolonged angioplasty or covered stent placement.

Pearls

- Atherosclerotic renal artery stenosis responds best to primary stenting, whereas fibromuscular dysplasia responds well to angioplasty and repeat angioplasty.
- Technique involves crossing the lesion with a hydrophilic guidewire, exchanging for an 0.018" wire for stent placement, which is aided by a long sheath.
- Balloon-mounted stents are used, which should not be larger than the normal renal artery, or there may then be risk of dissection and rupture. Stent placement may require predilatation with a small balloon.
- Complications include renal artery dissection, rupture, capsular perforation, and renal infarction due to emboli.

Suggested Reading

Blum U, Krumme B, Flügel P, et al. Treatment of ostial renal-artery stenoses with vascular endoprostheses after unsuccessful balloon angioplasty. *N Engl J Med.* 1997;336(7):459-465.

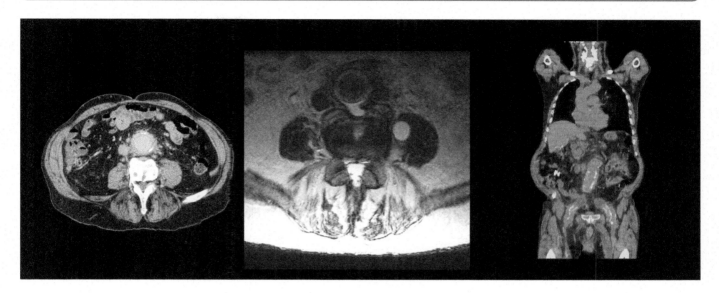

1. What imaging may be useful to diagnose an infected graft?

2. What is the incidence of graft infection?

3. How should graft infections be treated?

4. Can endovascular aneurysm repairs (EVARs) get infected?

5. What are the risk factors?

Case ranking/difficulty: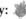

Answers

1. Computed tomography (CT) can demonstrate periaortic fluid and soft tissue collections and gas in the sac. Osteomyelitis in adjacent vertebrae may be seen. Hydronephrosis is a significant finding after abdominal aortic aneurysm (AAA) and also be an early sign of infection.

   Magnetic resonance (MR) may show high T2 signal in the sac, edema, collections, and can assess the lumbar spine and discs. Nuclear medicine scans such as In-111 or Tc-99m white blood cell scans; Ga-67 scans or PET scan can show active inflammation.

2. Aortic graft infection has been reported to occur in 1% to 6% of cases. Endovascular graft infection is less common.

3. Aggressive local treatment for groin infection can preserve the graft. If there is retroperitoneal sepsis, graft excision is required; axillo-bifemoral graft is used to revascularize the lower limbs.

4. Yes. The endovascular graft may need to be explanted.

5. An initial infected/mycotic aneurysm or aortoenteric fistula is a risk factor. Endovascular repair has been successful in these cases in conjunction with prolonged antibiotics.

   Simultaneous gastrointestinal surgery (eg, cholecystectomy), septicemia, and wound infection at the time of aneurysm repair are associated with graft infection.

Pearls

- Graft infection can present with both overt sepsis and low-grade infection.
- Graft explantation and revascularization through noninfected territory is required, such as excision of the aortic graft and revascularization of the legs with axillobifemoral graft, for example.

Suggested Reading

Orton DF, LeVeen RF, Saigh JA, et al. Aortic prosthetic graft infections: radiologic manifestations and implications for management. *Radiographics*. 2000;20(4):977-993.

35-year-old woman with left upper quadrant pain and hypotension after a horse riding accident

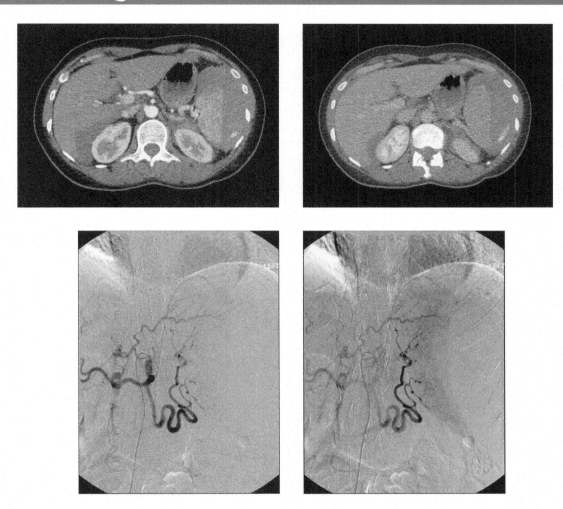

1. What are the indications for splenic artery embolization in trauma?

2. Which embolic material can be used?

3. What are the indications for splenic artery embolization?

4. What is a 6 Fr sheath and what equipment and devices can be placed through it?

5. What are disadvantages of standard coils compared to Amplatzer vascular plug (AVP) devices?

Case ranking/difficulty: 🏅

Answers

1. Embolization is indicated in a hemodynamically unstable patient or where there is evidence of active arterial contrast extravasation. Embolization is contraindicated in patients with other injuries that require laparotomy. Conservative management can be offered in the absence of contrast extravasation in a stable patient.

2. Coarse Gelfoam or coils are commonly used.

3. Aneurysms, pseudoaneurysms, hypersplenism, portal hypertension and splenic artery steal syndrome are indications.

4. For sheaths, French refers to the inner diameter, and for catheters, French refers to the outer diameter—so a 6 Fr sheath can accommodate a 6 Fr catheter. Larger AVPs may require up to a 7 Fr sheath, but a 14 mm plug will pass through a 6 Fr sheath. A 5 Fr catheter and a second buddy wire alongside it can also be used through a 6 Fr sheath in tandem.

5. AVP has a controlled release mechanism, can be repositioned, and is a single device often sufficient to cause occlusion in most situations.

Pearls

- Splenic embolization has a role in splenic trauma and can result in spleen salvage.
- Splenic artery embolization has a wide range of indications—excluding aneurysms and pseudoaneurysms, trauma, reducing splenic flow in steal and portal hypertension, and reducing splenic function in hypersplenism.

Suggested Readings

Bessoud B, Denys A, Calmes JM, et al. Nonoperative management of traumatic splenic injuries: is there a role for proximal splenic artery embolization? *AJR Am J Roentgenol.* 2006;186(3):779-785.

Madoff DC, Denys A, Wallace MJ, et al. Splenic arterial interventions: anatomy, indications, technical considerations, and potential complications. *Radiographics.* 2005;25(suppl 1):S191-S211.

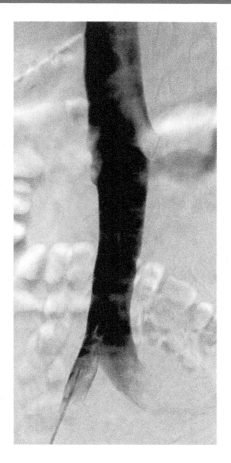

1. What is the study and what do you notice?

2. How are the renal veins visualized on a cavagram?

3. How would you inject iodinated contrast to perform a cavagram? What volume? What rate?

4. How would you inject carbon dioxide to perform a cavagram?

5. If carbon dioxide and iodinated contrast cannot be used, are there any other options?

Case ranking/difficulty:

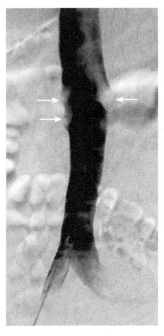

Cavagram.

It is also possible to inject through the filter sheath, but this would require opening the filter packaging, and so it might be more prudent to imaging first before committing to opening the filter. Hand injection does not fully opacify the cava.

4. Hand injection of 50 mL of CO_2 would be acceptable. Pump injection of CO_2 is not required.

5. Intravascular ultrasonography can be used to facilitate filter placement, or gadolinium can be used as an intravascular contrast agent.

Pearls

- Obtaining a high-quality cavagram is fundamental to safe inferior vena cava (IVC) filter placement.
- This allows the renal veins to be located, megacava to be excluded, anatomic variants to be noted, and the presence of caval thrombus to be assessed.
- Review of any cross-sectional studies prior to venography can also demonstrate anatomic variants.

Answers

1. There are two right-sided renal veins.

2. Renal veins can be identified on cavagrams by the inflow of unopacified blood into the cava. It is rare to directly visualize them as this would require significant reflux of contrast medium against the flow of blood.

3. Pump injection of iodinated contrast medium, 30 mL at 15 mL/s, would be acceptable through a pigtail catheter.

Suggested Reading

Zhu X, Tam MD, Bartholomew J, Newman JS, Sands MJ, Wang W. Retrievability and device-related complications of the G2 filter: a retrospective study of 139 filter retrievals. *J Vasc Interv Radiol.* 2011;22(6):806-812.

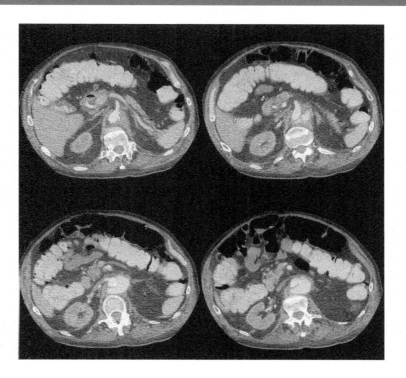

1. Endovascular repair is contraindicated due to infection, true or false?

2. What features raise suspicion of an underlying mycotic aneurysm?

3. What percentage of mycotic aneurysms are saccular?

4. What percentage of mycotic aneurysms are infrarenal?

5. Which microbe is the most common pathogen?

Case ranking/difficulty: 🍂

Category: Arterial system

Answers

1. A number of small series have reported successful outcomes with endovascular repair for thoracic, suprarenal, and infrarenal aortic mycotic aneurysms.

2. Rapid expansion, perianeurysmal soft tissue stranding, fluid collections, saccular configuration, and absence of signs of atherosclerosis raise the possibility of mycotic aneurysms.

3. In a report of a series of 7274 aneurysms treated at the Mayo Clinic, 58 were mycotic and 93% of these were saccular in nature.

4. The majority of mycotic aneurysms are thoracic, suprarenal, or juxtarenal. Only 30% are infrarenal.

5. *Staphylococcus aureus* may be more common in the Western world, but worldwide, salmonella is probably the most commonly implicated pathogen.

Pearls

- Rapid expansion, saccular aneurysms, perianeurysmal fluid collections or soft tissue stranding, lack of calcification or atherosclerosis, and significant intercurrent infections are signs that may be seen on imaging that are suggestive of mycotic aneurysm formation.
- Mycotic aneurysms occur where there is focal degeneration of the arterial wall due to bacterial infection, due to bacteremia or septic embolization, with microbes seeding into the intima or vasa vasorum.
- Mycotic aneurysms are associated with a high morbidity and mortality. Treatment involves antibiotic therapy, aggressive surgical debridement of infected tissue, and vascular reconstruction.

Suggested Reading

Macedo TA, Stanson AW, Oderich GS, Johnson CM, Panneton JM, Tie ML. Infected aortic aneurysms: imaging findings. *Radiology*. 2004;231(1):250-257.

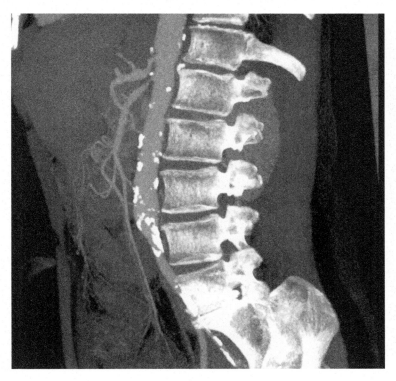 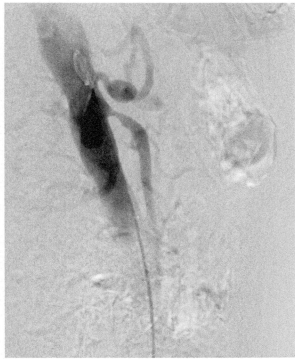

1. What is the classical presentation of chronic mesenteric ischemia?

2. What are the major branches of the superior mesenteric artery?

3. What are the different types of acute mesenteric ischemia, and which is commonest?

4. Which part of the colon is most at risk from chronic ischemia?

5. How can the diagnosis of chronic mesenteric ischemia be made?

Case ranking/difficulty:

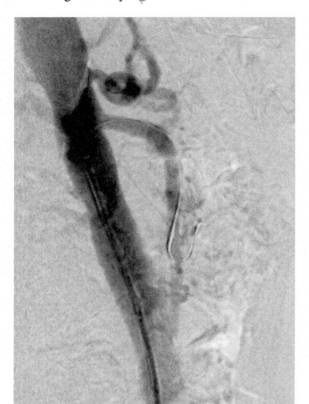

Lateral aortogram after stent placement.

Answers

1. Abdominal pain, weight loss, and a fear of eating in combination gives a history that can be attributed to chronic mesenteric ischemia.

2. Jejunal and ileal arteries are other named branches. The left colic artery is a branch of the inferior mesenteric artery (IMA, the hindgut artery).

3. SMA embolus is common, but ischemia can be nonocclusive or venous in nature.

4. The watershed area of the colon is at the splenic flexure.

5. Ultrasonography, computed tomography, magnetic resonance, or diagnostic angiography can demonstrate stenosis or occlusions but this must be interpreted in conjunction with the clinical scenario before high-risk intervention is considered.

Pearls

- Chronic mesenteric ischemia often presents with abdominal pain, weight loss, and fear of eating.
- The mantra is that 2 vessels are usually diseased as there are collateral pathways between the celiac trunk and SMA (via the pancreaticoduodenal arcades) and also between the SMA and IMA (via the colonic arcades).

Suggested Reading

Cognet F, Salem DB, Dranssart M, et al. Chronic mesenteric ischemia: imaging and percutaneous treatment. *Radiographics*. 2002;22(4):863-879; discussion 879-880.

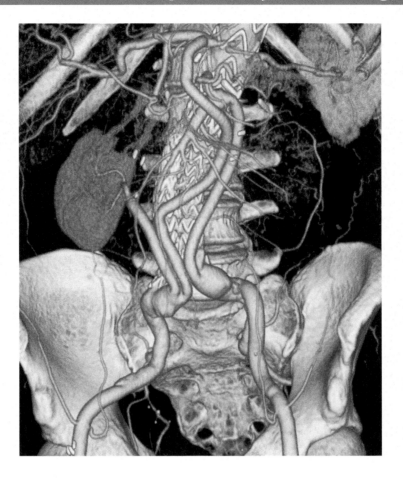

1. What is a "hybrid" repair?

2. What is an "elephant trunk"?

3. What is "debranching"?

4. In what other settings apart from thoracoabdominal aneurysm surgery lends itself to creative revascularization strategies?

5. What complication has happened in this case?

Case ranking/difficulty:

Category: Arterial system

Answers

1. Hybrid techniques refer to a combination of open surgery and endovascular repair and apply to complex thoracoabdominal repair.

2. After an arch repair, excess graft material is left in the native descending thoracic aorta. This is then used as a conduit for further repair, which can involve further surgery, endovascular aneurysm repair (EVAR), or hybrid techniques to complete the aortic repair at a second stage.

3. The origins of visceral branches are "sacrificed" or debranched.

   They are supplied by a visceral patch graft that comes from the lower aorta. This means that their origins can be sacrificed and the suprarenal aorta can be lined with the stent graft to exclude the aneurysm.

4. Transplantation also uses complex vascular grafts to reroute arterial, venous, and splanchnic supply, for example, with carotid or graft conduits from the iliacs, or aortic hoods slung from the aorta.

5. The left renal debranched graft has occluded.

Pearls

- Complex aortic repairs involving the arch and thoracoabdominal aorta is performed in a small number of high-volume centers of excellence around the world.
- A combination of surgical and endovascular techniques is used, often in a multistaged setting.
- In this case, treatment required stent graft placement in the thoracoabdominal aorta and retrograde vascularization of the debranched visceral arteries from grafts taken from the iliac arteries, a hybrid procedure, sometimes referred to as an "octopus" procedure.

Suggested Reading

Hughes GC, Barfield ME, Shah AA, et al. Staged total abdominal debranching and thoracic endovascular aortic repair for thoracoabdominal aneurysm. *J Vasc Surg.* 2012;56(3):621-629.

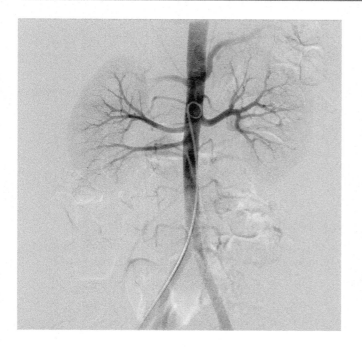 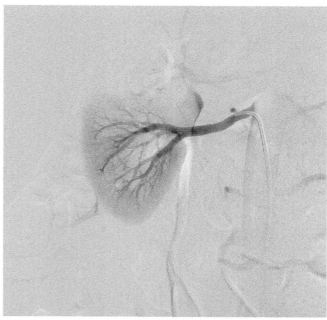

1. Review the angiogram, what do you notice?

2. What is the incidence of this abnormality?

3. Accessory renal arteries can arise from the inferior mesenteric artery (IMA)—true or false?

4. Accessory renal arteries can arise from iliac vessels—true or false?

5. Can accessory renal arteries arise from the common hepatic artery?

Case ranking/difficulty: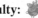

Answers

1. There is an accessory right renal artery.

2. It is very common, up to 30% or 40%.

3. True.

4. True.

5. This has not been reported.

Pearls

- Accessory renal arteries are common. Surgeons and interventionists must consider the presence of anatomic variation at all times.
- As well as directly affecting any renal intervention, many other arterial interventions can be affected by the presence of an accessory renal artery; for example, an ovarian artery can arise from this vessel.

Suggested Reading

Bordei P, Sapte E, Iliescu D. Double renal arteries originating from the aorta. *Surg Radiol Anat.* 2004;26(6):474-479.

A range of devices are pictured

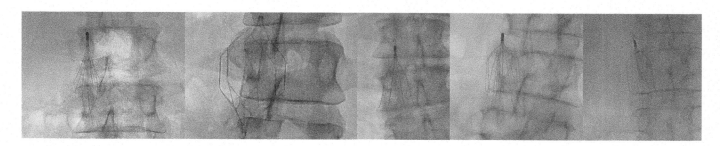

1. Name the filters—which of these are retrievable?

2. What factors affect retrieval success?

3. All filters are retrieved from a jugular route, true or false?

4. What is the rate of pulmonary embolism after filter placement?

5. What is the rate of caval occlusion after filter placement?

Case ranking/difficulty: 🐢

Answers

1. From left to right, these filters are the ALN, the OptEase, the Celect, a G2 and a G2X filter. All of these filters can be retrieved; the OptEase has the shortest manufacturer-recommended window of 23 days. OptEase filters have been removed at 60 days, the others after over 1 year.

2. Firstly, a filter should not be removed if there is a large thrombus in situ at time of retrieval. If so, the patient can be anticoagulated, and then return for retrieval at a later date. Filters that have tilted or migrated or fractured present some difficulties. Tilt poses a particular problem, as the hook can become endothelialized and incorporated into the cava wall.

3. The OptEase filter retrieval hook lies caudally, and so these filters are removed from a transfemoral access.

4. Post–filter placement pulmonary embolus (so-called breakthrough PE) occurs in about 1% of patients. This may be associated with some form of filter malfunction.

5. Caval occlusion can occur in around 1% of patients after filter placement.

Pearls

- Retrievable IVC filters can be removed using various retrieval devices such as snares or cones. These are often device specific. Most filters can be retrieved with snares. Advanced filter retrieval techniques are required if the filter is tilted and its retrieval hook/tip becomes endothelialized and incorporated into the caval wall. These techniques include angioplasty, self-made wire-loop snares to pull the filter off the caval wall, and even the use of endobronchial forceps to grab the filter, or laser-assisted retrieval. Retrievable filters can be left in situ to function as a permanent device. There is a generally a lower rate of filter retrieval. Active filter surveillance programs and better cross-disciplinary management should occur to improve filter retrieval, as devices left in situ when not required may expose the patient to unnecessary risk.

Suggested Readings

Berczi V, Bottomley JR, Thomas SM, Taneja S, Gaines PA, Cleveland TJ. Long-term retrievability of IVC filters: should we abandon permanent devices? *Cardiovasc Intervent Radiol.* 2007;30(5):820-827.

Minocha J, Idakoji I, Riaz A, et al. Improving inferior vena cava filter retrieval rates: impact of a dedicated inferior vena cava filter clinic. *J Vasc Interv Radiol.* 2010;21(12):1847-1851.

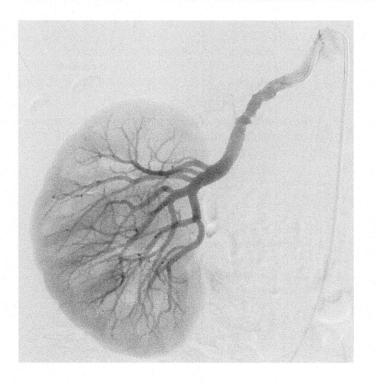 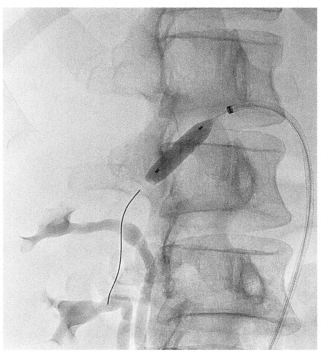

1. What is the diagnosis?

2. What else do you notice about the right kidney?

3. Which territories does this condition affect?

4. What is the association with aneurysmal disease?

5. What is the underlying pathology?

Case ranking/difficulty:

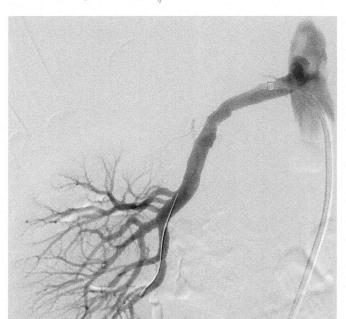

Postangioplasty image.

Answers

1. Fibromuscular dysplasia.

2. There is a Duplex system.

3. It affects the renal arteries in 60% to 85%. Case reports have shown it affecting coronary arteries, pulmonary arteries, and the aorta. It can also affect lower extremity and iliac vessels.

4. There is an association with aneurysm formation including intracerebral aneurysms, and so patients can present with subarachnoid hemorrhage. Macroaneurysms can occur in the renal arteries.

5. This is a noninflammatory, nonatherosclerotic condition. It can affect the media, intima, and adventitia with different combinations of fibroplasia and hyperplasia.

Pearls

- Fibromuscular dysplasia is a nonatherosclerotic noninflammatory process that causes stenosis, occlusion, aneurysms, and dissections in medium-sized vessels.
- It predominantly affects the renal arteries, but has cerebrovascular, visceral, and peripheral manifestations.
- Stenosis and the string of beads appearance occur as a result of focal, annular, repetitive, intimal, and medial pathologic changes.
- Angioplasty is the treatment of choice, but stenosis can be recurrent.

Suggested Reading

Meuse MA, Turba UC, Sabri SS, et al. Treatment of renal artery fibromuscular dysplasia. *Tech Vasc Interv Radiol.* 2010;13(2):126-133.

45-year-old man with declining renal function status post renal transplantation

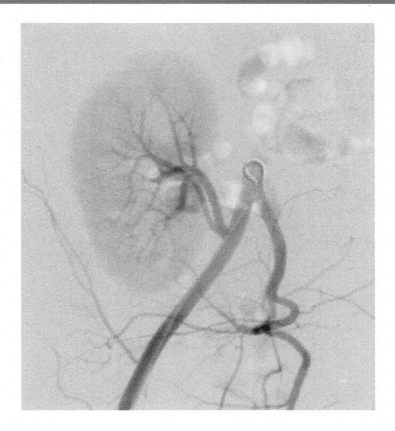

1. Review the angiogram. Is it normal?

2. How is the renal artery anastomosis formed? What are the common surgical variations?

3. List some causes for renal transplant failure.

4. What is the graft half-life for living donors?

5. How should transplant renal artery stenosis be treated?

Case ranking/difficulty:

Category: Arterial system

Answers

1. This is a normal angiogram of the renal transplant.

2. The renal artery is normally anastomosed to the external iliac artery. There can be multiple anastomoses. A Carrel patch involves placing a patch of donor aorta (with the multiple renal arteries) onto the external iliac artery.

3. Renal artery stenosis or thrombosis, renal vein thrombosis, rejection, and hydronephrosis can cause the graft to fail.

4. Currently, graft half-life for living donors is 20 years.

5. Transplant renal artery stenosis does respond to angioplasty. Other transplant interventions include percutaneous nephrostomy, ureteric stenting, biopsy, and drainage of collections and lymphoceles.

Pearls

• Noninvasive imaging with ultrasonography should be performed first. Angiography should be performed with a view to intervention. Iodinated contrast medium use can be minimized by performing the first runs with carbon dioxide. Carbon dioxide can be used to find the best oblique before formal imaging with iodinated contrast media.

Suggested Reading

Carrafiello G, Laganà D, Mangini M, et al. The role of interventional radiology in the management of kidney transplant complications. *Radiol Med.* 2005;110(3):249-261.

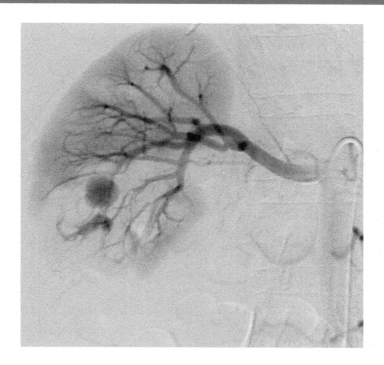

1. What is the incidence of hemorrhage requiring intervention after partial nephrectomy?

2. What angiographic signs are seen in hemorrhage?

3. Describe the intrarenal branching pattern of the renal artery.

4. What other renal interventions may also require embolization?

5. What embolic agents can be used?

Case ranking/difficulty: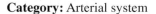

Category: Arterial system

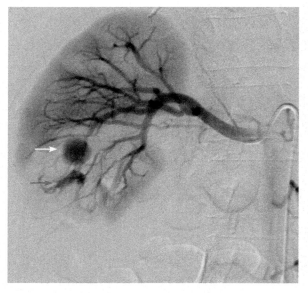

Angiogram shows pseudoaneurysm (white arrow) and extravasation (red arrow).

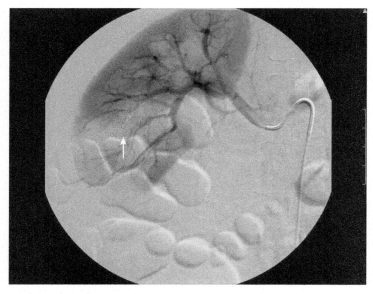

Postembolization angiogram (arrow indicates the coil).

Answers

1. This is reported in up to 2% of cases.

2. Active contrast extravasation, vessel irregularity, abnormal cut-off, and pseudoaneurysms might be seen. Arterial venous fistula can also be a complication after surgery. Arterial-caliceal fistula can also be seen.

3. This is variable, with no constant segmental organization. The main renal artery divides extrarenally into anterior and posterior divisions with 5 segmental branches—apical, upper, middle, lower, and posterior. Care must be taken to select the appropriate branch, and the target vessel often has a proximal origin. Oblique angiographic views can help to separate the branches. The goal of selective embolization is to preserve renal function.

4. Any renal intervention is associated with hemorrhage, including renal biopsy. Traumatic renal injuries can also be successfully treated with embolization.

5. Onyx and glue can be used in large pseudoaneurysms, but coils are the embolic agent of choice.

Pearls

- Partial nephrectomy is a common operation, and hemorrhage, which requires intervention, occurs in up to 2% of cases. Partial nephrectomy can be performed open, laparoscopically, or can be robotically assisted.
- Cryoablation is an alternative to partial nephrectomy performed for small renal cell carcinomas.
- Hemorrhage can have a delayed presentation, later than 2 weeks after surgery.

Suggested Readings

Baumann C, Westphalen K, Fuchs H, Oesterwitz H, Hierholzer J. Interventional management of renal bleeding after partial nephrectomy. *Cardiovasc Intervent Radiol.* 2007;30(5):828-832.

Montag S, Rais-Bahrami S, Seideman CA, et al. Delayed haemorrhage after laparoscopic partial nephrectomy: frequency and angiographic findings. *BJU Int.* 2011;107(9):1460-1466.

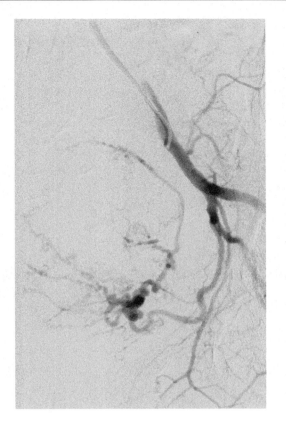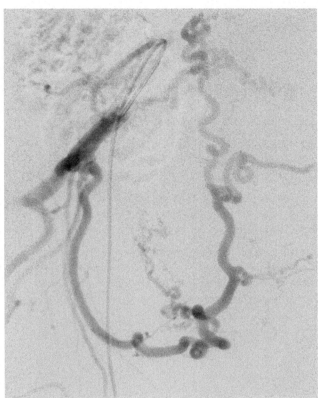

1. Review the angiograms, what do you see?

2. Which embolic agents would be appropriate?

3. What pre-procedural medications are required?

4. Can UFE be performed as a day-case procedure?

5. List 5 complications related to uterine fibroid embolization.

Case ranking/difficulty:

Answers

1. Both uterine arteries are hypertrophied and tortuous.

2. Spherical and nonspherical polyvinyl alcohol particles, smaller or larger than 500 μm, are widely used. There is some evidence to suggest that some particles are more advantageous than others, but there is no consensus.

3. Antiemetics, analgesia, and prophylactic antibiotics are important medications to offer the patient undergoing uterine artery embolizations.

4. Some operators do this, but the majority of operators offer post-procedural patient-controlled analgesia and an overnight stay. Some operators favor spinal anesthesia.

5. Complications include passage of fibroids, pyometrosis, and failure of the procedure to control symptoms. Postembolization syndrome and complications related to angiography can also occur.

Pearls

- Uterine fibroid embolization is a well-established procedure that provides symptomatic relief from fibroids.
- Prophylactic placement of bilateral occlusion balloons is a technique for providing access in the setting of high-risk placental deliveries allowing immediate access for internal iliac artery embolization.
- Uterine artery embolization can also be performed in a palliative setting in malignant conditions.

Suggested Reading

Bratby MJ, Belli AM. Radiological treatment of symptomatic uterine fibroids. *Best Pract Res Clin Obstet Gynaecol.* 2008;22(4):717-734.

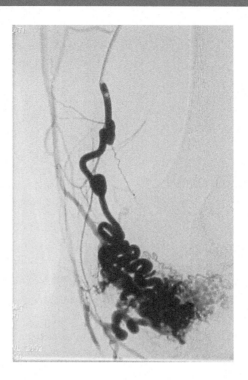

1. In what way can vascular malformations be classified?

2. What are the complications of high-flow arteriovenous malformations (AVMs)?

3. What are the anatomical features of a high-flow AVM?

4. What are the cardinal features of a venous malformation?

5. What are the cardinal features of soft-tissue hemangiomata?

Case ranking/difficulty:

Answers

1. Vascular lesions can be tumors or malformations. Malformations have been classified in several ways, eg, Mulliken and Glowacky. Single vessel type/ combined malformations, flow rate, and congenital/ present at birth can be useful ways to classify this complex range of lesions.

2. Lesions can be painful and there can be functional impairment due to mass effect. Lesions can ulcerate and hemorrhage. High-output cardiac failure is another complication.

3. High-flow AVMs have feeding arteries, a nidus, and draining veins. Ligation or embolization of the feeding artery is a poor treatment as the lesion easily revascularizes through smaller shunts. Intervention can be performed when the lesion is symptomatic or there are complications. Cosmesis is a relative indication.

4. Venous malformations grow in size with the patient, ultrasound shows venous lakes, and MRI can determine the extent of a lesion. They can be treated with sclerotherapy.

5. Vascular haemangiomata are present at birth, regress with age, and can be treated with propranolol. They are vascular tumors, not malformations.

Pearls

- Peripheral high-flow AVMs are rare entities and should be managed in centers of excellence with a dedicated multidisciplinary approach.
- Symptomatic patients can be offered embolization, which may be achieved in several stages. The goal of treatment is to eradicate the nidus, often through the use of liquid embolic agents.

Suggested Reading

Tan KT, Simons ME, Rajan DK, Terbrugge K. Peripheral high-flow arteriovenous vascular malformations: a single-center experience. *J Vasc Interv Radiol*. 2004;15(10):1071-1080.

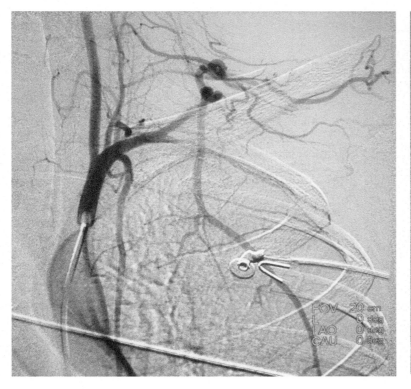 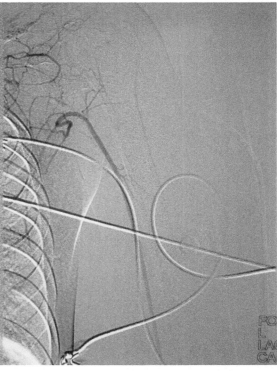

1. What are risk factors for upper extremity vascular injuries?

2. What are differences between upper and lower extremity vascular injuries?

3. Which is the commonest site of arterial injury in the arm?

4. Where can collateral pathways form in the upper limb?

5. What is the commonest anatomical variant?

Case ranking/difficulty: 🛡️

Answers

1. Young males and penetrating trauma are risk factors.

2. Lower limb vascular injury is associated with higher incidence of fasciotomy, is more likely due to blunt trauma, and is associated with more amputations and carries a higher mortality than upper limb trauma.

3. Forearm arterial injuries are commoner.

4. The chest wall and shoulder girdle arteries can provide collaterals. In this case, collateralization is seen from the costocervical trunk and chest wall. The profunda brachii gives radial and ulnar collaterals around the elbow. Collateralization of flow is seen readily.

5. High takeoff of the radial artery in the mid upper arm occurs in 15% of the population.

Pearls

- Upper extremity vascular trauma is often seen in conjunction with other injuries. Injuries to the subclavian artery are associated with high-impact blunt trauma to the thorax.
- The other upper limb arteries tend to be injured by penetrating injuries.
- Surgical options include open repair, bypass, or ligation. Sometimes conservative management is feasible because of collateral pathways. Endovascular repair with embolization of pseudoaneurysms or covered stent placement may be useful.

Suggested Reading

Franz RW, Goodwin RB, Hartman JF, Wright ML. Management of upper extremity arterial injuries at an urban level I trauma center. *Ann Vasc Surg.* 2009;23(1):8-16.

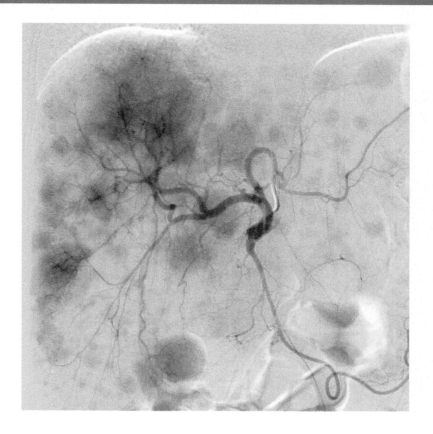

1. Where is the catheter?

2. List some tumors that are responsive to TACE.

3. More than 50% of melanoma patients will have a sustained partial response—true or false?

4. What is the 10-year mortality of ocular melanoma?

5. Hepatic metastases are the commonest site— true or false?

Case ranking/difficulty:

Category: Arterial system

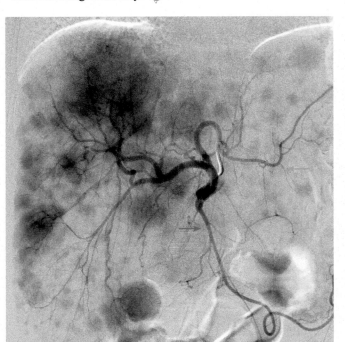

Common hepatic angiogram with liver metastases. Right hepatic artery (red arrow), left hepatic artery (green arrow), and the gastroduodenal artery (GDA; blue).

Answers

1. The catheter is in the common hepatic artery. There is massive hepatomegaly and so the left, right, and gastroduodenal arteries are seen.

2. Hepatocellular carcinoma (HCC), colorectal/ gastrointestinal stromal tumor (GIST)/neuroendocrine metastases are responsive to transarterial chemoembolization (TACE).

3. Some studies have shown that more than 50% of patients have a sustained partial response. The chemotherapeutic agent is cisplatin. Patients can undergo multiple rounds of TACE.

4. This is around 30% to 50%. Choroidal (uveal) melanoma is the commonest intraocular primary tumor.

5. True.

Suggested Reading

Huppert PE, Fierlbeck G, Pereira P, et al. Transarterial chemoembolization of liver metastases in patients with uveal melanoma. *Eur J Radiol.* 2010;74(3):e38-e44.

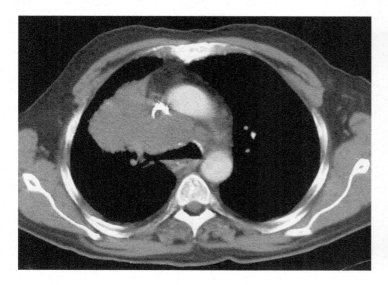 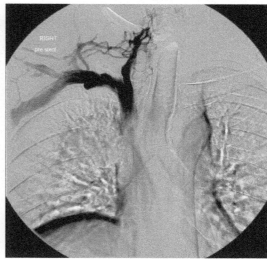

1. Superior vena cava (SVC) obstruction is always due to malignancy—true or false?

2. List 3 life-threatening complications of SVC stenting.

3. Symptoms take a number of weeks to settle—true or false?

4. What is the commonest underlying malignancy?

5. List some causes of nonmalignant SVC syndrome.

Case ranking/difficulty:

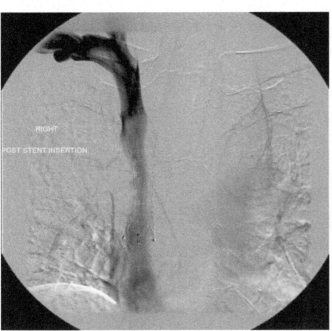

Poststent venogram.

4. Around 80% of SVC obstruction is due to a malignant process. Of the malignant cause, 75% is attributed to bronchogenic carcinoma (predominantly small cell) and 15% to non-Hodgkin lymphoma.

5. The most common cause for nonmalignant SVC syndrome is iatrogenic, due to previous and often multiple central venous interventions to place central venous catheters or cardiac implants.

Pearls

- SVC obstruction commonly presents with shortness of breath and facial swelling. The distressing syndrome can be rapidly reversed with stenting. If symptoms are not severe, the underlying cause can be treated with standard oncological treatment of the underlying malignancy.
- The stenosis or occlusion can be approached from jugular, femoral, or brachial approaches and a self-expanding stent can be placed.

Answers

1. False, SVC syndrome also occurs in dialysis patients as a result of multiple central venous catheters.

2. Massive pulmonary embolus can occur if there is a large burden of thrombus related to the obstruction; pericardial tamponade and SVC rupture can occur due to stent migration or a result of stent expansion. The procedural mortality rate is in the order of 2%.

3. Patients often experience immediate symptomatic benefit, and the vast majority improve in 24 to 72 hours.

Suggested Readings

Lanciego C, Chacón JL, Julián A, et al. Stenting as first option for endovascular treatment of malignant superior vena cava syndrome. *AJR Am J Roentgenol.* 2001;177(3):585-593.

Lanciego C, Pangua C, Chacón JI, et al. Endovascular stenting as the first step in the overall management of malignant superior vena cava syndrome. *AJR Am J Roentgenol.* 2009;193(2):549-558.

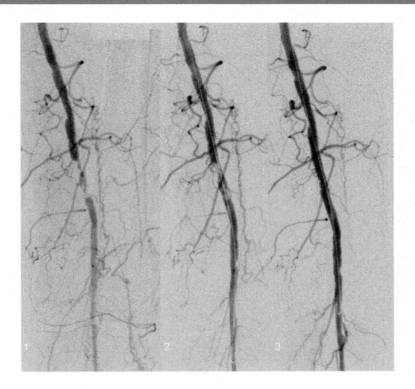

1. Describe the appearances in the 3 angiograms, what has been performed?

2. What SFA stents can be used?

3. What are potential complications particular to stent placement?

4. What options are available for treating intra-stent stenosis?

5. True or false—a covered stent graft requires an 8-Fr sheath?

Case ranking/difficulty: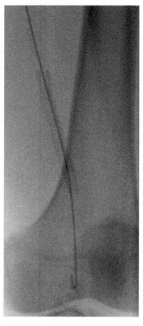

4. Angioplasty, cutting balloon angioplasty, and restenting are commonly used. Other techniques reported include cryoplasty, brachytherapy, laser debulking, and atherectomy.

5. False—Current generations of expanded polytetrafluoroethylene (ePTFE)-covered nitinol stent grafts are 6 Fr and can be placed over a 0.018" wire.

Superficial femoral artery (SFA) stent.

Pearls

- Heavily calcified lesions and lesions that fail to respond to angioplasty may benefit from stent placement.
- There is a growing range of choice for SFA stent placement, which includes nitinol stents, covered nitinol stent grafts, and drug-eluting stents. Long-term data from randomized controlled trials are awaited.
- Stent fractures may lead to restenosis and occlusion.

Suggested Readings

Ansel GM, Lumsden AB. Evolving modalities for femoropopliteal interventions. *J Endovasc Ther.* 2009;16(suppl 2):II82-II97.

Scheinert D, Scheinert S, Sax J, et al. Prevalence and clinical impact of stent fractures after femoropopliteal stenting. *J Am Coll Cardiol.* 2005;45(2):312-315.

Answers

1. Initial angiogram demonstrates a tight superficial femoral artery (SFA) stenotic lesion. There is a residual stenosis post angioplasty, and so a stent is placed with good result.

2. A covered stent graft, nitinol or stainless steel bare metal stents, and drug-eluting stents can be used.

3. Fracture can lead to restenosis and occlusion and even pseudoaneurysm formation.

Another range of devices is shown

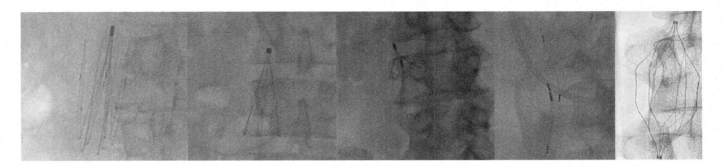

1. Name the filters. Which are retrievable?

2. What anatomical locations have IVC filters been inadvertently placed?

3. Name some indications for permanent inferior vena cava (IVC) filter placement.

4. List some complications of IVC filters.

5. IVC filters can be placed at the bedside using intravascular ultrasonography (IVUS)—true or false?

Case ranking/difficulty: 🏵

Answers

1. These are all permanent IVC filters. From left to right, they are the Venatech filter, the Greenfield filter, a Simon Nitinol filter, a Bird's Nest filter, and the TrapEase filter.

2. Filters have mistakenly been placed in the aorta, right atrium, below the confluence of the iliac veins, even in a paralumbar vein, and the spinal canal—these complications have all been reported in the vascular surgery literature. Operators should be familiar with the deployment sheaths and techniques that are particular to each individual filter.

3. Indications for IVC filter placement are for protection against pulmonary embolism (PE). Patients with iliofemoral deep vein thrombosis (DVT) and massive PE are at risk from further thromboembolic disease. Patients may have contraindications to anticoagulation—due to active bleeding or a history of intracranial hemorrhage. Patients can also develop venous thromboembolism (VTE) despite being anticoagulated. Perioperative candidates or patients with malignancy are also candidates for IVC filter placement. Permanent IVC filter placement can occur in any of the above situations, where it is likely that risk of PE from VTE is long-term and where the patient is unlikely to return to, or receive anticoagulation. Decisions to implant and retrieve filters should be coordinated and have multidisciplinary involvement.

4. Filters can migrate, fracture, and penetrate the caval wall. These events can be symptomatic, and fractured filters have embolized to the heart and have required retrieval or open-heart surgery. There may be an

association with increased DVT post–filter placement, as well as caval stenosis and caval thrombosis. Access site thrombosis, access complications, and complications associated with venography and contrast medium can also occur.

5. Intravascular ultrasonography–guided IVC filter placement is particularly advantageous in critically ill patients who may be at risk of transfer to the interventional suite from an intensive care setting.

Pearls

- Permanent IVC filters include the Venatech, TrapEase, Simon Nitinol, Greenfield and Bird's Nest filter. There is a growing trend for retrievable filters to be left in situ to function as a permanent device, but there are little data regarding the long-term safety of some of these devices.

Suggested Readings

Decousus H, Leizorovicz A, Parent F, et al. A clinical trial of vena caval filters in the prevention of pulmonary embolism in patients with proximal deep-vein thrombosis. Prévention du Risque d'Embolie Pulmonaire par Interruption Cave Study Group. *N Engl J Med.* 1998;338(7):409-415.

Grassi CJ, Swan TL, Cardella JF, et al. Quality improvement guidelines for percutaneous permanent inferior vena cava filter placement for the prevention of pulmonary embolism. *J Vasc Interv Radiol.* 2003;14(9 pt 2):S271-S275.

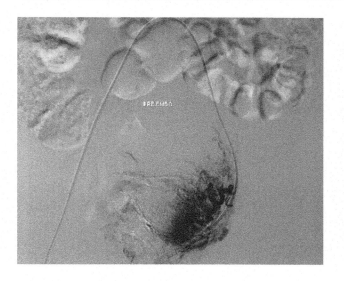
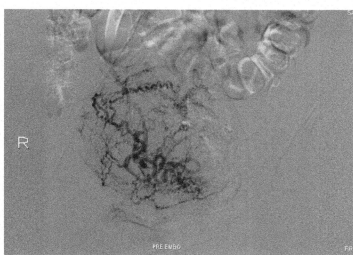

1. What catheters can be used to select the internal iliac arteries?

2. You identify persistent enhancing fundal fibroid in pelvic gadolinium-enhanced magnetic resonance (MR) images of a 38-year-old woman 3 months after bilateral uterine artery complete embolization. What is the possible reason for failure of procedure?

3. What are the complications after uterine artery embolization (UAE)?

4. When the uterine artery is absent, it is often replaced by what?

5. What is the clinical success of UFE and is pregnancy possible afterwards?

Case ranking/difficulty:

Category: Arterial system

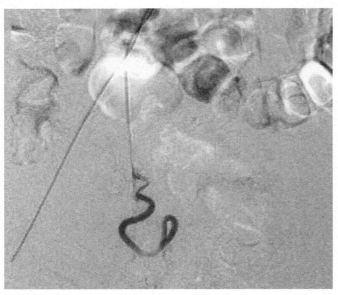

Selective angiogram of the left uterine artery after embolization.

Answers

1. This is commonly performed using Cobra or ultra-long reverse-curve catheters such as a Roberts catheter. Standard catheters, glide catheters, or microcatheters can be used to select the uterine arteries, a matter of operator preference, but larger host catheters may be occlusive, which can affect the embolization process, and are more likely to cause vessel spasm.

2. Clinical success approaches 90% but ovarian arteries that give significant fibroid supply can be present.

3. Serious complications include intrauterine infection, uterine ischemia or necrosis, and expulsion of pedunculated submucosal fibroids. Major complications occur in about 1% of patients.

4. In 1% of the population, the uterine artery is absent and is often replaced by the ipsilateral ovarian artery.

5. Pregnancy can occur after uterine fibroid embolization (UFE) but the long-term effects are not understood. UFE helps 90% of patients with fibroids, and around 70% of those with adenomyosis.

Pearls

- In 1% of the population, the uterine artery is absent and is often replaced by the ipsilateral ovarian artery. Outcomes of women seeking to become pregnant after uterine embolization are not well defined.

Suggested Reading

Spies JB, Scialli AR, Jha RC, et al. Initial results from uterine artery embolization for symptomatic leiomyomata. Presented at Radiologic Society of North America, Chicago, November 29, 1998.

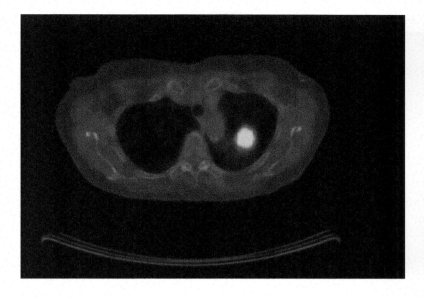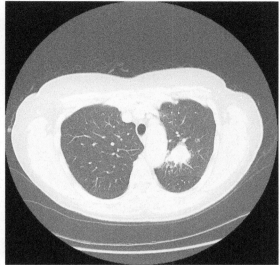

1. How would you biopsy this lesion—prone or supine?

2. What can make CT biopsy challenging?

3. What are the common complications?

4. How would you biopsy a cavitating lesion?

5. What is FEV1 and what is its significance here?

Case ranking/difficulty:

Category: Gastrointestinal system

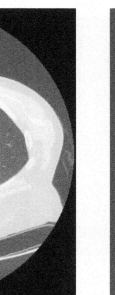

The biopsy was performed in the prone position crossing the fissure.

Sagittal view.

Answers

1. Prone is shorter but will cross the fissure theoretically, increasing the risk of pneumothorax. Anterior approach is very deep, which may be more challenging as the lesion may move, and there may be an increased risk of hemorrhage. I decided to come from behind.

2. Bony landmarks and the shoulder girdle can make access difficult, and respiration motion can also be a problem.

3. Hemoptysis and pneumothorax are common.

4. Aim to sample the wall of the lesion, not the center.

5. The FEV1 is the forced expiratory volume that can be expired in 1 second and is an important lung function test. Patients with an FEV1 of <1 may not tolerate a large pneumothorax, and the biopsy may be contraindicated.

Pearls

- CT-guided procedures are performed by all radiologists, but many interventional radiologist find themselves doing a large share of biopsy and drainage procedures.
- Core cutting biopsy or fine-needle aspiration cytology can be performed.
- Coaxial needles offer the capability of taking multiple samples with only 1 breach of the visceral pleura.

Suggested Reading

Yankelevitz DF, Davis SD, Chiarella DA, Henschke CI. Pitfalls in CT-guided transthoracic needle biopsy of pulmonary nodules. *Radiographics*. 1996;16(5):1073-1084.

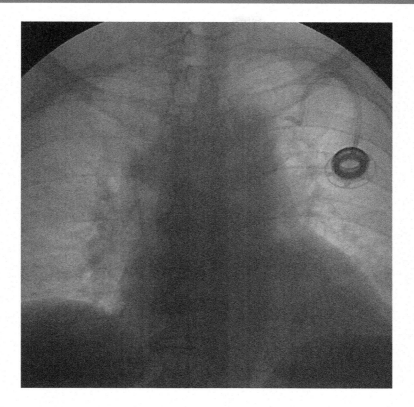

1. What has happened to the port and why?
   What would you do?

2. List some common intravascular foreign bodies
   that require retrieval.

3. Inferior vena cava (IVC) filters have
   been successfully retrieved from the right
   ventricle—true or false?

4. Diagnostic catheters have known to become
   knotted and then require special retrieval
   techniques—true or false?

5. Intravascular bullet embolization can occur
   after gunshot wounds—true or false?

Case ranking/difficulty:

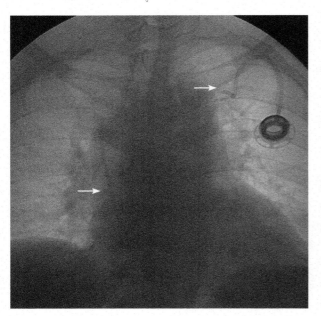

Spot fluoroscopic image demonstrating a broken port.

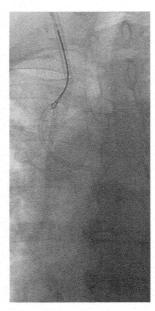

Successful retrieval of the broken catheter.

Answers

1. The port has broken as a result of the 1st rib and clavicle causing the material to fatigue. Percutaneous retrieval using an intravascular snare should be performed.

2. Inferior vena cava (IVC) filters, central venous lines, VP shunts, guidewires, misplaced coils, and stents are common items that require retrieval.

3. True. Several mechanisms are thought to lead to infrarenal IVC filters migrating en-bloc into the heart. Operator error, placement of a filter into a megacava, the sail phenomenon (where a large thrombus hits the filter causing it to migrate), and guidewire entrapment from jugular central vein access have all been reported to lead to IVC filter entrapment.

4. True. Knotted catheters have been reported as have special techniques to unknot them.

5. Intravascular bullet embolization is indeed a well-recognized phenomenon.

Pearls

- Intravascular foreign body retrieval is another important IR technique.
- Filters are the most commonly retrieved device.
- Broken catheters, misplaced stents, and coils also require retrieval.

- There are many different types of snare devices available; the most commonly used is probably the "gooseneck" snare. These can be used through directional catheters. Other snare devices have leaflets as opposed to the "lasso" shape. There are some commercially available coil retrieval devices. Dormia baskets can be useful.
- Retrieval devices may also need to be improvised (eg, self-made wire-loop snare), or borrowed from other departments (eg, endobronchial forceps).
- The filter literature is full of novel and advanced techniques that can also be applied to other intravascular foreign body retrievals. Another challenging situation is if a reverse curve diagnostic catheter gets knotted, and there are several reported techniques discussing how to "unknot" a catheter!

Suggested Readings

Gabelmann A, Kramer S, Gorich J. Percutaneous retrieval of lost or misplaced intravascular objects. *AJR Am J Roentgenol*. 2001;176(6):1509-1513.

Ronsivalle J, Statler J, Venbrux AC, Arepally A. Intravascular bullet migration: a report of two cases. *Mil Med*. 2005;170(12):1044-1047.

Wolf F, Schernthaner RE, Dirisamer A, et al. Endovascular management of lost or misplaced intravascular objects: experiences of 12 years. *Cardiovasc Intervent Radiol*. 2008;31(3):563-568.

45-year-old man with a left arm brachiobasilic arteriovenous (AV) fistula with prolonged bleeding after dialysis

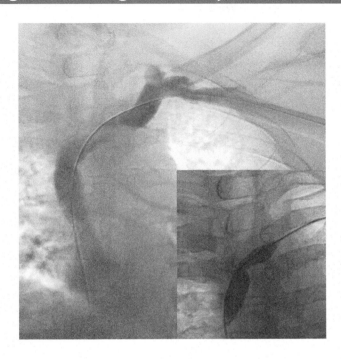

1. What do you see in the image? What has been the result of angioplasty?

2. What would you do next?

3. List 5 modes of renal replacement therapy.

4. List some risk factors for the development of central vein stenosis.

5. What is a high-pressure balloon? What is the "mean burst pressure" and what is the "rated burst pressure"?

Case ranking/difficulty: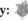

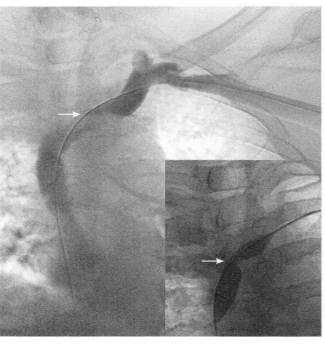

Venogram, and inset, result of balloon angioplasty.

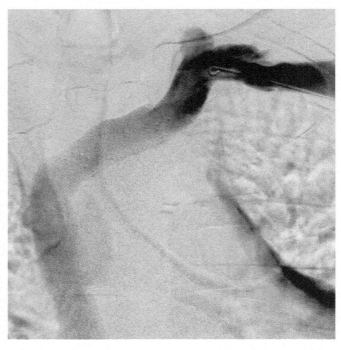

Post–stent placement venogram.

Answers

1. There is a left brachiocephalic vein stenosis. There is residual "waisting" of the angioplasty balloon.

2. Use of a high-pressure balloon, cutting balloon, or stent are options after initial failed angioplasty.

3. Transplant, dialysis with central catheter, dialysis with a native fistula, dialysis through a vascular graft, and peritoneal dialysis.

4. The main association is with previous subclavian central venous access procedures for intravenous access or cardiac device implantation.

5. High-pressure balloons are made of nylon or polyethylene terephthalate (PET). High-pressure balloons are noncompliant as controlled and repeatable force/pressure/diameter characteristics are required. Low-pressure compliant balloons are made from silicone; these are used for molding or occlusion. The mean burst pressure is the pressure above which 50% of the balloons might rupture. The rated burst pressure is the pressure below which 99.9% of balloons will not rupture. There are drug-eluting balloons, and many other forms of balloons in development that can, for example, deliver thermal energy or laser.

Pearls

- Angioplasty is used as the primary treatment for central vein stenosis. Primary angioplasty has a longer primary patency than primary stenting.
- Stenting should be reserved for angioplasty-resistant lesions. There is some evidence that primary stenting with polytetrafluoroethylene (PTFE)-covered stents is beneficial in specific situations (eg, primary stenting of the venous anastomosis in grafts).

Suggested Readings

Haskal ZJ, Trerotola S, Dolmatch B, et al. Stent graft versus balloon angioplasty for failing dialysis-access grafts. *N Engl J Med.* 2010;362(6):494-503.

Ozyer U, Harman A, Yildirim E, Aytekin C, Karakayali F, Boyvat F. Long-term results of angioplasty and stent placement for treatment of central venous obstruction in 126 hemodialysis patients: a 10-year single-center experience. *AJR Am J Roentgenol.* 2009;193(6):1672-1679.

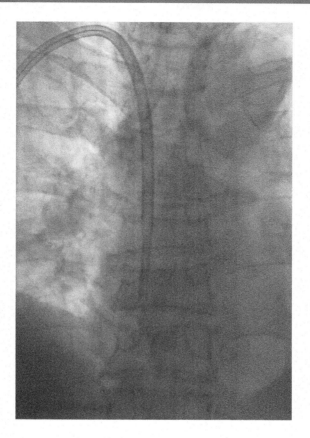

1. What catheter has been sited?

2. What else do you notice about this patient?

3. What are the complications associated with plasmapheresis?

4. What flow rates are typically required for dialysis?

5. List some factors that may reduce line sepsis.

Category: Venous system

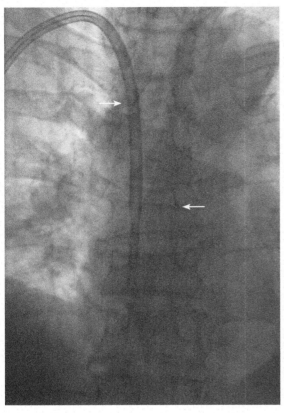

Post line placement. Note the vertebral collapse associated with the underlying condition.

3. Catheter-related bloodstream infections (CRBSI) or catheter dysfunction due to fibrin sheath formation can occur, as well as those complications associated with central venous access. Hypocalcaemia may occur due to the use of citrate.

4. 300 mL/min.

5. Meticulous catheter care is the main factor. Sterile conditions for placement, antibiotic impregnated catheters, and antibiotic locking solutions may also reduce CRBSI. Use of catheters with the minimal number of required lumens and ports is also associated with lower infection rates.

Pearls

• Plasmapheresis (also known as apheresis) or plasma exchange can be performed through dual-channel large-bore dialysis catheters. Catheters can be tunneled or nontunneled depending on the number of treatments that are expected to be given.

• Plasma exchange is used in the treatment of autoimmune and hematologic diseases and results in the rapid removal of circulating autoantibodies or proteins responsible for hyperviscosity syndromes. It can therefore be used in myeloma, Waldenström macroglobulinemia, thrombotic thrombocytopenic purpura (TTP), and myasthenia gravis. Blood is withdrawn and circulated through a cell separator that removes the plasma but returns the remainder of the blood in conjunction with a plasma substitute.

Answers

1. A tunneled dialysis catheter has been sited. Note the dual channels—arterial and venous ports. The tips of dialysis catheters have different designs; for example, split-tip catheters are popular. These catheters are commonly made from polyurethane or silicone and have large lumens and specialized tip design to allow large flow rates.

2. The combination of vertebral collapse and dialysis catheter suggests that the patient has myeloma and is due for plasmapheresis, or alternatively could have developed renal failure and requires dialysis.

Suggested Reading

Trerotola SO. Hemodialysis catheter placement and management. *Radiology*. 2000;215(3):651-658.

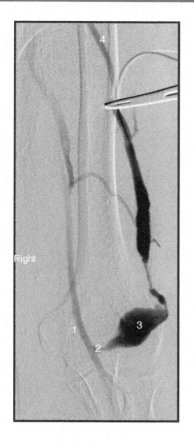
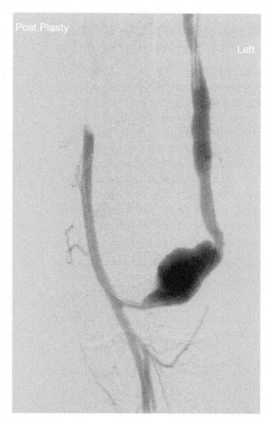

1. Name the locations/vessels labelled 1 through 4.

2. How can the arterial anastomosis be imaged?

3. List different types of accesses that allow dialysis.

4. What types of interventional procedures may be performed on fistulas?

5. What kind of balloons can be used on fistulas?

Case ranking/difficulty: 🎖️   **Category:** Venous system

Answers

1. 1. Brachial artery. 2. Anastomosis. 3. Perianastomotic/
    proximal cephalic vein. 4. Distal/outflow cephalic vein.

2. The AV anastomosis can be imaged with ultrasound. At
    fistulogram, the anastomosis can be directly visualized
    with an angiogram performed from the brachial artery
    (direct brachial artery access, best done with a 3-Fr inner
    dilator from a micropuncture set) or from the venous
    side. Imaging the anastomosis from the venous side
    can involve injecting while the operator compresses
    the outflow (manually with fingers or a hemostat, or
    sometimes with a blood pressure cuff), or by passing a
    catheter and guidewire into the artery and then injecting
    contrast medium through the catheter (as is done in the
    postangioplasty image in this case).

3. Native arteriovenous fistulas, AV synthetic grafts, central
    venous tunneled dialysis catheters, and peritoneal
    dialysis are options.

4. Angioplasty, stenting, thrombolysis, and coil embolization
    of collaterals can be performed to maintain fistula
    function.

5. Standard, high-pressure, and cutting angioplasty balloons
    can be used on fistulas.

Pearls

- Ultrasound surveillance often detects stenoses before
  they become clinically apparent, or indeed before
  they progress to an occlusion. It is an important part
  of providing a fistula service. Also, ultrasonography
  helps the interventionist to plan the procedure and
  access points.
- Native AV fistulas are preferential to synthetic grafts,
  which, in turn, are preferential to tunneled dialysis
  catheters for long-term dialysis access.

Suggested Reading

Zangan SM, Falk A. Optimizing arteriovenous fistula
  maturation. *Semin Intervent Radiol.* 2009;26(2):144-150.

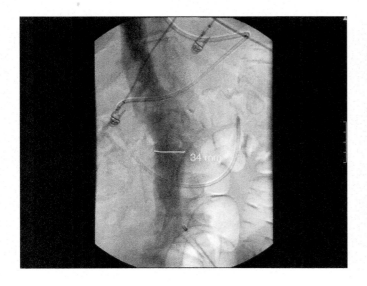 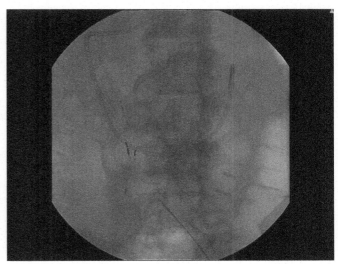

1. What does the cavagram show?

2. What is the maximum caval size that a Bird's Nest filter can be used in?

3. What other conditions are associated with megacava?

4. In the setting of megacava, how can filters be used to protect against PE?

5. What is the incidence of megacava?

Case ranking/difficulty: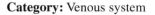

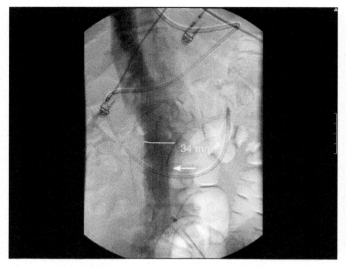

Cavagram, caval width 34 mm.

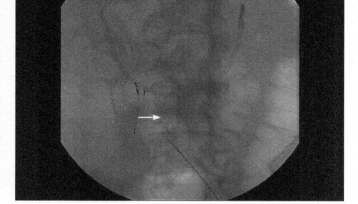

Bird's Nest inferior vena cava (IVC) filter.

Answers

1. Megacava occurs when the cava is 28 mm or more. Cavagrams may underestimate the true caval size.

2. 40 mm (A megacava is when the IVC is more than 28 mm).

3. Severe TR is associated with megacava.

4. Bilateral placement of filters into each common iliac vein filters is indicated if the cava is >40 mm.

5. Series have reported an incidence of up to 3% based on measurements of the cava at filter placement.

Pearls

- A megacava is defined as being more than 28 mm in size. Some devices can be placed into cavas at 30 or 32 mm (always check manufacturer recommendations). A Bird's Nest filter can be placed into a cava up to 40 mm (per manufacturer guidelines); other options for caval filtration include placing 2 filters, 1 in each common iliac vein. There are case reports of en bloc filter migration into the heart, and the cava has been shown to have dynamic changes in size with respiration and valsalva, so device choice in large cavas is important.

Suggested Reading

Nicholson AA, Ettles DF, Paddon AJ, Dyet JF. Long-term follow-up of the Bird's Nest IVC filter. *Clin Radiol.* 1999;54(11):759-764.

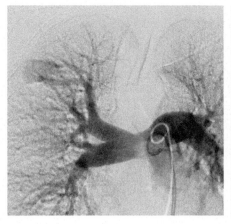 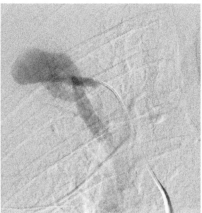 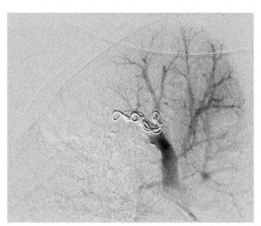

1. Are pulmonary arteriovenous malformations more likely to be sporadic, or associated with hereditary hemorrhagic telangiectasia?

2. Where else can lesions exist in HHT?

3. The majority of pulmonary AVMs have one feeding vessel—true or false?

4. What complications lead to increased mortality?

5. What are the indications for embolization?

Case ranking/difficulty:    **Category:** Arterial system

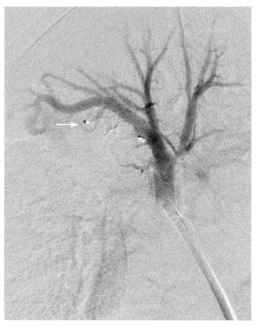

Image after deployment of an Amplatzer vascular plug (AVP).

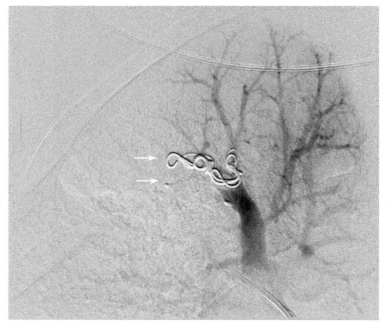

Final image after coil and Amplatzer vascular plug (AVP) embolization.

Answers

1. About 15% of patients with pulmonary AVMs do not meet the diagnostic criteria for HHT.

2. Mucosal lesions can cause epistaxis. AVMs can also occur in the liver and brain.

3. Around 80% of pulmonary AVMs are simple, and 20% are complex.

4. Pulmonary AVMs can rupture. There can be brain abscesses, and strokes can occur because of paradoxical emboli.

5. Enlargement, paradoxical embolus, hypoxemia, and AVMs with feeding vessels of greater than 3 mm diameter are indications for treatment.

Pearls

- Pulmonary AVMs can be solitary or multiple. They are associated with Osler-Weber-Rendu syndrome/hereditary hemorrhagic telangiectasia. Patients are at risk of hemoptysis and septic cerebral emboli.
- These lesions can be treated with embolization. AVPs and coils are commonly used. Treatment is successful in the vast majority of cases with regression/involution of the AVM. Lesions can persist because of recanalization, or due to interval growth of previously nonvisualized feeding vessels. These lesions may need secondary intervention.

Suggested Reading

Pollak JS, Saluja S, Thabet A, et al. Clinical and anatomic outcomes after embolotherapy of pulmonary arteriovenous malformations. *J Vasc Interv Radiol.* 2006;17(1):35-44; quiz 45.

38-year-old woman presents with back pain and macroscopic hematuria. At cystoscopy, a blood clot in the bladder and bleeding from the right ureteral orifice were detected

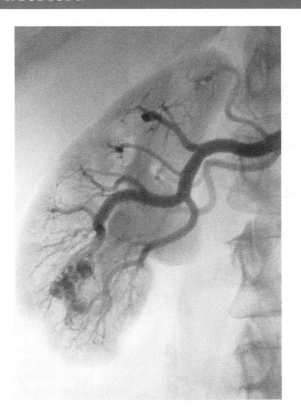

1. What is the diagnosis?

2. How can this condition present?

3. Describe the branching pattern of the renal artery.

4. Which are acceptable management strategies?

5. Which embolic material might be preferred?

Case ranking/difficulty:    **Category:** Arterial system

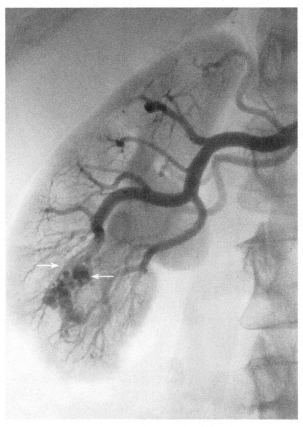

Right renal angiogram showing an AVM with multiple feeding arteries.

Answers

1. This is a congenital cirsoid AVM. Polyarteritis nodosa causes small aneurysms.

2. It can present with macroscopic hematuria, heart failure, and hypertension, with renal colic due to the passage of clots, or be an incidental finding on CT.

3. Segmental arteries divide into lobar arteries, which in turn become interlobar, interlobular, and then afferent arterioles.

4. Conservative management, embolization, and nephrectomy may all be indicated.

5. Ethanol or glue would be preferred to treat the nidus.

Pearls

- Congenital AVMs in the renal circulation can be classified into cirsoid or cavernous subtypes, which are less common. Cirsoid AVMs have a classical corkscrew appearance. Cavernous AVMs have a single feeding artery, a dilated channel, and a single draining vein.
- Acquired arteriovenous fistulas account for two-thirds of renovascular lesions in this category. These can occur after biopsy, surgery, or idiopathic where an aneurysm may erode into a vein.

Suggested Reading

Chimpiri AR, Natarajan B. Renal vascular lesions: diagnosis and endovascular management. *Semin Intervent Radiol.* 2009;26(3):253-261.

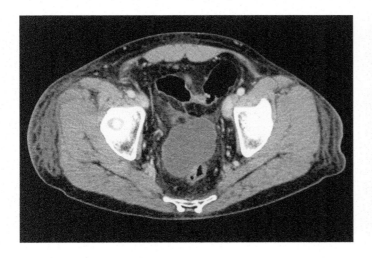
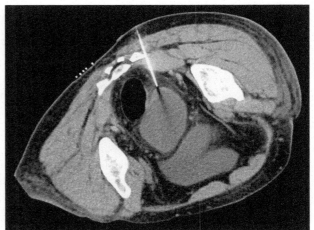

1. Describe the anatomy of the piriformis muscle.

2. Which is better—transpiriformis or infrapiriformis access, and why?

3. Describe the Seldinger technique for drain placement.

4. Describe the trocar technique for drain placement.

5. What is the angled gantry technique?

Category: Gastrointestinal system

Answers

1. Piriformis arises from the ventral aspect of the lateral border of the sacrum, passes through the greater sciatic foramen, and inserts onto the greater tuberosity.

2. The gluteal vessels and sacral plexus lie anterior to the piriformis, so a subpiriformis approach is best, but if this cannot be avoided, then the access should be as close to the sacrum as possible.

3. Needle access into the cavity is obtained, and then a wire is placed through the needle and coiled within said cavity. The access wire can then be used to serially dilate the tract and then the drain is inserted over-the-wire.

4. This is performed as a direct puncture, with a 3-part drain—needle, metal stiffener, and plastic drain. The drain is inserted directly into the cavity, and then the drain is advanced or "stripped" forward over the metal stiffener to form in the cavity.

5. If a path to the target is not available due to interposition of bowel, the CT gantry can be angled, and an inferior-to-superior path, for example, at 10 or 15 degrees can be planned.

Pearls

- A medial subpiriformis window is a safe route into the pelvis via a transgluteal approach, as the neurovascular bundle is not at risk.
- In this case, however, piriformis had to be transgressed but attention was paid to the location of the sciatic nerve.

Suggested Reading

Harisinghani MG, Gervais DA, Hahn PF, et al. CT-guided transgluteal drainage of deep pelvic abscesses: indications, technique, procedure-related complications, and clinical outcome. *Radiographics.* 2002;22(6):1353-1367.

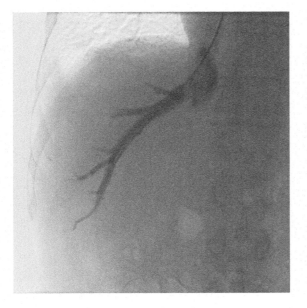
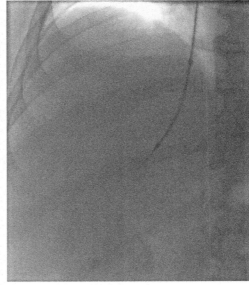

1. List some indications for transjugular liver biopsy.

2. Transjugular biopsy samples are better than percutaneous samples—true or false?

3. Describe the venous drainage of the liver.

4. What other access and biopsy sites are possible?

5. List some complications of transjugular liver biopsy.

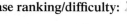

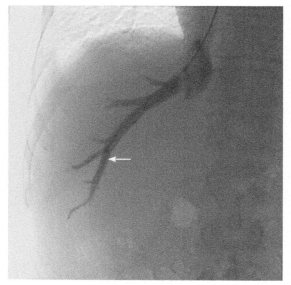

Hepatic venogram.

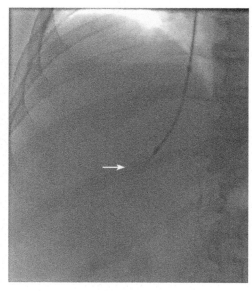

Core biopsy needle placed coaxially through the sheath.

Answers

1. Ascites, coagulopathy, and the need for pressure measurements are the main indications for transjugular liver biopsy.

2. Transjugular cores are 18G but fragment in up to 33% of cases. Nevertheless, technical success is toward 100% and histologic diagnosis is made in 96% of cases. The key indicator of a satisfactory biopsy is the number of complete portal tracts in each core. Six to 11 portal tracts are required, depending upon indication. Multiple passes are needed to ensure adequate samples are obtained.

3. There is a right, middle, and left hepatic vein. The caudate lobe often drains directly into the cava. (This can be encountered during adrenal vein sampling when seeking out the right adrenal vein). There is also anatomic variation, with a right inferior accessory vein being common.

4. Left internal jugular approach is feasible. Similarly, biopsy can be taken from the left hepatic vein. Transjugular biopsy can be performed in transplant livers but the operator should be familiar with the anatomy of the surgical anastomosis ("piggyback" vs end-to-end, for example).

5. Capsular perforation with perihepatic hematoma, inadequate biopsy specimens, and biopsy of nontarget tissue including kidney can occur.

Pearls

- Transjugular biopsy can be performed when ascites or coagulopathy precludes percutaneous liver biopsy.
- Right heart and wedged and free hepatic pressures can be measured to evaluate for the presence of right heart failure and portal hypertension.
- Transjugular liver biopsy is performed via a jugular approach. A catheter is used to access a hepatic vein, usually the right or middle hepatic vein. The catheter is then exchanged for a sheath that allows a long core biopsy needle to be passed coaxially. The sheath is then rotated anticlockwise/anteriorly if in the right hepatic vein, or clockwise/posteriorly if in the middle hepatic vein and biopsies are obtained.

Suggested Reading

Behrens G, Ferral H, Giusto D, Patel J, Van Thiel DH. Transjugular liver biopsy: comparison of sample adequacy with the use of two automated needle systems. *J Vasc Interv Radiol.* 2011;22(3):341-345.

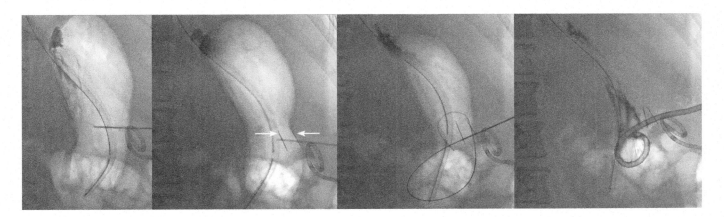

1. Name some indications for gastrostomy tube placement.

2. What can be done if the tube falls out?

3. What are the complications of gastrostomy?

4. What can be done if the transverse colon appears to be in the way?

5. What can be done if the patient has ascites?

Answers

1. Enteral nutrition in patients with head and neck cancer and neurologic disease are common indications. Gastrostomy tubes can also be placed for decompression in palliation of proximal obstruction. Gastrostomy access can also be used to place duodenal stents for gastric outlet obstruction.

2. Tubes can be replaced. If the tract is mature, this is not urgent. If a tract is recent, this should be treated as a relative emergency. Attempts made within 24 hours are much more successful than those left more than 1 day (in one study, mean success occurred at 1.1 days, mean failure at 2.7 days).

3. Leak is seen in up to 1%. Local infection at the entry is common and self-limiting.

4. Gastrostomy can also be performed under CT guidance if there is a difficult access window. An intercostal approach can also be used if the stomach lies above the subcostal margin.

5. The ascites can be drained at the same time, and then the gastrostomy tube can be placed. Placement of an epigastric drain near the site of the planned gastrostomy is recommended, and the ascitic drain should be left in situ for 2 weeks until the gastrostomy tract has matured.

Pearls

- Interventional radiology has an important role in provision of nutritional support. Gastrostomy can be placed endoscopically (ie, percutaneous endoscopic gastrostomy [PEG]), percutaneously (ie, radiologically inserted gastrostomy [RIG], gastrostomy tube [G-tube]), or surgically.
- Endoscopy can be associated with increased risk because of potential respiratory complications. In patients with head and neck cancer, endoscopy may be difficult. There are a range of gastric tubes, such as those with pigtails or "buttons."
- Nutrition should be enteral when there is a functional gastrointestinal (GI) tract. Parenteral nutrition via a Hickman line is for patients with a nonfunctioning GI tract or when diversion is required.
- Gastrostomy can also be placed via a "venting" tube for palliation of upper GI tract obstruction and which then obviates the need for a nasogastric tube. Gastrostomy access can also be placed to facilitate other interventions such as placement of a duodenal stent.

Suggested Reading

Nijs EL, Cahill AM. Pediatric enteric feeding techniques: insertion, maintenance, and management of problems. *Cardiovasc Intervent Radiol.* 2010;33(6):1101-1110.

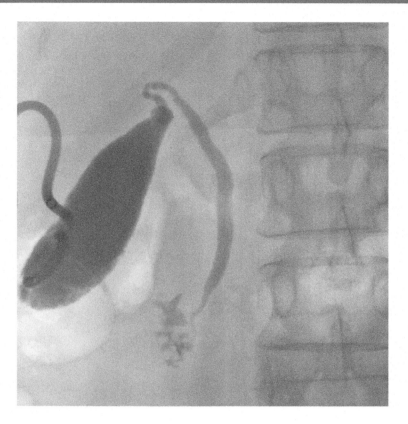

1. What are the indications for percutaneous cholecystostomy?

2. It should be performed with ultrasonography and fluoroscopy—true or false?

3. How and when should the tube be removed?

4. What are the complications of percutaneous cholecystostomy?

5. What should be done once the tube is inserted?

Case ranking/difficulty: 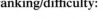   **Category:** Gastrointestinal system

Answers

1. Cholecystostomy is used as a temporizing measure in critically ill patients with acute cholecystitis who are unfit for surgery.

2. False, some operators just use ultrasonography.

3. The tube can be removed at surgery. If patients with stones are deemed unfit for surgery, or if the acute event was due to acalculous cholecystostomy, then the tube can be removed. The tube should be capped 48 hours prior to removal, as a clinical test for cystic duct obstruction. Removal can be performed after 2 weeks. Some operators will only remove the tube after performing a tractogram to check for tract maturation and to exclude any potential leak of bile into the peritoneum. If this is seen, a drainage tube can be reinserted and the tractogram repeated in a few weeks.

4. Complications include hemobilia, gallbladder perforation, and biliary peritonitis due to bile leak. Vagal stimulation can occur at time of placement. Tube dislodgement can also be a problem.

5. A bile aspirate can be obtained and the gallbladder decompressed. All tubes should be secured in place. Cystic duct patency should not be tested at tube placement, as contrast injection can increase risk of sepsis due to bacterial translocation. Clinical improvement is generally seen after 24-48 hours.

Pearls

- Percutaneous cholecystostomy is an important drainage procedure in critically ill patients who develop cholecystitis who do not respond to conservative treatment and are not fit for surgery.
- Transhepatic or direct gallbladder punctures can be performed.

Suggested Reading

Ginat D, Saad WEA. Cholecystostomy and transcholecystic biliary access. *Tech Vasc Interv Radiol.* 2008;11(1):2-13.

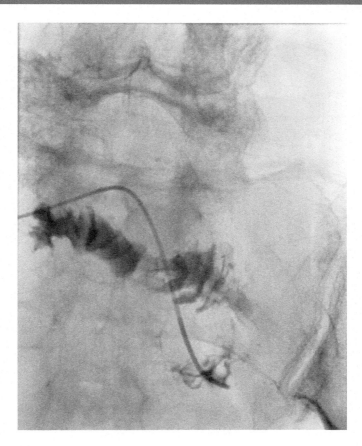

1. What is the most appropriate step to replace this tube?

2. Fresh tracts should be explored urgently—true or false?

3. Describe how you would reaccess the gastrointestinal tract.

4. What other techniques can help with replacing the tube?

5. If the tube is blocked, it should be exchanged—true or false?

Case ranking/difficulty:

Category: Gastrointestinal system

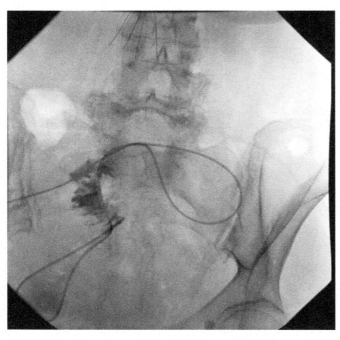

Tube inserted.

Answers

1. The tract should be probed and a new tube inserted.

2. Fresh tracts will close easily and access can be lost, so they should be treated urgently.

3. Attempts should initially be made with a glidewire to access the gastrointestinal tract through the preexisting hole. If this fails, a short catheter can be used and contrast injected to demonstrate the path. Care should be taken to avoid creating false passages.

4. Inserting a tube over a glidewire can be challenging, so a nonhydrophilic or stiff wire may be required. The same tube should be inserted, as the patient and patient's carers are happy with and able to care for the tube.

5. Tubes can be unblocked using injections of saline or dissolvents, or mechanically by passing a wire through the tube.

> ### Pearls
>
> - Feeding tubes can become dislodged.
> - Fresh tracts should be urgently reexplored to save the access.
> - Mature tracts can be easily reaccessed.
> - Tube maintenance and tube exchanges are important procedures.

Suggested Reading

Nijs EL, Cahill AM. Pediatric enteric feeding techniques: insertion, maintenance, and management of problems. *Cardiovasc Intervent Radiol.* 2010;33(6):1101-1110.

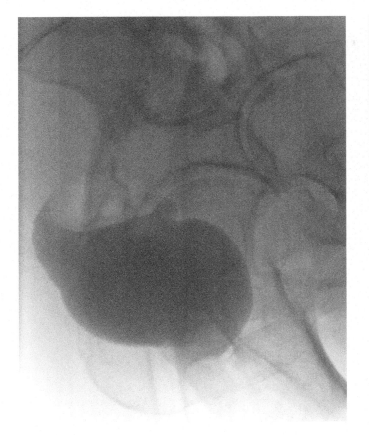
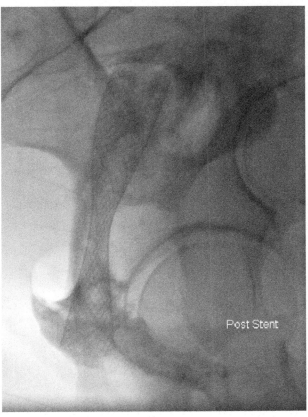

1. List indications for colonic stent placement.

2. What long-term complications can occur for stents placed as definitive palliative treatment?

3. What are the potential advantages of stenting as a bridge to surgery?

4. Can stents be placed with radiologic guidance into the descending colon?

5. Can stents be placed into the transverse colon under radiologic guidance?

Case ranking/difficulty: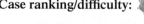

Category: Gastrointestinal system

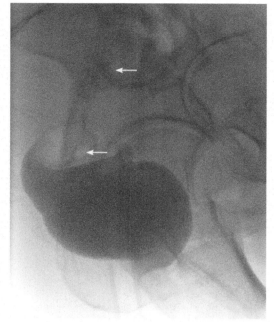

Lateral proctogram, which demonstrates a large tumor.

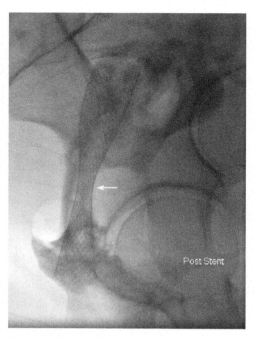

Poststent image. The stent is centered across the stricture.

Answers

1. Stents can be placed to deal with the acute obstructive episode as a bridge to surgery or placed as definitive palliative treatment.

2. Stent migration, perforation, reobstruction due to tumor ingrowth, and tenesmus can occur.

3. Stenting as a bridge to surgery allows patients physiological status and fluid balance and nutritional status to be optimized prior to surgery. Surgery can then be performed in one stage, as a temporary stoma is not required because the obstruction has been dealt with.

4. Colon stents can be placed under radiologic guidance into the descending colon; however, long redundant colonic loops can make this challenging. Combined procedures with an endoscopist are often successful in this setting.

5. Yes. This has also been reported.

Pearls

- Stenting allows for the initial management of the obstruction.
- The patient can be optimized for surgery, and as the obstruction has resolved, a primary anastomosis can be fashioned without the need for a temporary stoma.

- Colonic stenting can be performed per-rectally with catheters and sheaths. Combined procedures with endoscopy can also be performed, which is particularly useful for lesions that are more proximal.
- Catheters and sheaths can be negotiated around multiple bends, and the redundant loops that form can be reduced with catheter rotation or retraction. Use of a larger sheath and catheter allows contrast to be injected both proximal and distal to the lesion to facilitate stent placement. Self-expanding metal stents, for example, 20 × 60 or 20 × 90 mm Wallstents, can be used.
- Complications include perforation and stent migration.

Suggested Readings

Katsanos K, Sabharwal T, Adam A. Stenting of the lower gastrointestinal tract: current status. *Cardiovasc Intervent Radiol.* 2010;34(3):462-473.

Shrivastava V, Tariq O, Tiam RN, Nyhsen C, Marsh R. Palliation of obstructing malignant colonic lesions using self-expanding metal stents: a single-center experience. *Cardiovasc Intervent Radiol.* 2007;31(5):931-936.

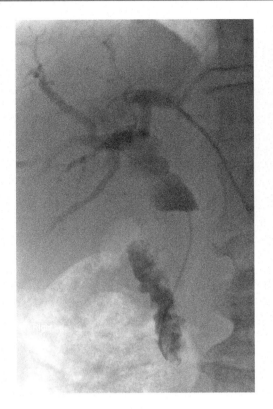 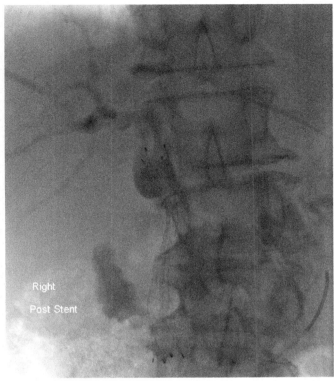

1. Review the images—what is being deployed?

2. What endobiliary stents can be used?

3. What are the complications of biliary stent placement?

4. Balloon dilatation is always required after stent placement—true or false?

5. Covered biliary stents can be removed—true or false?

Case ranking/difficulty: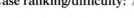

Answers

1. A self-expanding metallic stent is being deployed.

2. Self-expanding nitinol stents are straightforward to deploy. Self-expanding stainless steel stents such as a Wallstent may shorten significantly, and precise placement needs attention. Covered stents are available, and may be associated with better patency rates and reduced reintervention rates due to tumor ingrowth. Balloon-expanding stents can be used when stenting across a short intra-hepatic stricture is required.

3. Stent migration, tumor ingrowth, tumor overgrowth, and obstruction of other ducts can result from biliary stenting, as well as all the usual complications associated with percutaneous transhepatic cholangiography (PTHC).

4. False. Stents continue to expand over the next 24 hours in general. Pre-stent placement balloon dilatation of the stricture is sometimes required to facilitate passage of the stent device, which may range from 6 to 10 Fr.

5. True. Retrieval of covered metallic biliary stents has been reported in the setting of managing bile leaks.

Pearls

- A self-expanding nitinol stent is used in this case. Self-expanding stainless steel stents (eg, Wallstents) are also available, as are covered stents (eg, Viabil). Balloon-expandable stents can be used when precise placement of a stent across a short intrahepatic ductal stricture is required.
- Common bile duct (CBD) stents can be placed for lower strictures. Right and left hepatic duct "kissing stents" can be placed, or a left-to-right hepatic duct stent can be placed in conjunction with a right-sided CBD stent to maximize hepatic drainage.

Suggested Reading

Krokidis M, Fanelli F, Orgera G, Bezzi M, Passariello R, Hatzidakis A. Percutaneous treatment of malignant jaundice due to extrahepatic cholangiocarcinoma: covered Viabil stent versus uncovered Wallstents. *Cardiovasc Intervent Radiol.* 2010;33(1):97-106.

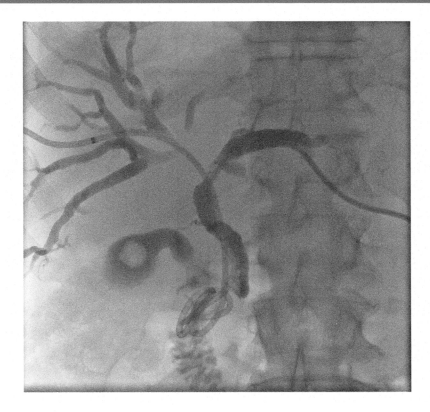

1. Review the image. Where are the strictures?

2. What is the Bismuth classification in this case?

3. What treatment options are available for cholangiocarcinoma?

4. What is the lifetime risk of developing cholangiocarcinoma in patients with primary sclerosing cholangitis?

5. What is the risk of cholangiocarcinoma occurring in a choledochal cyst?

Case ranking/difficulty:

Category: Gastrointestinal system

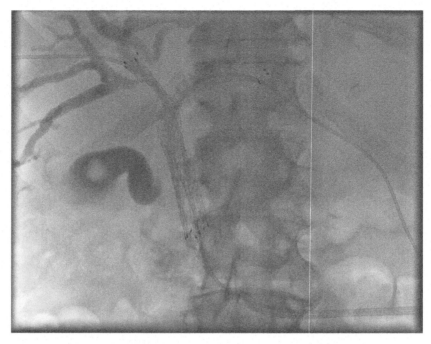

Post stenting.

Answers

1. There are strictures involving the right and left intrahepatic ducts and also the proximal common hepatic duct.

2. This is a type 4 Bismuth lesion.

3. Tumors can be resected. Liver transplantation is curative. Chemoradiation is another treatment modality. Percutaneous transhepatic cholangiography (PTHC) has several roles—diagnosis and biopsy, mapping out anatomy for resection, placement of biliary drains to aid resection, and placement of plastic or metal stents for palliation.

4. Lifetime risk is reported to be 5% to 15%.

5. A malignant transformation rate of 5% is quoted.

Pearls

- Hilar cholangiocarcinoma is known as the Klatskin tumor. This is most commonly an infiltrative adenocarcinoma that grows along the bile ducts.
- The Bismuth classification is used to describe the involvement of the hepatic ducts. Type 1 occurs below the confluence, type 2 involves the confluence, type 3 involves the common hepatic duct and the left or right duct, and type 4 is multifocal or involves the CHD and both left and right ducts.
- Risk factors include intraductal stones, bile duct adenomas, bile duct papillomatosis, ulcerative colitis, primary sclerosing cholangitis, smoking, Caroli disease, and choledochal cysts.

Suggested Reading

Khan SA, Davidson BR, Goldin R, et al. Guidelines for the diagnosis and treatment of cholangiocarcinoma: consensus document. *Gut*. 2002;51(suppl 6):VI1-VI9.

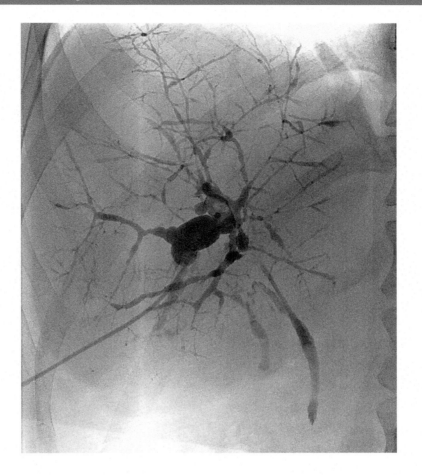

1. What is the diagnosis?

2. What other conditions are associated with this diagnosis?

3. What is the management of this condition?

4. Discuss the epidemiology of this condition.

5. How can a PTC be performed and give a contraindication and a complication.

Case ranking/difficulty: **Category:** Gastrointestinal system

Answers

1. This is PSC.

2. Cholangiocarcinoma, colorectal carcinoma, and ulcerative colitis (UC) are associations. PSC can progress to cirrhosis. Other rare associations include retroperitoneal fibrosis, fibrosing mediastinitis, orbital pseudotumor, Sjögren's syndrome and Riedel's thyroiditis.

3. Medical management, endoscopic retrograde cholangiopancreatography (ERCP) or percutaneous stent placement, and ultimately transplantation are used in the treatment of PSC.

4. Males are more commonly affected and it can present in the early 20s. Around 5% of those with UC may develop PSC. Ten percent to 15% of those with PSC develop cholangiocarcinoma. Liver failure develops at around 10 to 12 years from diagnosis.

5. Left- or right-sided approaches can be taken. Ascites is a relative contraindication. Postprocedure sepsis occurs in around 10%. Prophylactic antibiotics should be given. Most procedures can be performed using sedoanalgesia.

Pearls

- PSC is a chronic liver disease that results from inflammation and fibrosis of the bile ducts. There are associations with cholangiocarcinoma and ulcerative colitis.
- ERCP and percutaneous transhepatic cholangiography are useful diagnostically and therapeutically.
- Liver transplantation is the definitive treatment.

Suggested Readings

Ahrendt SA, Pitt HA, Kalloo AN, et al. Primary sclerosing cholangitis: resect, dilate, or transplant? *Ann Surg.* 1998;227(3):412-423.

Mueller PR, Harbin WP, Ferrucci JT, Wittenberg J, vanSonnenberg E. Fine-needle transhepatic cholangiography: reflections after 450 cases. *AJR Am J Roentgenol.* 1981;136(1):85-90.

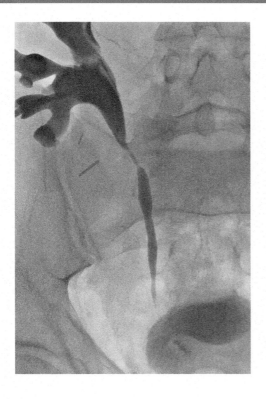 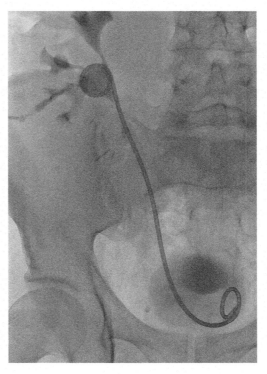

1. What are the graft half-lives for living and cadaveric renal transplants?

2. List 10 medical issues related to renal transplant patients and allograft function.

3. How can renal allograft dysfunction be monitored?

4. What is the incidence of acute renal artery thrombosis?

5. What is the incidence of major complications in nephrostomy placement?

Case ranking/difficulty: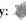

Answers

1. The graft half-life for a living donor is 20 years, and for a cadaveric donor, it is 12 years.

2. Rejection (hyperacute, acute, chronic), nephrotoxicity of immunosuppression, wound complications, arterial thrombosis, renal vein thrombosis, ureteric stenosis/obstruction, urine leak, and lymphocele. Infectious disease and malignancy can also be caused by immunosuppression. Metabolic bone disease is also another risk.

3. Serial creatinine measures are the first sign of dysfunction. Ultrasound-guided percutaneous allograft biopsy is commonly required.

4. This occurs in 1% of grafts.

5. Major complications such as hemorrhage or vascular injury occur in 1% to 4%, and septic shock can occur in 1% to 9% of patients.

Pearls

- Urologic complications related to renal transplantation occur in up to 12.5% of cases and they include leak, ureteric stenosis, ureteric necrosis, and stone formation.
- Ureteric stenosis is thought to occur as a result of different mechanisms. Stenotic lesions can be ischemic (because of poor anastomotic technique and excessive hilar dissection) or also result from a leak that leads to periureteric fibrosis.
- Early intervention can result in preservation of graft function.

Suggested Readings

Dalgic A, Boyvat F, Karakayali H, Moray G, Emiroglu R, Haberal M. Urologic complications in 1523 renal transplantations: the Baskent University experience. *Transplant Proc.* 2006;38(2):543-547.

Kaskarelis I, Koukoulaki M, Georgantas T, et al. Ureteral complications in renal transplant recipients successfully treated with interventional radiology. *Transplant Proc.* 2008;40(9):3170-3172.

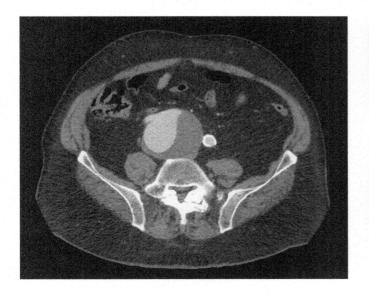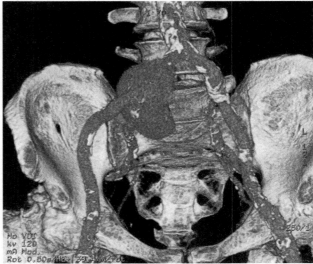

1. What are other, non-degenerative causes of common iliac artery (CIA) aneurysms?

2. When is the treatment of a CIA aneurysm indicated?

3. What factors need to be considered in planning endovascular repair?

4. How would you manage a 4 cm CIA aneurysm with an origin 1 cm below the aortic bifurcation, with 1 cm of normal CIA above the iliac bifurcation?

5. What is the mortality of open repair of an iliac artery aneurysm?

Case ranking/difficulty: 🐾

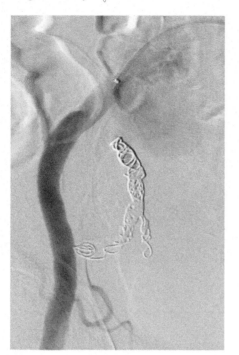

S/p Right IIA coiling.

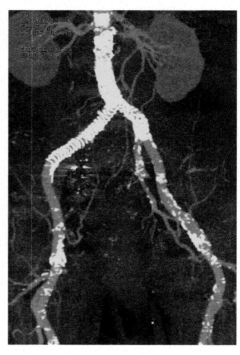

S/p EVAR.

Answers

1. Trauma during pregnancy and collagen vascular diseases are other recognized causes of iliac aneurysms.

2. Symptomatic and large CIA aneurysms are at risk of rupture. It is felt that aneurysms at 3.5 cm should be considered for elective repair. Regular surveillance is recommended as some aneurysms may grow at a fast rate.

3. Size and aneurysmal change in the abdominal aorta, length of the proximal and distal landing zones in the CIA, involvement of the internal iliac artery, and caliber of the access vessels need to be considered.

4. As the proximal and distal landing zones are short (<1.5 cm), there is a risk of endoleak. A full bifurcated EVAR with coiling of IIA and extension into the right external iliac artery (EIA) to ensure a seal at both ends of the aneurysm would be required. Branched iliac graft would also be possible, which would preserve the right internal iliac artery.

5. Mortality has been reported to be up to 11%, reflecting the complex nature of surgery deep in the pelvis.

Pearls

- Isolated iliac aneurysms account for 2% to 7% of abdominal aneurysmal disease.
- Proximal and distal landing zones, aortic disease, internal iliac disease, and the presence of bilateral disease all have an impact on what treatment options should be considered.

Suggested Reading

Uberoi R, Tsetis D, Shrivastava V, Morgan R, Belli AM, Belli AM. Standard of practice for the interventional management of isolated iliac artery aneurysms. Cardiovasc *Intervent Radiol*. 2011;34(1):3-13.

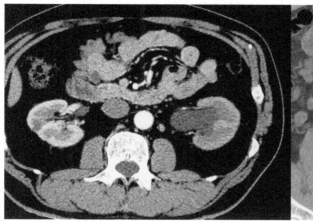 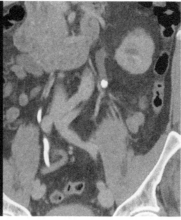 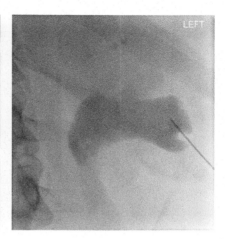

1. Where is the optimal access?

2. How can you decide if you have accessed an anterior or posterior calyx?

3. 21/22G needle access is safer than 18G access—true or false?

4. Antegrade JJ stent is best performed through a lower pole access—true or false?

5. Upper pole accesses have higher complication rate—true or false?

Category: Genitourinary system

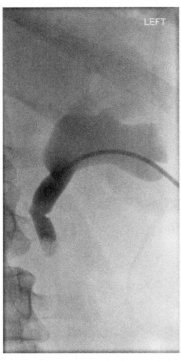

Obstructing upper ureteric calculus again demonstrated.

Answers

1. The avascular plane of Brodel lies between the anterior and posterior arterial arcades posterolaterally and is an optimal access point. Lower pole or upper pole or midpole calyceal accesses are favorable, depending on the indication; for example, stone access would depend on stone burden and location, and planning to convert to antegrade JJ stent may be best via a midpole access.

2. Posterior calices appear en-face, and anterior calices are likely tangential. Contrast will pool anteriorly, and air will fill the posterior calices in a prone patient.

3. There is no evidence to suggest one technique is safer than another. Small bore Chiba access and then 0.018" needle access followed by Neff set dilation to facilitate 0.035" wire access is one technique. Direct access with a 3-part 18G needle allows direct access with 0.035" wires.

4. A lower pole access may lead to a steep curve around the pelvis into the ureter. A mid- or upper pole access facilitates access into the ureter and makes JJ stent placement easier.

5. Upper pole accesses are required for complex stone treatments and may have higher complication rates due to pleural transgression.

Pearls

- Percutaneous nephrostomy placement is a core interventional radiology procedure.
- Several techniques are used. Fluoroscopic guidance, ultrasonographic guidance, or a combination of both can be used. Ultrasonography may be more beneficial than a landmark technique when the kidney is malrotated or if there is a horseshoe kidney. Nephrostomy can also be placed under computed tomographic guidance. Nephrostomy can be aided by intravenous pyelogram. This can be particularly useful if the system is nondilated.

Suggested Reading

Dyer RB, Regan JD, Kavanagh PV, Khatod EG, Chen MY, Zagoria RJ. Percutaneous nephrostomy with extensions of the technique: step by step. *Radiographics.* 2002;22(3):503-525.

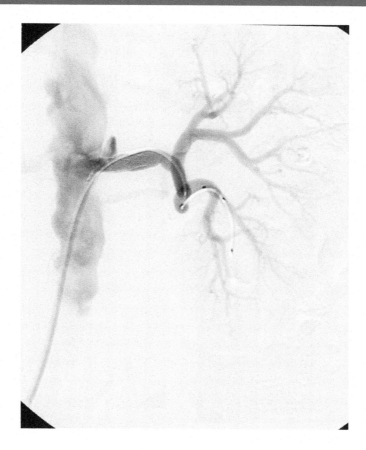

1. Review the angiogram that has been obtained after stent placement—what has happened?

2. What is the management?

3. List some ideal properties of a stent system.

4. Compare and contrast balloon-mounted and self-expanding stents.

5. Consider the advantages and disadvantages of stent grafts.

Case ranking/difficulty:

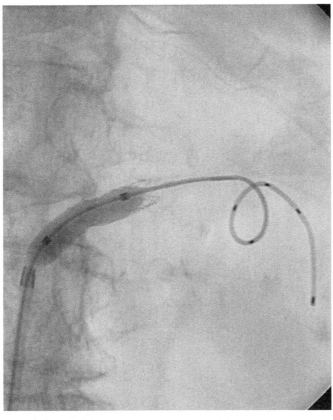

A covered stent was placed and fully dilated with a 5-mm-diameter balloon.

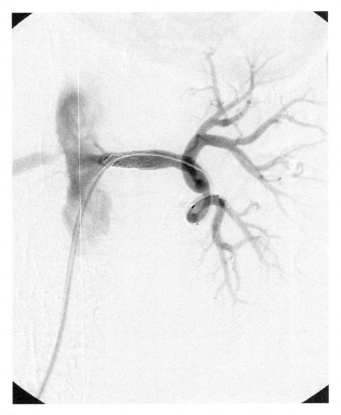

The contrast extravasation has resolved with good flow through the left renal artery.

Answers

1. There is a small area of contrast extravasation seen after stent placement.

2. This can be managed with a covered stent.

3. A good expansion ratio means that the device can be smaller, or low-profile. High radial strength is desirable as the expanded stent must resist compression. Stents should also be flexible, easily deployed, and visible.

4. Balloon-expandable stents are mounted on balloons and are deployed by balloon dilatation. They tend to have high radial force. They can be crushed and reocclude, where they may be compressed by external forces or in areas of tortuosity. Both balloon-mounted stents and self-expanding stents can be of equal profile at a given size, but smaller balloon-mounted stents are available.

5. Stent grafts may have a larger delivery system than uncovered stents of an equivalent size. They can be used to treat ruptures as in this case, or ruptures of iliac arteries. They are also used to treat aneurysms, for example, aortic aneurysms or popliteal aneurysms.

Pearls

- Rupture is not common but can be a life-threatening complication. Selection of the proper-size balloon should be considered carefully prior to the procedure. In patients with severe calcific atherosclerosis, extra care must be paid to avoid the risk rupture and plaque dislodgement.
- Placement of a covered stent can quickly control the bleeding.
- As a rule that applies to many procedures, the wire should be always in place during angioplasty in case any complication occurs.

Suggested Reading

Martin LG, Rundback JH, Sacks D, et al. Quality improvement guidelines for angiography, angioplasty, and stent placement in the diagnosis and treatment of renal artery stenosis in adults. *J Vasc Interv Radiol.* 2002;13(11):1069-1083.

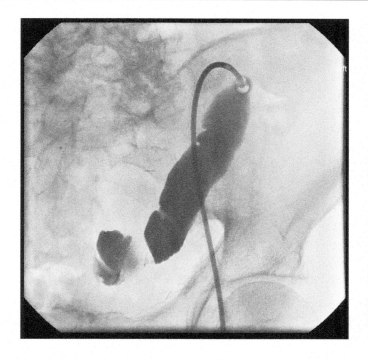
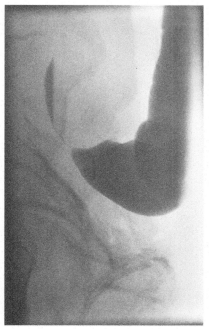

1. Ureteroileal anastomotic obstruction occurs in what percentage of patients following ureteric diversion surgery?

2. How would you manage a stenosis at the ileal conduit?

3. What are possible surgical strategies for urinary diversion?

4. Urinary diversion surgery is always performed due to malignant disease—true or false?

5. What is the risk of malignancy after ureterosigmoidostomy?

Case ranking/difficulty: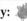

Category: Genitourinary system

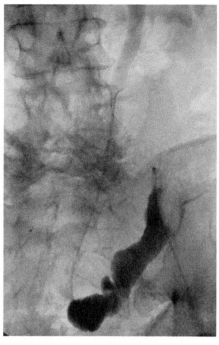

Retrograde access crosses the stenosis.

Answers

1. Anastomotic obstruction occurs in up to 15% of patients.

2. Nephrostomy, nephrostomy and antegrade stent, nephrostomy and antegrade nephroureteral catheter, and retrograde nephroureteral catheter would be interventional options. Surgical revision may also be required. Nephrostomy, however, would not be an ideal long-term solution as the patient would have to care for both the nephrostomy catheter and their stoma.

3. There are multiple possible ways of reconstructing the urine output and these include implantation of both ureters into an ileal conduit, left to right ureteroureterostomy, bladder hitch with ureteric implantation, and neobladder formation. It is of paramount importance to understand the surgical anatomy prior to performing any procedure. Implantation of ureters into the sigmoid colon is now largely historical because of possible malignant transformation.

4. Other reasons would include trauma or congenital abnormalities such as bladder exstrophy.

5. There is a risk of developing sigmoid carcinoma, 20 to 30 years after urinary diversion. A 24% risk at 10 years is quoted.

Pearls

- Anastomotic stenosis between the ureter and ileal conduit can occur because of recurrent disease or be postsurgical.
- The stenosis can be accessed retrogradely via the ileal conduit, or antegrade via percutaneous nephrostomy access.

Suggested Reading

Alago W, Sofocleous CT, Covey AM, et al. Placement of transileal conduit retrograde nephroureteral stents in patients with ureteral obstruction after cystectomy: technique and outcome. *AJR Am J Roentgenol.* 2008;191(5):1536-1539.

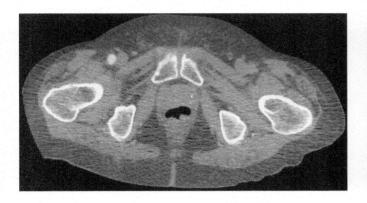 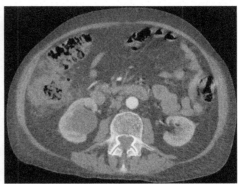

1. What 2 diagnoses can you make?

2. What are causes of arterial embolism?

3. What other embolic syndromes can occur?

4. What is a paradoxical embolus?

5. What is the emergency management of venous air embolism?

Case ranking/difficulty:

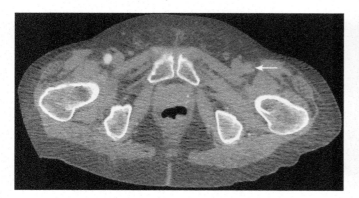

Computed tomographic angiography (CTA) shows nonopacification of the left common femoral artery.

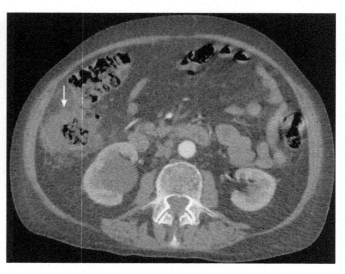

CTA shows colorectal carcinoma.

Answers

1. The patient has acute arterial embolus and a colorectal carcinoma.

2. Emboli can come from several sources. AF is the commonest cause. Foreign bodies, and malignant and septic emboli can also be causes. Atrial myxoma is also another source.

3. Other classical descriptions of emboli include fat, amniotic fluid, and air as sources.

4. These patients frequently present with neurologic impairment. Emboli pass through a patent foramen ovale, which can be seen in up to 35% of people.

5. Patients with suspected massive air embolus should be managed in the left lateral decubitus position—this prevents air passing though the right heart into the pulmonary arteries. Oxygen, intubation, air aspiration, and hyperbaric oxygen therapy can reduce morbidity.

Pearls

• Acute limb ischemia can occur in the setting of malignant disease and outcomes of intervention are reasonable.
• The SFA, brachial and popliteal arteries are sites where this has been reported. In-patient mortality was 12%, limb loss 37%, and 1-year survival 44%.
• Embolectomy is the main treatment option.

Suggested Reading

Tsang JS, Naughton PA, O'Donnell J, et al. Acute limb ischemia in cancer patients: should we surgically intervene? *Ann Vasc Surg.* 2011;25(7):954-960.

86-year-old woman with back pain and a lumbar vertebral compression fracture

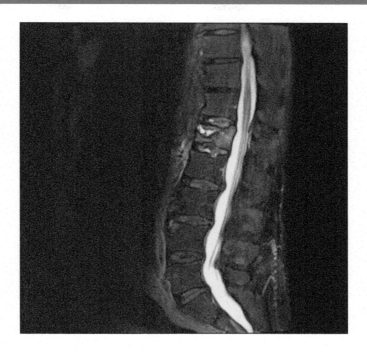

1. What treatment might be appropriate for the lesion shown?

2. Which are indications for kyphoplasty?

3. What are known complications?

4. How would you perform the procedure?

5. What cement and how much would you inject?

Case ranking/difficulty: 🌢

Category: Lymphatic system

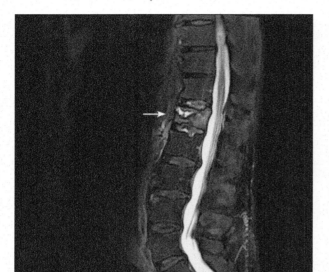

Vertebral compression with fracture cleft and edema.

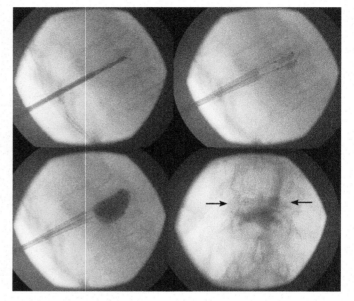

Kyphoplasty is performed with restoration of the superior endplate.

Answers

1. Osteoporotic compression fractures are common and can be treated with vertebroplasty or kyphoplasty. Malignant lesions can be treated in conjunction with ablative techniques.

2. Acute fractures and malignant or myelomatous lesions can respond well to treatment. Complete vertebral collapse and high lesions above T4 are contraindications to treatment.

3. Cement leak and embolization can cause significant complications.

4. Combination of anteroposterior and lateral screening is important to facilitate accurate access into the vertebral body without transgression of the medial wall of the pedicle. Balloon inflation and curetting creates a stable cavity into which cement can be injected. Lumbar accesses can be obtained using a parapedicular or transpedicular approach. Extrapedicular accesses are required for thoracic lesions, and these are more challenging.

5. Procedures can be performed under local anesthesia. Polymethylmethacrylate (PMMA) cement is most commonly used. One to 3 mL of cement can result in effective treatments.

Pearls

- Kyphoplasty involves cement augmentation in combination with high-pressure balloon treatment to restore vertebral body height.
- Vertebroplasty and kyphoplasty can be used to treat painful benign and malignant vertebral compression fractures.
- Access is obtained into each used of the vertebral body using either a transpedicular or parapedicular approach. Kyphoplasty balloons are used along with curetting to produce a large cavity into which cement is injected under fluoroscopic control.

Suggested Reading

Kasperk C, Grafe IA, Schmitt S, et al. Three-year outcomes after kyphoplasty in patients with osteoporosis with painful vertebral fractures. *J Vasc Interv Radiol.* 2010;21(5):701-709.

57-year-old man with active retroperitoneal hemorrhage following renal biopsy

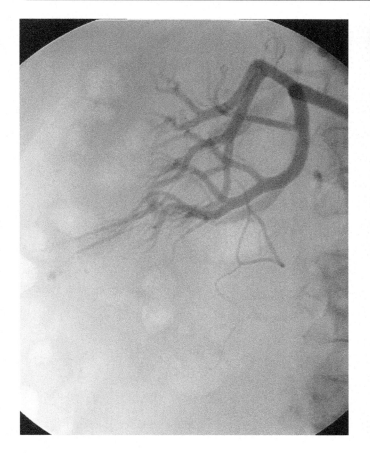 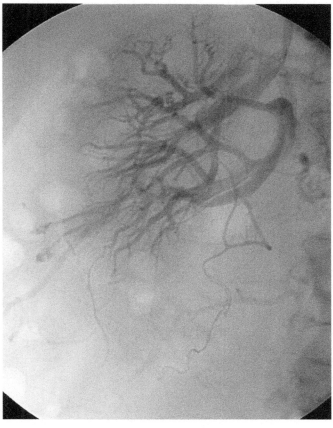

1. What is a pseudoaneurysm?

2. What features are common to both AVF and AVM?

3. What are the causes of AVFs?

4. Why is alcohol a poor choice of embolic agent in this setting?

5. How many days after surgery is the mean presentation?

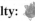
Case ranking/difficulty: **Category:** Arterial system

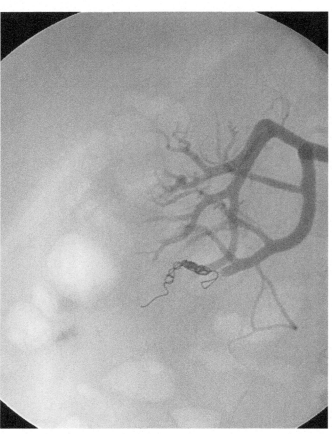

Right renal arteriogram after coil embolization shows resolved contrast extravasation and cessation of the early venous drainage.

Answers

1. Renal pseudoaneurysm is a rare vascular lesion that arises when an arterial injury within the kidney leads to contained hemorrhage. The associated hematoma forms outside the arterial wall and is typically surrounded by a layer of fibrous inflammatory tissue and blood clot. These lesions are unstable and their rupture can lead to life-threatening hemorrhage.

2. Renovascular malformations include congenital arteriovenous malformations (AVMs) and arteriovenous fistulas (AVFs). AVMs are congenital communications between arteries and veins with a vascular nidus that bypasses the capillary bed. Congenital AVMs are rare and subclassified into cirsoid, angiomatous, and aneurysmal types. Congenital AVMs are different from iatrogenic or traumatic AVF, which are characterized by a single direct communication between an artery and a vein without an intervening vascular nidus. These lesions

may present with a wide range of signs and symptoms that vary from hypertension to renal masses. Imaging is valuable in the detection and characterization of AVM and AVF. The presence of arteriovenous shunting characterizes AVM and AVF.

3. AVFs can be idiopathic, iatrogenic, or associated with malignancy.

4. One aim of selective embolization is to preserve renal function. Alcohol is used to infarct the kidney, which will result in permanent kidney damage. The common application is devascularization prior to surgical nephrectomy for renal cell carcinoma, or removal of a failed transplant.

5. Patients diagnosed with a renal arterial pseudoaneurysm presented at a mean of 15 days after surgery and 85% had gross hematuria at presentation. Almost all of the patients with renal arterial pseudoaneurysm were treated with embolization with a high success rate.

Pearls

- Iatrogenic renal vascular injury can occur after partial nephrectomy or biopsy and lead to hematuria or retroperitoneal hematoma. Pseudoaneurysm and arteriovenous fistula are associated complications.
- Angiography and embolization is the reference standard for both diagnosis and treatment in the acute setting, although computed tomographic scan can be used if symptoms are not severe or the diagnosis is uncertain.
- Renal pseudoaneurysm has been reported to occur in various clinical scenarios, including after renal trauma, surgery and percutaneous procedures, as well as inflammatory and neoplastic processes within the kidney.

Suggested Readings

Hyams ES, Pierorazio P, Proteek O, et al. Iatrogenic vascular lesions after minimally invasive partial nephrectomy: a multi-institutional study of clinical and renal functional outcomes. *Urology*. 2011;78(4):820-826.

Jain S, Nyirenda T, Yates J, Munver R. Incidence of renal artery pseudoaneurysm following open and minimally invasive partial nephrectomy: a systematic review and comparative analysis. *J Urol*. 2013;189(5):1643-1648.

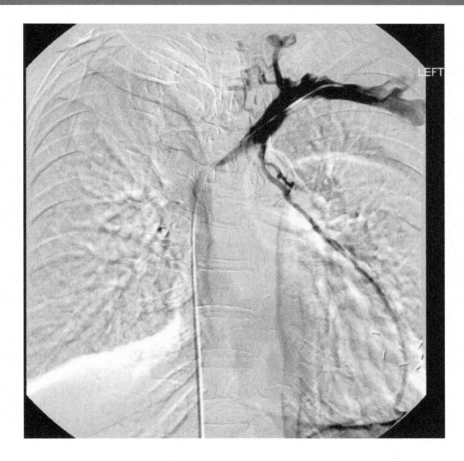

1. Name the vein seen passing inferiorly in the image.

2. List some causes of SVC obstruction.

3. Describe the azygous and hemiazygous veins.

4. List some complications of central line placement.

5. Why is knowledge of venous drainage of the thorax important clinically?

Case ranking/difficulty:

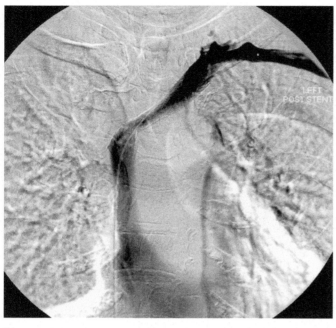

S/p stent.

Answers

1. It is the superior pericardial vein.

2. Small cell carcinoma, central venous catheter placement, mediastinal fibrosis, radiotherapy, and a retrosternal thyroid are potential causes of SVC obstruction.

3. The azygous vein begins at L1 as a continuation of the ascending lumbar vein, passes through the diaphragm, and runs to the right of the vertebral column. The hemiazygous vein drains the lower intercostal spaces.

4. Insertion site thrombosis, line-related sepsis, arterial misplacement, cardiac tamponade, and pneumothorax are known complications.

5. Venous drainage of the thorax is important in many clinical scenarios, including access, sampling, and obstructions.

Pearls

- Misplaced central venous catheters can cause cardiac tamponade, and hyperosmolar solutions such as those used for total parenteral nutrition can cause venous erosion.

Suggested Reading

Kapur S, Paik E, Rezaei A, Vu DN. Where there is blood, there is a way: unusual collateral vessels in superior and inferior vena cava obstruction. *Radiographics*. 2010;30(1):67-78.

72-year-old man with a known endoleak seen on a computed tomographic (CT) angiogram

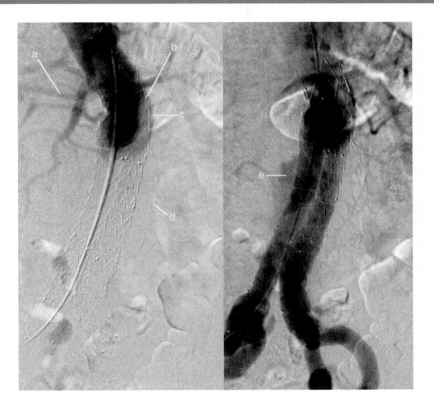

1. Review the early and late phases of the angiogram and label (a) to (e)!

2. Regarding angiography—what aids endoleak detection?

3. Which are valid treatment options available to the vascular surgeon?

4. Which are endovascular options here?

5. What are endostaples?

Case ranking/difficulty: 🌰

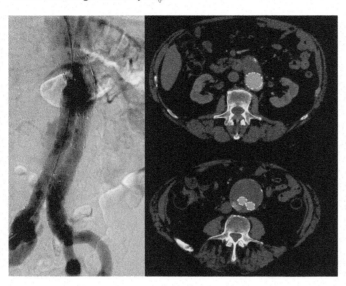

Angiogram with corresponding findings at CTA.

Answers

1. A is the right renal artery, B is the top of the endograft, C is contrast outside the graft consistent with a type 1 endoleak, D is the aortic sac, and E is delayed filling in the sac.

2. Catheter position above the graft may result in filling of the visceral branches. Placing the catheter in the top of the graft can help detect type 1 endoleaks. Also, angiography performed within the graft underneath an inflated molding balloon would help characterize endoleaks as flow from the neck would be blocked by the inflated balloon.

3. Ligation, tying, or reinforcement of the neck at open surgery or laparoscopically is possible. Graft explant and open repair is another surgical option.

4. Endovascular options include Palmaz stent or aortic cuff placement, conversion to a fenestrated graft, chimney technique with a cuff, or endostapling.

5. Staples penetrate the stent and aortic wall and are designed to improve the seal. There are a range of endostapling devices—some use balloon-mounted systems; others use angulated catheters to facilitate wall apposition and staple placement. There are little robust outcome data as yet.

Pearls

- Angiography is not required to detect endoleaks as they are readily visible on CTA. Like contrast-enhanced ultrasonography, angiography may have a role in classifying the leak.
- It may also help with planning to see in great detail as to how much neck is available for cuff placement and may direct subsequent management.

Suggested Reading

Donas KP, Kafetzakis A, Umscheid T, Tessarek J, Torsello G. Vascular endostapling: new concept for endovascular fixation of aortic stent-grafts. *J Endovasc Ther.* 2008;15(5):499-503.

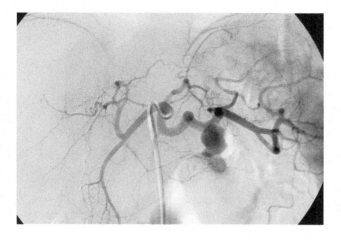
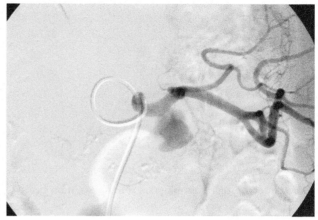
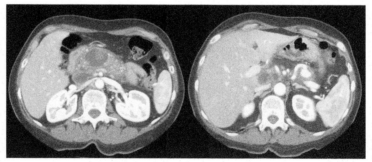

1. What do the angiograms show?

2. What does the CT show?

3. What is the unifying diagnosis?

4. How is definitive diagnosis of this condition made?

5. What mechanisms lead to GI bleeding in the setting of chronic pancreatitis?

Case ranking/difficulty: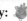

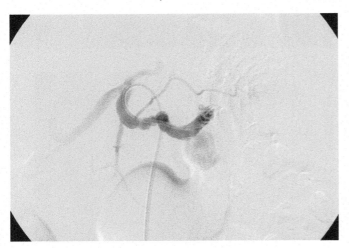

Postembolization of splenic arteriogram shows resolution of the pseudoaneurysm.

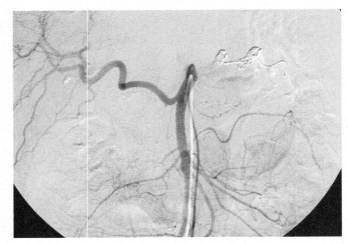

Selective superior mesenteric artery (SMA) injection reveals no collateral to the splenic arterial pseudoaneurysm. There is a replaced right hepatic artery.

Answers

1. There is a large splenic artery pseudoaneurysm and evidence of a replaced right hepatic artery (the common hepatic artery gives rise to a gastroduodenal artery [GDA] and a left hepatic artery [LHA]).

2. There is chronic pancreatitis, hemorrhage into cysts, and splenic artery pseudoaneurysm.

3. Hemosuccus pancreaticus is defined as blood entering the gastrointestinal tract through the pancreatic duct, resulting in a rare and elusive form of gastrointestinal bleeding.

4. Angiography represents the optimal imaging modality for suspected hemosuccus pancreaticus, although objective demonstration of a communication of intravascular contrast between a peripancreatic vessel and the pancreatic duct or pseudocyst is exceedingly unusual.

5. Gastrointestinal hemorrhage is an infrequent, but well-known, complication of chronic pancreatitis. Gastric varices can occur secondary to splenic vein thrombosis. Hemorrhage into pseudocysts can occur and pseudoaneurysms can be found in several arterial territories.

Pearls

- Hemorrhage into the pancreatic duct and then into the gastrointestinal tract through the ampulla of Vater is known as "hemosuccus pancreaticus," a distinctly unusual complication that often poses difficult diagnostic and therapeutic problems.
- It is usually a life-threatening situation. The characteristic finding is intermittent epigastric pain followed by gastrointestinal hemorrhage, which occurs 30-40 minutes later.

Suggested Readings

Sakorafas GH, Sarr MG, Farley DR, Que FG, Andrews JC, Farnell MB. Hemosuccus pancreaticus complicating chronic pancreatitis: an obscure cause of upper gastrointestinal bleeding. *Langenbecks Arch Surg.* 2000;385(2):124-128. [Review]

Sandblom P. Gastrointestinal hemorrhage through the pancreatic duct. *Ann Surg.* 1970;171(1):61-66.

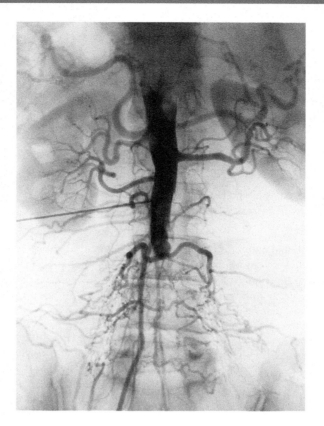

1. What is the diagnosis?

2. How was this image obtained?

3. What other access could be used to obtain this arteriogram?

4. According to the Trans-Atlantic Inter-Society Consensus for the Management of Peripheral Arterial Disease (TASC II), what category is this lesion?

5. Which are treatment options?

Case ranking/difficulty:

Answers

1. This is Leriche, or Leriche's, syndrome.

2. Prone or lateral positioning is required for a translumbar aortogram. The translumbar access needle was felt to reduce complications like dissection. Direct aortic access is still required but in a different setting—percutaneous access into aortic sacs is a useful procedure.

3. A brachial angiogram.

4. The Leriche syndrome is categorized as a type D aortoiliac lesion by the TASC II, with surgery as the recommended treatment of choice.

5. Depending on the location, extent, and nature of the aortoiliac obstruction and the patient's comorbidities, all are potential options. If the patient is not fit for laparotomy, extraanatomic grafts are an option. If the patient is particularly frail, endovascular recanalization has been performed successfully.

Pearls

- Leriche syndrome is a variant of atherosclerotic diseases, which specifically involves young, male patients. Aortoiliac occlusive disease obviously also occurs in older patients with atherosclerosis.
- It classically presents with the triad of erectile dysfunction, buttock claudication, and absent femoral pulses.
- Aortobifemoral or axillobifemoral grafts are the mainstay of treatment but endovascular therapy has been performed with placement of a long length of stent—with passage through a long-occluded segment aided by having both a transfemoral and a transbrachial wire.

Suggested Reading

Krankenberg H, Schlüter M, Schwencke C, et al. Endovascular reconstruction of the aortic bifurcation in patients with Leriche syndrome. *Clin Res Cardiol.* 2009;98(10):657-664.

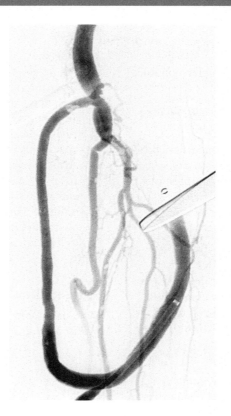

1. What is the anatomy of the dialysis access shown?

2. What critical issue is seen here?

3. What are the treatment options?

4. Which is the key factor for successful declotting of a thrombosed dialysis graft?

5. What are causes of early graft re-occlusion?

Case ranking/difficulty: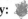

Answers

1. The arterial anastomosis of the forearm loop is taken from the brachial artery and the venous outflow passes to the medial aspect of the arm—this is a brachiobasilic forearm loop AV graft.

2. There is a stenosis at the arterial anastomosis, but note the filling defects seen in the distal arteries.

3. Depending on the extent of the emboli, the treatment can range from intravenous heparin infusion to surgical embolectomy. Mechanical or aspiration thrombectomy using balloon or guiding catheter is an effective and quick method to remove the clot. Intraarterial thrombolysis should be considered if mechanical thrombectomy fails.

4. Progressive luminal narrowing or any cause of significant flow reduction can cause graft thrombosis and occlusion. The venous anastomosis is the commonest cause for AV grafts going down. Although all of the above are important, identifying the cause is the most important.

5. Studies report an early failure rate of up to 20% of grafts. Early-thrombosing grafts respond poorly to percutaneous intervention, with subsequent patency rates lower than those reported for grafts treated equivalently for thrombosis later in their natural history. Patients with early graft failure also often have underlying medical comorbidities that may predispose to graft failure.

Pearls

- Stenosis of arterial anastomosis of the AV dialysis graft can reduce the flow through the shunt and eventually cause thrombosis.
- Evaluation of the arterial anastomotic stenosis can be performed by placement of a diagnostic catheter beyond the anastomosis, which minimizes the risk of pushing thrombus from graft into the artery beyond the anastomosis.
- In an occluded graft, direct injection through the antegrade sheath while occluding the outflow to cause reflux of the contrast medium can push the intragraft clots into the artery through the arterial anastomosis of the graft and is an improper technique.

Suggested Reading

Morgan R, Belli AM. Percutaneous thrombectomy: a review. *Eur Radiol.* 2002;12(1):205-217.

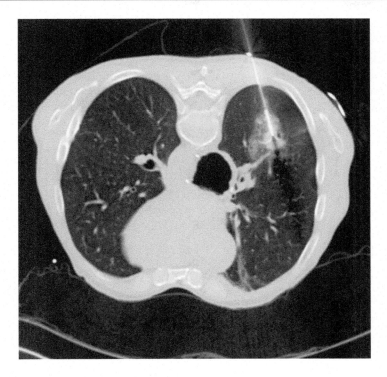
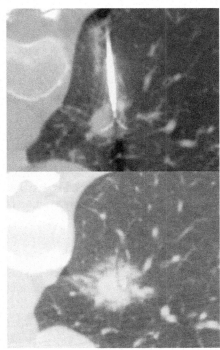

1. What are the indications for lung RFA?

2. What are complications?

3. What are signs of recurrence?

4. In the liver, what is the effect of a lesion being close to the portal vein?

5. Pacemakers and ICDs are contraindications— true or false?

Case ranking/difficulty: 🗡

Answers

1. Primary lung lesions and solitary or multiple metastases can be treated. They can be treated with curative or palliative intent. Metastases can be treated in multiple stages to preserve and maintain viable lung tissue in the long term.

2. Complications can be related to needle placement and collateral damage in the ablation zone.

3. Lesions may ultimately shrink and cavitate, but can look larger at 3 months. Lesion growth or positron emission tomographic (PET) scan avidity at 6 months is felt to indicate recurrence.

4. Like in the lungs, metastases can also be treated to preserve normal tissue volume. The portal vein can act as a "heat sink," which means the lesion does not reach critical temperature, but advanced techniques can be employed such as balloon occlusion.

5. Interactions with cardiology hardware can occur—devices may need to be reprogrammed and temporary pacing equipment should be available.

Pearls

- Image-guided radiofrequency ablation of tumors is yet another treatment that many interventional radiologists can offer. Standard needle placement techniques are used to access liver, lung, and renal lesions.

Suggested Reading

Pereira PL, Salvatore M. Standards of practice: guidelines for thermal ablation of primary and secondary lung tumors. *Cardiovasc Intervent Radiol*. 2012;35(2):247-254.

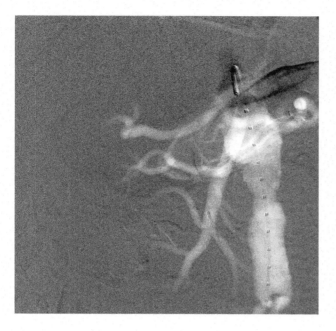 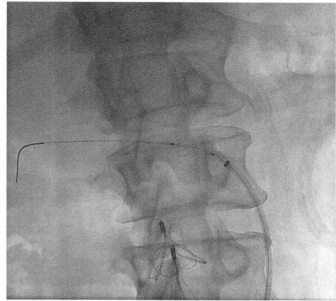

1. When is angioplasty better than stenting?

2. What are advantages and disadvantages of carbon dioxide as a contrast agent?

3. What is "carbon dioxide lock"?

4. What happens to the CO_2 physiologically?

5. How can high-quality CO_2 angiograms be obtained?

Case ranking/difficulty: 🌑

Category: Arterial system

Answers

1. Fibromuscular dysplasia generally responses to angioplasty well.

2. Because of the lower density and viscosity (400 times less than that of iodinated contrast material), CO_2 has an inferior imaging quality compared to ionic or nonionic contrast material. However, it is cheap, allergy-free, and nontoxic.

3. Large and repeat boluses can cause a gaseous blockage in the SMA origin and cause visceral ischemia.

4. After injection, CO_2 dissolves rapidly in blood and is excreted by the lungs in first-pass fashion. This excretion mechanism is so efficient that there is no apparent cumulative dose limit for CO_2. Even large and repeated doses of CO_2 gas have no effect on arterial pH, P_{CO_2}, or P_{O_2}.

5. High-quality CO_2 angiography does not require specialized injectors or imaging equipment, but an understanding of the unique features of CO_2 with close attention to technique is needed. CO_2 acts by displacing blood from the vessels of interest. Manual injections through small catheters can easily achieve this objective because the viscosity of CO_2 gas is extremely low compared to liquids. High frame rates are needed to track the bolus, and postprocessing of angiograms may be required to see the whole vessel.

Pearls

- Contrast-induced nephropathy is a major concern in patients with chronic renal insufficiency, particularly in patients who are found at angiography not to have significant renal artery stenosis despite a suggestive clinical picture and a noninvasive workup.
- CO_2 can be used as an alternative to iodinated agents for contrast angiography in patients with renal insufficiency and allergies to iodinated contrast material.

Suggested Readings

Caridi JG, Stavropoulos SW, Hawkins IF Jr. CO_2 digital subtraction angiography for renal artery angioplasty in high-risk patients. *AJR Am J Roentgenol.* 1999;173(6):1551-1556.

Spinosa DJ, Matsumoto AH, Angle JF, Hagspiel KD, Cage D, Bissonette EA, Koenig KG, Ayers CR, McConnell K. Safety of CO_2- and gadodiamide-enhanced angiography for the evaluation and percutaneous treatment of renal artery stenosis in patients with chronic renal insufficiency. *AJR Am J Roentgenol.* 2001;176(5):1305-1311.

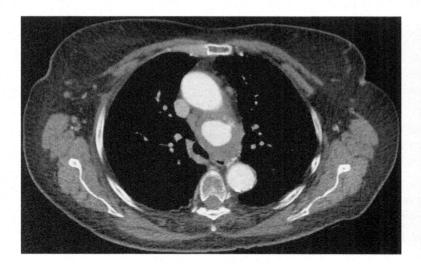
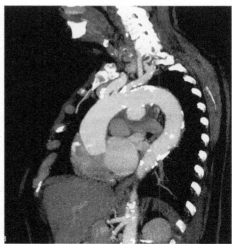
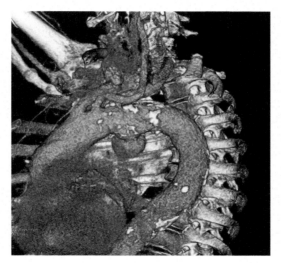

1. What is the pathology?

2. Can it be stented?

3. How much stent oversizing is recommended in TEVAR?

4. List the Crawford classification of thoracoabdominal aneurysms.

5. What are the indications for TEVAR?

Case ranking/difficulty:

Answers

1. This is a saccular aneurysm of the aortic arch. It is degenerate and presents with a chronic history. In the setting of an acute presentation and trauma, a pseudoaneurysm would be more likely.

2. It is a difficult case. There is less than 1 cm of landing zone even if planning to cover the left subclavian, and so left common carotid origin might also need to be overstented.

3. TEVAR does not need oversizing or balloon molding in dissection, but this is recommended to treat aneurysms.

4. The modified Crawford classification groups thoracoabdominal aneurysms based on the involvement of the proximal and distal descending aorta, suprarenal aorta, and infrarenal aorta.

   Type 1: from distal to the left subclavian extending to above the renals; type 2: from the left subclavian to below the renals; type 3: from the mid descending thoracic aorta at the sixth intercostal space to below renals; type 4: total abdominal affecting the suprarenal abdominal aorta to the bifurcation; and type 5: from the sixth intercostal space to just above renals.

5. Indications for TEVAR include descending aneurysm at 6.5 or above, symptomatic aneurysms, complicated dissection, post dissection aneurysm formation, trauma, rupture, and fistula formation. TEVAR may also be indicated in mycotic aneurysms if this is felt to be a life-saving strategy.

Pearls

- TEVAR is indicated to treat descending thoracic aneurysm that are greater than 6.5 cm in diameter. It is also indicated to treat saccular aneurysms and any symptomatic aneurysm that may be causing mass effect, compression, and is certainly indicated in the acute setting of trauma and rupture.
- It can be a moot point as to what is a penetrating ulcer, saccular aneurysm, or pseudoaneurysm. Pathologic definitions are clear concerning aneurysms and pseudoaneurysm—that is, which layers of the arterial wall are involved. Clinically, this is largely determined by the presentation.

Suggested Reading

Heijmen RH, Deblier IG, Moll FL, et al. Endovascular stent-grafting for descending thoracic aortic aneurysms. *Eur J Cardiothorac Surg.* 2002;21(1):5-9.

40-year-old man presents for arch aortogram, and another man has a computed tomographic angiogram

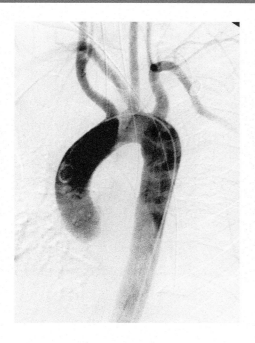 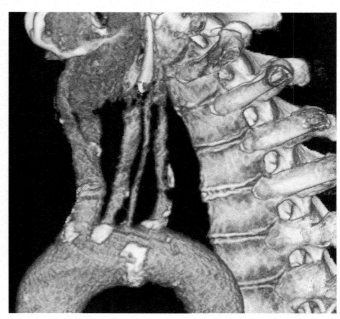

1. Which of the following is the commonest arch variant?

2. What is the sequence of arch vessel origins with an aberrant right subclavian?

3. What are the determinants of arch 'sidedness' and rings?

4. What are the right-sided aortic arch variants?

5. What are the key features and characteristics of a double arch?

Case ranking/difficulty: 🍂

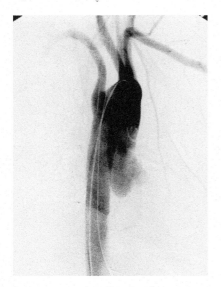

Arch aortogram showing the aberrant artery.

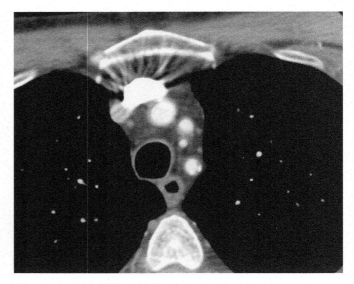

Direct vertebral origin from the arch.

Answers

1. The bovine arch is the most common variant.

2. Sequence of branches is the right CCA, then left CCA, then left subclavian followed finally by the right subclavian.

3. Sidedness is defined by which main bronchus (or both) is crossed by the arch. A ring can be caused by the pulmonary vasculature. Compression can occur without a ring, and rings surround both the trachea and esophagus.

4. Mirror image right aortic arch, right AA with retroesopheal left subclavian, right AA with diverticulum of Kommerell, right AA with left descending aorta, and right AA with retroesophageal innominate are described.

5. Double arch with right-sided dominance is most common. Double arches occur due to persistence of both left and right fourth arches and left and right dorsal aortas. Yes, there is such a thing as a persistent fifth aortic arch. This is a very complicated area of anatomy/embryology.

Pearls

- The 3 most common arch variants are bovine arch, direct aortic origin of the left vertebral artery, and an aberrant right subclavian artery.
- Arch variants are complicated, and deep understanding requires investigation in the pediatric, cardiovascular, and embryologic literature.

Suggested Reading

Kellenberger CJ. Aortic arch malformations. *Pediatr Radiol.* 2010;40(6):876-884.

47-year-old woman with jaundice and deranged liver function tests presents for a procedure

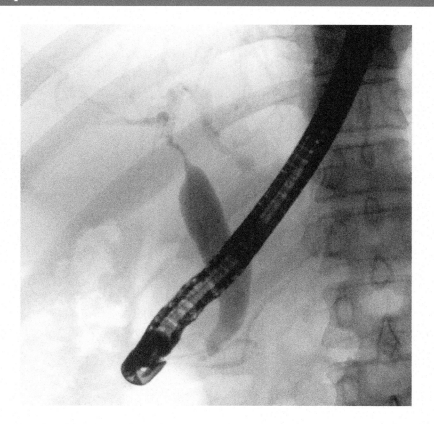

1. What are the indications for ERCP?

2. What procedures can be performed via ERCP?

3. What are the complications of ERCP?

4. What are contraindications to ERCP?

5. What is the incidence of ERCP-related complications?

Category: Gastrointestinal system

Answers

1. ERCP is a very useful diagnostic and therapeutic modality and can be used for stones, pancreatitis, malignancy, and trauma—a wide range of conditions that affect the biliary tree, pancreas, and ampulla of Vater.

2. Stent placement, sphincterotomy, brush biopsy, and common bile duct (CBD) clearance can all be performed via ERCP.

3. Sphincterotomy can lead to hemorrhage. Post-ERCP pancreatitis tends to be mild and occurs in up to 5% of patients.

4. ERCP may be technically possible in patients who have had Billroth 2 surgical reconstruction or pancreaticoduodenectomy—aided by balloon-assisted techniques.

5. Hemorrhage occurs in 1% to 2% and can be managed endoscopically; rarely is angiography or surgery required. Perforation occurs in 0.3% to 0.6% and tends to be retroperitoneal in nature. The risk of cholangitis is 1% to 3%. ERCP pancreatitis occurs in 5% to 30% and tends to run a mild course.

Pearls

- ERCP is the first line for treating CBD disease but is challenging with previous bypass surgery. Duodenal diverticulum and extrinsic compression may make ERCP challenging.
- Emergency biliary drainage procedures may be required for acute cholecystitis, acute cholangitis, and transplant biliary obstruction, but proper medical management such as broad-spectrum antibiotics and fluid resuscitation is vital.
- Percutaneous transhepatic cholangiography, ERCP, endoscopic ultrasonography (EUS), and surgery are complementary techniques and best practice involves multidisciplinary input.

Suggested Reading

Uberoi R, Das N, Moss J, Robertson I. British Society of Interventional Radiology: Biliary Drainage and Stenting Registry (BDSR). *Cardiovasc Intervent Radiol.* 2012;35(1):127-138.

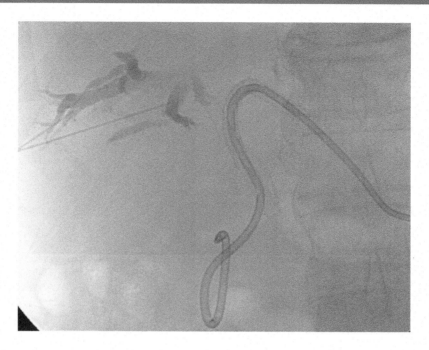

1. Five foreign objects are seen—what are they?

2. What is the commonest cause of stent occlusion?

3. What are the complications of metallic biliary stents?

4. What are the disadvantages of balloon-expandable stents in the biliary system?

5. How would you proceed to deploy a self-expanding biliary stent after achieving a suitable bile duct access?

Case ranking/difficulty: 🦡

Answers

1. Two metallic stents, a left-sided internal-external biliary drain, and 2 cholangiogram access needles are seen, one central and another definitive peripheral access.

2. Tumor ingrowth between the struts of the stent can cause re-occlusion. Tumor ingrowth was observed in only 6.5% of metal prostheses with a narrow woven mesh (eg, Wallstent), whereas prostheses with larger spaces between the struts (eg, Gianturco stent) had ingrowth rates of up to 50%.

3. Stents can occlude due to tumor ingrowth and bile encrustation. Stents can also migrate.

4. Balloon-expandable stents are mounted on angioplasty balloon, and the inherent rigidity can make it difficult to advance the stent around acute angles in the biliary system, and this can result in the endoprosthesis being displaced from its position over the balloon unless it is protected within a sheath. Another drawback of balloon-expandable stents in the biliary tree is the difficulty of achieving sufficient overlap of short endoprostheses around acute angles. Another disadvantage is that, unlike self-expandable stents, balloon-expandable devices do not continue to expand following their release, making it

necessary to achieve complete dilatation of the stricture before stent insertion, which is not always possible.

5. Primary stenting can be achieved through a 6-Fr sheath. Predilatation can make stent insertion easier. For strictures at the hilum of the liver or the mid common duct it is preferable to use a long endoprosthesis that will have its proximal end peripherally in an intrahepatic duct and its lower end 2-3 cm below the stricture.

Pearls

- Internal biliary stents can occlude, commonly due to tumor ingrowth. Metallic stents are normally placed for palliative indications, but if the patient's life expectancy is more than 6 months, an internal/external biliary catheter should be placed.

Suggested Reading

Adam A. Metallic biliary endoprostheses. *Cardiovasc Intervent Radiol*. 1994;17(3):127-132.

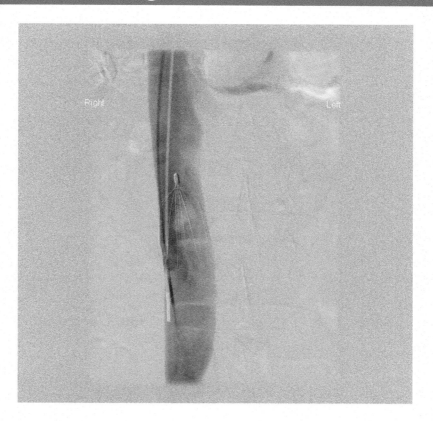

1. Would you proceed to remove the filter?

2. What is the incidence of breakthrough pulmonary embolism (PE) (ie, PE occurring after IVC filter placement?)

3. What is the potential risk of using J wires in a cava that contains a filter?

4. What is the incidence of thrombus in IVC filters?

5. What is the prognosis and natural history of IVC filter thrombus?

Case ranking/difficulty:

Category: Venous system

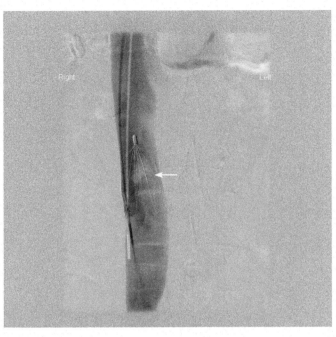

Preretrieval cavagram.

Answers

1. The thrombus seen here would preclude filter retrieval. The filter could be removed in the future after the clot has resolved.

2. Significant PE can occur in up to 1% of patients after filter placement.

3. J wires or pigtail catheters can get entrapped in the filter.

4. One large series looking at computed tomographic scans after IVC filter placement found an incidence of thrombus in the filter of 18.6%.

5. IVC filter thrombus is thought to be benign—it rarely leads to caval occlusion, anticoagulation is thought to have little effect on regression, there is no increased risk of PE, and it may well regress spontaneously.

> ### Pearls
>
> • A large thrombus in the IVC filter is a contraindication to its removal.
> • Careful technique is recommended for performing a preretrieval cavagram—as J wires and pigtail catheters can become stuck in, or can displace the filter. Straight wires and straight flush catheters may be used.

Suggested Readings

Ahmad I, Yeddula K, Wicky S, Kalva SP. Clinical sequelae of thrombus in an inferior vena cava filter. *Cardiovasc Intervent Radiol.* 2010;33(2):285-289.

Wang SL, Timmermans HA, Kaufman JA. Estimation of trapped thrombus volumes in retrievable inferior vena cava filters: a visual scale. *J Vasc Interv Radiol.* 2007;18(2):273-276.

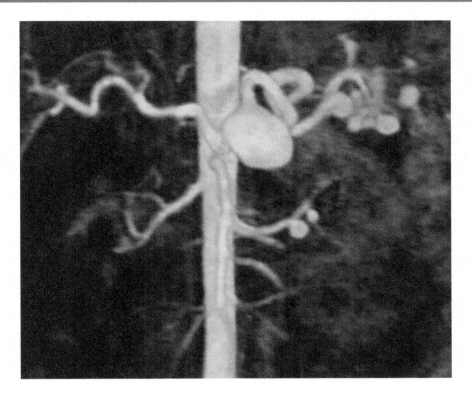

1. What is the imaging technique?

2. What is the diagnosis?

3. How can this condition be treated?

4. Discuss key epidemiological and clinical features of splenic artery aneuryms.

5. What are the biological and clinical features of Ehler's Danlos syndrome?

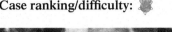
Case ranking/difficulty:

Category: Arterial system

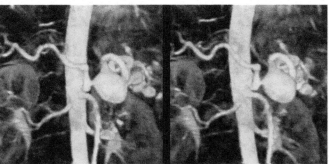

Different oblique views.

Answers

1. This is a reconstruction from a contrast-enhanced magnetic resonance angiogram.

2. There are multiple visceral artery aneurysms.

3. Conservative management, surgical treatment, or endovascular options that include embolization, stent placement, and direct sac puncture techniques. Stents include covered stents and remodeling stent systems.

4. Rupture rate is 2%, and mortality of a rupture is up to 40%. Aneurysms over 2 cm in size should be considered for treatment. They are associated with portal hypertension, and rapid growth can occur during pregnancy.

5. It is an autosomal dominant condition where there is loss of type 3 collagen fibers. Type 4 is associated with aortic and intracranial aneurysms.

Pearls

- Visceral aneurysms are increasingly diagnosed as incidental findings on imaging performed for some other reason, but still 1 in 5 of these presents as an emergency.
- The goal of intervention radiologic (IR) therapy is to exclude the aneurysm from the circulation and so prevent growth and rupture, while at the same time attempting to preserve the underlying circulation.
- Treatment can therefore involve stent graft placement, embolization with coils. plugs or liquid embolics, or even with direct sac injections in specific situations.

Suggested Readings

Belli AM, Markose G, Morgan R. The role of interventional radiology in the management of abdominal visceral artery aneurysms. *Cardiovasc Intervent Radiol.* 2012;35(2): 234-243.

Spiliopoulos S, Sabharwal T, Karnabatidis D, et al. Endovascular treatment of visceral aneurysms and pseudoaneurysms: long-term outcomes from a multicenter European study. *Cardiovasc Intervent Radiol.* 2011;35(6):1315-1325.

45-year-old man who had a failed right lower quadrant renal transplant presents for embolization

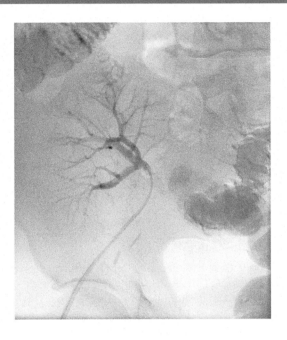 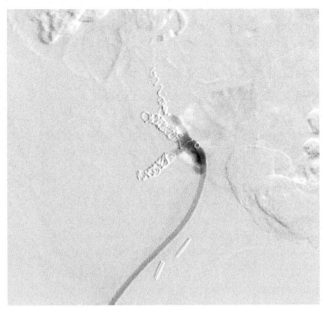

1. What is the main reason to perform renal artery embolization for the failed renal transplant?

2. What embolic agents can be used for renal transplant embolization?

3. What complications are best treated with surgical transplant nephrectomy?

4. What are the most common indications for embolization in patients after renal transplantation?

5. Post-embolization syndrome in renal transplant allograft includes which symptoms?

Case ranking/difficulty: 🦡

Answers

1. Patient may not be able to tolerate a failed graft left in situ after immunosuppression has been discontinued. Percutaneous embolotherapy is an alternative for ablating symptomatic nonfunctional renal allografts.

2. Alcohol, coils, particles and AVPs can be used for renal transplant embolization.

3. Transplantectomy is the best treatment if there are some associated complications such as allograft infection, neoplasia, or high risk of graft rupture.

4. In the post–renal transplant patient, percutaneous biopsies of the allograft is often necessary when there is indication of graft failure—arteriovenous fistulas and pseudoaneurysms can occur as a result of renal biopsy and are common indications for embolization in renal transplantation patients.

5. Postembolization syndrome is the most common side effect and can present with localized tenderness and fever.

Pearls

- Graft intolerance syndrome occurs where patients have ongoing immunologic intolerance to a failed graft. Allograft nephrectomy has been the conventional therapy. Percutaneous embolotherapy is an alternative for ablating the symptomatic nonfunctioning renal transplant.
- Preoperative embolization can also be performed, which can aid resection, typically when resection can be challenging because of inflammation and scarring and where there is concern with bleeding.

Suggested Readings

Delgado P, Diaz F, Gonzalez A, et al. Intolerance syndrome in failed renal allografts: incidence and efficacy of percutaneous embolization. *Am J Kidney Dis.* 2005;46(2):339-344.

Delgado P, Diaz F, Gonzalez A, et al. Transvascular ethanol embolization: first option for the management of symptomatic nonfunctioning renal allografts left in situ. *Transplant Proc.* 2003;35(5):1684-1685.

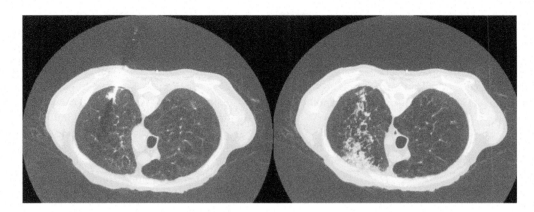

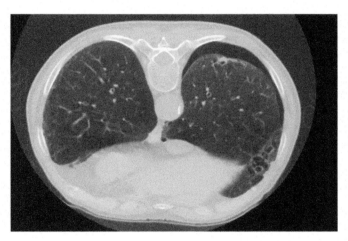

1. What factors may decrease pneumothorax rates?

2. Which factors are associated with increased risk of hemorrhage?

3. What percentage of pneumothoraces required chest tube placement?

4. What is the reported incidence of pneumothorax?

5. Which patients are at higher risk?

Case ranking/difficulty: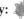

Answers

1. Aiming to only breach the visceral pleural once, and use of smaller coaxial needles may reduce the incidence of pneumothorax. Large lesions and lesions that abut the pleura are associated with a lower risk of pneumothorax.

2. Smaller, central lesions are associated with increased risk of hemorrhage—surrounding normal lung does not tamponade the hemorrhage as compared to larger lesions, which abut the pleural surface. Surprisingly, the presence of a pleural effusion is associated with a lower risk of hemorrhage.

3. Large series have reported a risk of around 6%.

4. It depends how it has been measured—eg, symptomatic versus all pneumothoraces. Bottom line is that it is common.

5. Smokers, those with emphysema, and older patients are at higher risk.

Pearls

- Pneumothorax is a common complication. Some operators utilize breath-holding during needle placement or use fluid menisci in needles. There are no robust data to suggest that needle size affects pneumothorax rate. Crossing the pleura multiple times may increase risk. It is possible to anesthetize the pleura without crossing it.
- It is also sometimes useful to be able to create an iatrogenic pneumothorax or indeed pleural effusion as a protective mechanism during radiofrequency ablation (RFA) and this can be done with a 21G needle.
- Hemoptysis due to pulmonary hemorrhage is common and tends to be self-limiting.

Suggested Reading

Wu CC, Maher MM, Shepard JA. Complications of CT-guided percutaneous needle biopsy of the chest: prevention and management. *AJR Am J Roentgenol*. 2011;196(6):W678-W682.

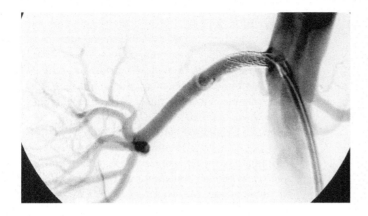 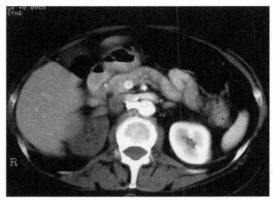

1. What are complications of renal stent placement?

2. What is the commonest pathology for which renal artery stenting is performed?

3. What are the associations of atherosclerotic renal artery stenosis?

4. What are the possible treatments for renal artery stenosis?

5. What are the current accepted indications for renal artery intervention in atherosclerotic renal artery stenosis?

Case ranking/difficulty: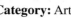

Answers

1. Stents can fracture and migrate. They can cause renal artery rupture. Neo-intimal hyperplasia can occur, leading to stenosis and thrombosis.

2. Atherosclerotic stenosis is the most common indication for renal artery stenting. Fibromuscular dysplasia responses well to angioplasty. Renal artery aneurysm and arteriovenous (AV) fistula are most commonly treated with embolization.

3. This is associated with atherosclerotic disease in the usual vascular territories—coronary, carotid, and lower extremity territories.

4. Treatment options include medical therapy or revascularization, which can be performed surgically or percutaneously. Surgical revascularization techniques for RAS have included endarterectomy, extraanatomic bypass grafting, and aortorenal bypass grafting.

5. Flash pulmonary edema and bilateral renal artery stenosis with renal impairment are still accepted indications for stenting.

Pearls

- Acute thrombotic occlusion of the renal artery is a serious but rare complication occurring after renal artery angioplasty and stenting.
- Thrombosis can be treated with thrombolysis, thrombectomy, or placement of an additional stent. The kidney can tolerate total acute ischemia for about 90 minutes before becoming nonviable. The collateral circulation can maintain kidney viability for weeks or even months after occlusion of a previously normal renal artery in some cases. Nevertheless, acute thrombotic occlusion is an emergent condition and there is very limited time window to salvage the kidney.
- Acute thrombotic occlusion of renal artery stent is an emergency and intervention should start as soon as possible.

Suggested Reading

Morris CS, Bonnevie GJ, Najarian KE. Nonsurgical treatment of acute iatrogenic renal artery injuries occurring after renal artery angioplasty and stenting. *AJR Am J Roentgenol.* 2001;177(6):1353-1357.

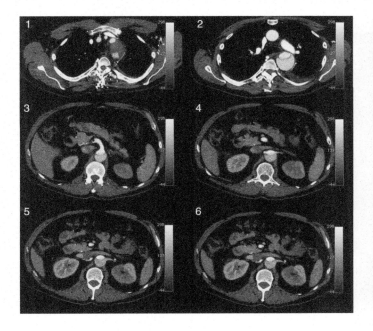

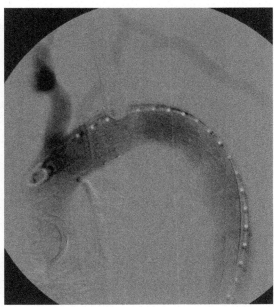

1. Review the collated computed tomographic (CT) images. Which vessels arise from the true lumen?

2. Can this patient be treated with thoracic endovascular aortic repair (TEVAR)?

3. How can you distinguish between the true lumen and the false lumen?

4. Why are stents not oversized and not post-dilated in dissection?

5. What are the outcomes of an uncomplicated type B dissection?

Case ranking/difficulty:

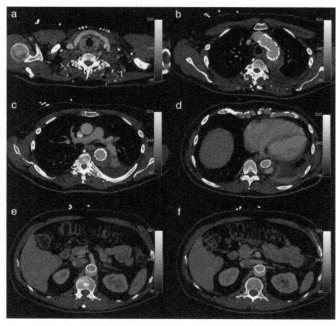

Post stent computed tomography (CT): (a) carotid–subclavian bypass; (b) stent in arch; (c, d) residual flow in the FL; (e, f) patent visceral branches.

Answers

1. All the visceral vessels, bar the inferior left renal artery, originate from the true lumen (TL).

2. Yes, but the intramural hematoma surrounds the origin of the left subclavian artery. If there is sufficient landing zone behind the left common carotid, then TEVAR can be performed by covering the left subclavian artery.

3. The false lumen is larger; and note the curvature of the lumen and see how the FL has sharp edges/acute angles. Transesophageal ultrasonography during the procedure can determine the wire position.

4. No oversizing is required, as the goal of TEVAR in complicated type B dissection is to restore intimal integrity and hold the proximal TL open. Balloon dilatation risks causing retrograde type A dissections. Actually, the TEVAR reconstruction can be built from top or below—careful planning and familiarity with stenting systems is very important. Distal tapering can be accepted, as the FL will thrombose and remodel over time.

5. Type B dissections can become complicated, aneurysmal, or stable. Aneurysms >6 cm have a risk of rupture that outweighs open repair and may be considered for TEVAR or open repair.

Pearls

- TEVAR has a role for acute complicated aortic dissection—that is, acute dissection with ischemia, rupture, pain, hypertension, and progressive false lumen with true lumen occlusion.
- The goal of TEVAR is to restore the intimal integrity by covering the intimal entry point with the stent functioning to hold open the proximal true lumen.
- TEVAR has a role for trauma, aneurysms, and acute complicated type B dissections and can be life saving in the setting of aortoenteric and aortobronchial fistulas.

Suggested Reading

Criado FJ. Aortic dissection: a 250-year perspective. *Tex Heart Inst J*. 2011;38(6):694-700.

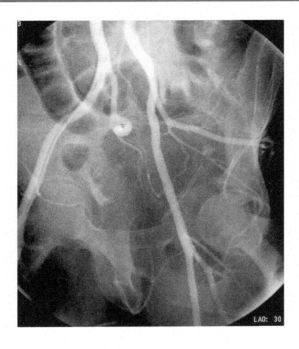 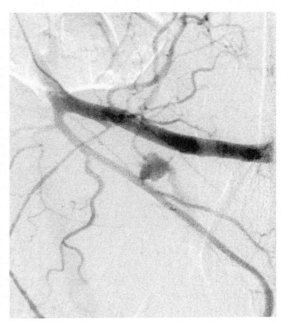

1. What are causes of gluteal artery injury?

2. Can "gluteal compartment syndrome" occur?

3. Major vascular injury should be treated within what time frame?

4. In major trauma, what should happen first—skeletal fixation or definitive vascular repair?

5. Which artery is most likely to be affected by trauma?

Case ranking/difficulty: **Category:** Arterial system

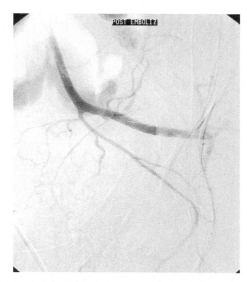

Postembolization image shows resolution of the pseudoaneurysm.

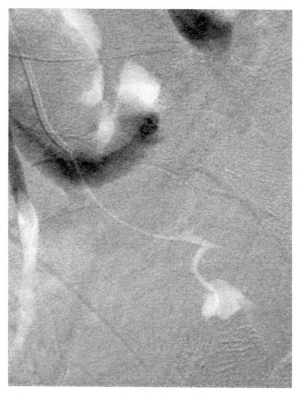

Superselective catheterization of the bleeding branch of the superior gluteal artery confirms the bleeding point.

Answers

1. Blunt and penetrating trauma, hip, and pelvic fractures can cause gluteal arterial injuries.

2. Gluteal compartment syndrome is extremely rare and occurs in conjunction with laceration of the gluteal artery.

3. Major vascular injury such as vessel transection means the limb requires revascularization within 4 to 6 hours or irreversible damage may be sustained after this time period.

4. If there is major trauma then an on-table angiogram should be performed. Next, fasciotomy should be considered. Then arterial shunting can be performed. Then there is time for external fixation, followed by definitive vascular repair (www.trauma.org). Immediate vascular repair may be affected by subsequent orthopedic manipulation. Ischemic damage can occur early because of compartment syndrome.

5. Popliteal artery is a common site for trauma and is affected by knee dislocation and lower extremity fractures.

Pearls

- Gluteal artery injury is uncommon; most of them are related to blunt or penetrating trauma and are rarely in iatrogenic etiology. Physical examination may reveal a small pulsatile mass over the buttock associated with overlying bruit.
- The mainstay of diagnosis is angiography, but these aneurysms may not be visible on an aortic flush angiogram, and selective angiography may be required to delineate the abnormality.
- The superior gluteal artery is more commonly injured than the inferior gluteal artery.
- Microcatheter selective embolization is the treatment of choice.

Suggested Readings

Agarwal M, Giannoudis PV, Syed AA, Hinsche AF, Matthews SJ, Smith RM. Pseudoaneurysm of the inferior gluteal artery following polytrauma: diverse presentation of a dangerous complication: a report of two cases. *J Orthop Trauma*. 2003;17(1):70-74.

Culliford AT, Cukingham RA, Worth MH Jr. Aneurysms of the gluteal vessels: their etiology and management. *J Trauma*. 1974;14(1):77-81.

McMillan WD, Smith ND, Nemcek A Jr, Pearce WH. Transcatheter embolization of a ruptured superior gluteal artery aneurysm: case report and review of the literature. *J Endovasc Surg*. 1997;4(4):376-379. [Review]

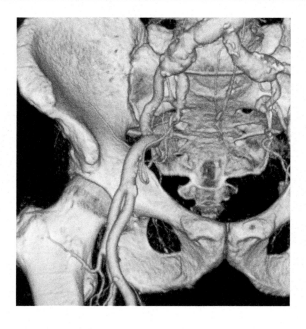 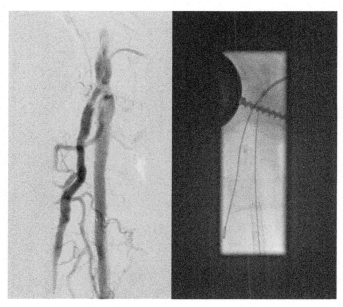

1. Where should the common femoral artery be accessed in an antegrade puncture?

2. What do you notice on the left image. Why is this important?

3. If you gain access into the common femoral artery but the wire passes into the profunda, what can be done?

4. How often is the femoral bifurcation above the middle of the femoral head?

5. What are the risks of access related complications?

Case ranking/difficulty:

Category: Arterial system

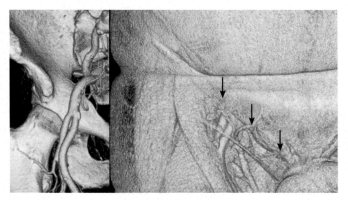

Note that the common femoral artery is seen above the inguinal ligament.

Answers

1. Antegrade access in a hostile groin is not always straightforward. The aim is to access the common femoral over the middle third as this facilitates hemostasis. Ultrasonography should be used.

2. There is a high femoral bifurcation. Direct access into the profunda must be avoided. Access above the inguinal ligament carries a risk of retroperitoneal hemorrhage. In this case, a direct superficial femoral artery (SFA) stick may be the best option.

3. Avoid placing a glidewire through a needle as the hydrophilic coating can shear off. A directional catheter can be pulled back while a wire is sounded until the SFA is accessed but there is a risk of losing access in a deep groin. A 2-wire technique may be preferable—a Brite-tip sheath is inserted over the wire into the profunda. A second wire is placed into the back of the sheath and used to sound the SFA as the sheath is pulled back (2 wires can be placed coaxially through a 5-Fr sheath). If access is lost, then the sheath can simply be reinserted

over the "safety" wire that is sitting in the profunda. A left anterior oblique angiogram opens up the left femoral bifurcation.

4. High femoral bifurcations can occur in up to 10%.

5. Low punctures risk pseudoaneurysm formation, and high punctures carry a risk of retroperitoneal hemorrhage, and major complications occur in up to 1%.

Pearls

- The ideal femoral access is obtained over the middle third of the femoral head, which aids compressive hemostasis. High punctures have increased risk of retroperitoneal hemorrhage. Low punctures have increased risk of pseudoaneurysm formation.
- High femoral artery bifurcation can be problematic if an antegrade femoral artery access is acquired. Blind access, use of landmark techniques, or fluoroscopy cannot account for anatomic variations and can result in direct access into the SFA or profunda.
- Review of any preprocedural imaging and ultrasound-guided access is recommended.
- If the wire preferentially passes into the profunda, then many techniques exist to convert this to an SFA access, such as using a Brite-tip sheath and 2 wires, or a directional catheter.

Suggested Reading

Tam MD, Lewis M. The effect of skin entry site, needle angulation and soft tissue compression on simulated antegrade and retrograde femoral arterial punctures: an anatomical study using Cartesian co-ordinates derived from CT angiography. *Surg Radiol Anat.* 2012;34(8): 751-755.

57-year-old man with onset of hypotension and back pain on table during iliac angioplasty

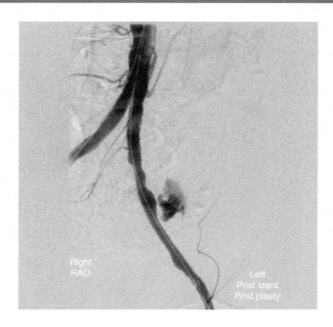

1. List 5 causes of iliac artery rupture.

2. What are risk factors for rupture during iliac intervention?

3. What is your management plan?

4. What is the incidence of iatrogenic iliac rupture during PTA?

5. What safety considerations can be put in place for improving iliac angioplasty outcomes?

Case ranking/difficulty:

Category: Arterial system

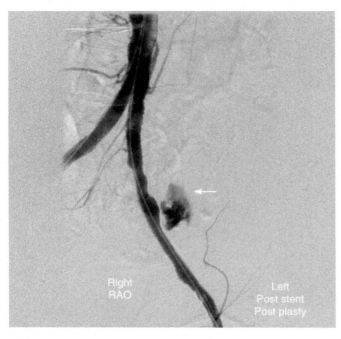

Angiogram performed after iliac angioplasty and stent placement.

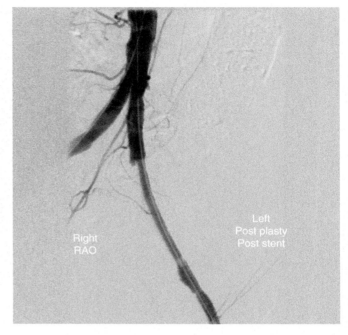

Final angiogram after placement of a covered stent.

Answers

1. Iatrogenic after iliac intervention, trauma, mycotic aneurysm, iliac aneurysm, and spontaneous rupture in connective tissue disease.

2. Heavily calcified vessels, use of oversized devices, diabetics, and patients taking corticosteroids are risk factors.

3. Immediate balloon tamponade, fluid resuscitation, and vascular surgery consultation should be conducted. Then, a covered stent should be placed across the rupture site, which tends to be successful. If there is persistent hemorrhage, open surgery may be required.

4. A series of 657 iliac interventions reported a rupture rate of 0.8%.

5. Safety considerations include pre-procedural check list, team communication, debriefing and operator self audit (eg BIAS registry) are important. As are appropriate stocking and availability of equipment, hemodynamic monitoring, intravenous access and communication with the patient during the procedure are important.

   The BIAS registry (British Society of Interventional Radiology Iliac Artery Angioplasty-Stent III registry) is used in the United Kingdom which is an important national database and excellent model for audit and outcome data.

Pearls

- Iliac rupture is a life-threatening complication and occurs in around 0.5% of cases (1 in 200).
- It is therefore highly likely that an interventional radiologist will encounter this complication during their career.
- Immediate replacement of the angioplasty balloon to tamponade the rupture is required, followed by placement of a covered stent. Balloon-expandable and self-expanding stent grafts are available. The operator must have immediate access to these devices and be familiar with their use and sheath requirement.

Suggested Readings

Chatziioannou A, Mourikis D, Katsimilis J, et al. Acute iliac artery rupture: endovascular treatment. *Cardiovasc Intervent Radiol.* 2007;30(2):281-285.

Uberoi R, Milburn S, Moss J, Gaines P, Gaines P; BIAS Registry Contributors. British Society of Interventional Radiology Iliac Artery Angioplasty-Stent Registry III. *Cardiovasc Intervent Radiol.* 2009;32(5):887-895.

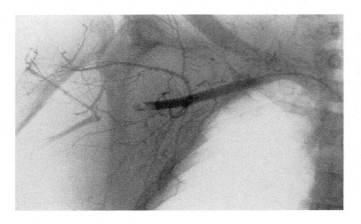
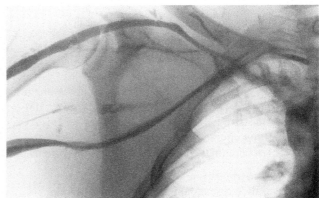

1. What are the common etiologies of axillary artery transection?

2. A patient has a knife in situ. The emergency department (ED) resident asks you if this should be removed as he is worried about artifact in the computed tomography (CT) he has ordered. What is your advice?

3. What are signs of arterial injury?

4. When is open surgery mandated?

5. Which muscle is an important landmark for the subclavian artery?

Case ranking/difficulty:

Answers

1. Although not common, shoulder injury (such as dislocation and humeral neck fracture) has been reported as the most common etiology of transection of axillary artery.

2. Foreign objects should only be removed in the operating room (OR) as probing of the wound in the ED could lead to massive hemorrhage should a clot be disturbed. CT before going to the OR will help to rule out other thoracic/abdominal/spinal injuries in stable patients.

3. Occlusion, truncation, caliber change, stenosis, extravasation, pseudoaneurysms, and AV fistula formation are signs of arterial injury.

4. Open surgery is necessary if there are open fractures, foreign bodies, infection risk, neurological involvement, or complete transection of the artery.

5. Scalenus anterior divides the subclavian into 3 parts. The first part gives rise to the internal mammary, vertebral, and the thyrocervical trunk. The middle part gives off the costocervical trunk. The third distal part gives off the dorsal scapular artery.

Pearls

- Axillary artery transection occurs as a result of blunt trauma, commonly in motor vehicle accidents, or following anterior shoulder dislocation. Transection of the axillary artery is often associated with a severe brachial plexus lesion, and requires emergent treatment. Endovascular repair and hybrid procedures combining open and endovascular techniques can offer reliable solutions to these challenging problems.

Suggested Readings

Kelley SP, Hinsche AF, Hossain JF. Axillary artery transection following anterior shoulder dislocation: classical presentation and current concepts. *Injury.* 2004;35(11):1128-1132.

Witz M. Transected axillary artery: unusual blunt trauma. *J Trauma.* 2003;54(1):203.

45-year-old man who is status post living donor right lobe liver transplant. He presents with elevation of liver enzymes

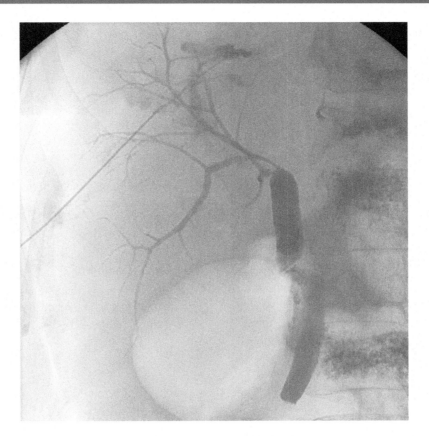

1. What is seen on the cholangiogram?

2. What are the risks of biliary complications in live and deceased donor livers?

3. What is the incidence of biliary complications?

4. What is a split-liver transplant?

5. What is the management of an anastomotic stricture?

Case ranking/difficulty:

Answers

1. There is no leak or obstruction, but there is stenosis. The cystic duct stump in the native common duct can also be seen.

2. Many studies have shown a higher incidence of biliary tract complications in living donor liver transplants (LDLTs) as compared to deceased donor liver transplants (DDLTs). Bile leaks were the most common complication due to LDLT (17.1%); however, stricture was the most common complication due to DDLT (7.5%).

3. Large series have reported overall biliary complications after living donor transplantation to range from 15% to 35%.

4. A split liver transplant increases the pool of cadaveric transplants, where segments 4 to 8 are used for an adult transplant and segments 2 and 3 for a pediatric recipient.

5. ERCP is first line. If percutaneous drainage is required, strictures can be treated with balloon dilatation and sequential up-sizing of internal-external drains. Ultimately, surgical revision may be required.

Pearls

- Biliary complications are the most important source of complications after liver transplantation, and an important cause of morbidity and mortality.
- Many studies have shown a higher incidence of biliary tract complications in living donor liver transplantation compared with cadaveric transplants.
- The most common biliary complications after liver transplantation include bile leaks, anastomotic and intrahepatic strictures, stones, and ampullary dysfunction.

Suggested Reading

Duailibi DF, Ribeiro MA. Biliary complications following deceased and living donor liver transplantation: a review. *Transplant Proc*. 2010;42(2):517-520.

45-year-old woman with occluded aorta and iliac arteries unfit for major surgery

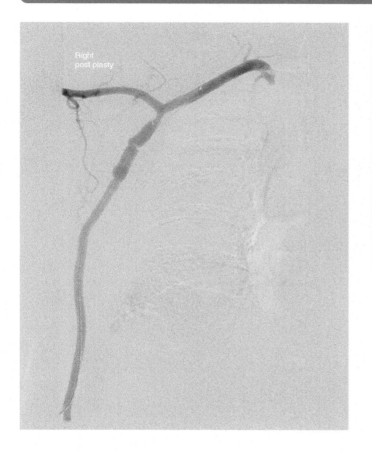

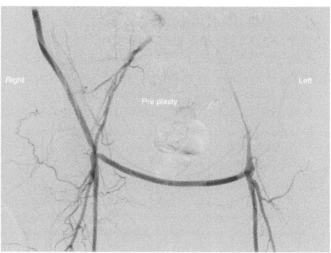

1. What are the indications for axillobifemoral grafts?

2. What are graft-related complications?

3. What is the role of ultrasound surveillance?

4. How and where would you access the graft for intervention?

5. What is the 5-year patency?

Case ranking/difficulty:

Answers

1. This graft is an option when the patient is unfit for aortobifemoral repair or has an infected aortic graft or an aortoduodenal fistula.

2. The graft can develop stenoses, occlusions, or become infected. Steal syndrome can occur. Brachial plexus injury is possible at time of surgery.

3. Ultrasonographic surveillance should be performed regularly so that anastomotic stenoses can identified and treated before they lead to thrombotic graft occlusion.

4. Accessing the graft at a rib means that this can then be used to aid manual hemostasis. A vertical puncture will allow "turning" of the catheter to deal with both proximal and distal anastomoses. Multiple views are required to delineate the anatomy, particularly at the femoral anastomoses. Prophylactic antibiotics are commonly used to reduce the risk of graft infection, but there is no strong evidence base.

5. The right axillary artery is favored as it is less likely affected by occlusive disease. Five-year patency is around 20% to 40%.

Pearls

- The axillobifemoral graft is an important extraanatomic graft.
- It allows revascularization of the lower limbs, bypassing any thoracoabdominal pathology and obverting the need for a major thoracotomy or laparotomy.
- One indication is therefore the revascularization of the lower limbs in the setting of aortoiliac occlusive disease. It is also useful in patients with infected aortic grafts and aortoenteric fistulas.

Suggested Reading

El-Massry S, Saad E, Sauvage LR, et al. Axillofemoral bypass with externally supported, knitted Dacron grafts: a follow-up through twelve years. *J Vasc Surg*. 1993;17(1):107-114; discussion 114-115.

65-year-old man with history of previous multiple arterial bypass surgeries

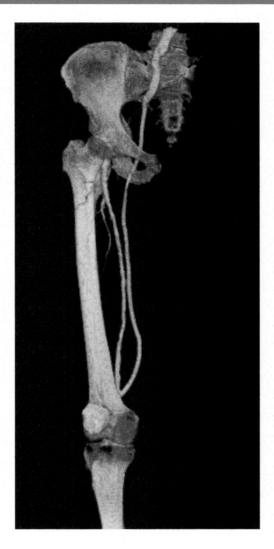

1. List commonly used extra-anatomic grafts.?

2. The graft leaves the pelvis through the greater sciatic foramen—true or false?

3. The graft requires a laparotomy—true or false?

4. What is the reported 5-year graft patency?

5. What is the 5-year limb salvage rate after obturator graft?

Case ranking/difficulty:

Category: Arterial system

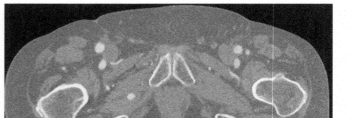

Note the position of the graft on cross-sectional imaging.

Pearls

- The obturator graft is an important alternative for lower limb revascularization in the setting of sepsis in the groin.
- Infection and the need to revascularize a limb can occur with (a) groin sepsis with sinus or abscess formation, (b) in situ infected graft material, and (c) infected pseudoaneurysm formation.
- The volume-rendered images demonstrate an obturator bypass graft. It is important to understand the options available for revascularization and to identify these grafts on cross-sectional imaging—their appearances can be strange to the novice because of their extraanatomic locations.

Volume rendered computed tomographic angiogram, lateral view.

Suggested Reading

Patel A, Taylor SM, Langan EM, et al. Obturator bypass: a classic approach for the treatment of contemporary groin infection. *Am Surg.* 2002;68(8):653-658; discussion 658-659.

Answers

1. Extra-anatomical grafts are important options for vascular surgeons. These include axillary bifemoral, femoral to femoral crossover grafts. Carotid subclavian bypasses are useful in thoracic aortic intervention. This case shows an obturator graft.

2. This graft leaves the pelvis through the obturator foramen.

3. The graft, if taken from the external iliac arty, can be formed through a lower abdominal extraperitoneal incision.

4. Five-year graft patency is reported at 80%.

5. Obturator by-pass is an effective operation and has a limb salvage rate of 60% at 5 years.

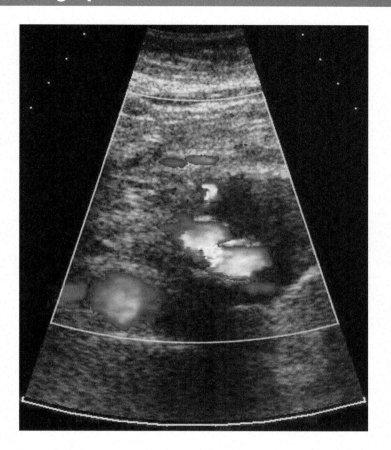

1. What ultrasound features can be seen?

2. Which other structures can be seen?

3. What features would you adjust to ensure optimized ultrasound images?

4. What is contrast-enhanced ultrasonography (CEUS)?

5. How are microbubbles excreted and what is their clinical role?

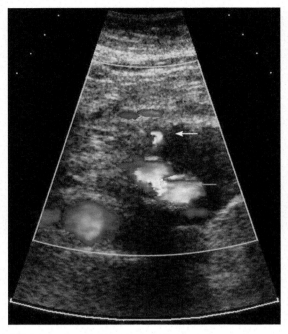

Color Doppler of EVAR.

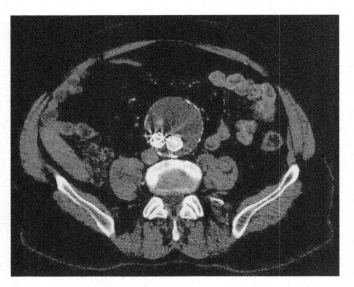

Computed tomographic (CT) corroboration.

Answers

1. There is a type 2 endoleak.

2. The sac, graft limbs, and an endoleak can be seen. Surrounding structures such as the cava and inferior mesenteric vessels are also identified.

3. Appropriate transducer selection, use of color scale and gain, and tissue compression are important.

4. CEUS requires injection of microbubbles, which arrive as a bolus in the intravascular space.

5. They are excreted via the lungs and do not leave the intravascular space. Low–mechanical index (MI) imaging is required. CEUS can demonstrate endoleaks where other modalities fail and can be particularly useful in differentiating between the different types of endoleak.

Pearls

- Ultrasonography is a useful tool for post-EVAR surveillance. This is particularly useful in patients with impaired renal function and can obviate the need for contrast-enhanced CT. Ultrasonography is however operator dependent, and patient factors such as obesity and bowel gas can make ultrasonography less sensitive.
- Ultrasonography can determine sac size and identify endoleaks.

Suggested Reading

Mirza TA, Karthikesalingam A, Jackson D, et al. Duplex ultrasound and contrast-enhanced ultrasound versus computed tomography for the detection of endoleak after EVAR: systematic review and bivariate meta-analysis. *Eur J Vasc Endovasc Surg.* 2010;39(4):418-428.

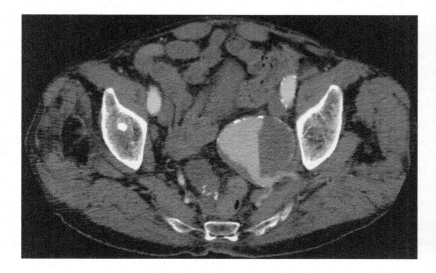 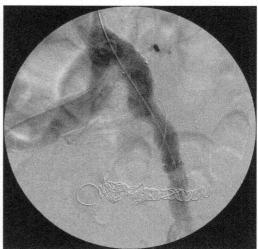

1. A 4 cm internal iliac artery aneurysm arises 1 cm below the iliac bifurcation. What is your management plan?

2. Which plane tends to best show the right IIA origin on conventional pelvic angiography?

3. What is the incidence of buttock claudication after iliac artery embolization?

4. What is the advantage of open surgery?

5. Regarding iliac aneurysms—which is the most common?

Case ranking/difficulty:

Answers

1. The distal branches should be embolized. If the length of trunk is less than 1 cm, then stent graft across the IIA origin should be considered. If more than 1 cm, then it is possible to also embolize the trunk, for example, with a plug.

2. A left anterior oblique (LAO) projection best opens up the right iliac bifurcation. Of course this is variable, and review of preprocedural computed tomography (CT) using maximum-intensity projections (MIPs) or volume-rendered (VR) images may help show the best angle.

3. About 20% of patients can experience buttock claudication after IIA embolization—this can improve over time.

4. Open surgery with sac excision will remove the underlying mass effect—whereas though sac reduction can occur after endovascular repair, this may occur over a longer time period.

5. Common iliac artery (CIA) aneurysm account for about 70% of iliac aneurysms, internals about 30%. External aneurysms are rare—and this is thought to be because the external iliac artery (EIA) has a different developmental origin compared to the CIA and IIA.

Pearls

- Isolated internal iliac aneurysms are rare but rupture carries a high mortality rate.
- Treatment options for IIA aneurysms are dependent upon the length of normal arterial trunk above the aneurysm. If long, then the distal branches can be embolized and coils or a plug placed in the trunk. If short, a stent graft should be placed across the IIA origin.

Suggested Reading

Sakamoto I, Sueyoshi E, Hazama S, et al. Endovascular treatment of iliac artery aneurysms. *Radiographics*. 2005; 25(Suppl 1):S213-S227.

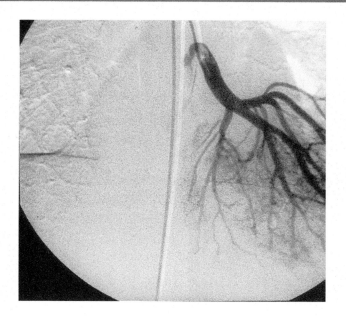

1. What is the diagnosis?

2. The blood supply of this lesion is commonly
   derived from where?

3. What is the most common association?

4. What are the differences between intralobar
   and extralobar subtypes?

5. What are treatment options here?

Case ranking/difficulty:

Category: Arterial system

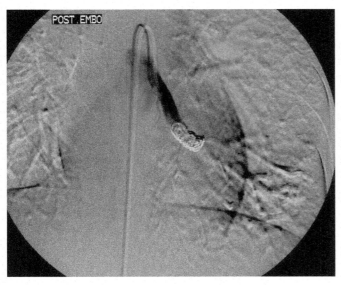

Angiogram after embolization shows complete occlusion of anomalous artery.

Pearls

- Sequestrated lung is a mass of lung tissue without connection with the bronchial tree with a systemic arterial supply.
- It can be extralobar or intralobar.
- Intralobar sequestration is more common and occurs within lung tissue, sharing lung pleura and drains via pulmonary veins. It tends to present in adolescence with recurrent pneumonia.
- Extralobar type is located outside the normal lung, with its own pleura, and has aberrant systemic venous drainage. This can be seen on antenatal imaging and presents in infancy with pneumonia.

Suggested Reading

Lee BS, Kim JT, Kim EA, et al. Neonatal pulmonary sequestration: clinical experience with transumbilical arterial embolization. *Pediatr Pulmonol.* 2008;43(4): 404-413.

Answers

1. Pulmonary sequestration. There is a mass of lung tissue that is supplied by a large branch from the descending thoracic aorta. Scimitar syndrome (venolobar syndrome) describes anomalous pulmonary drainage of the right lung into the inferior veno cava (IVC).

2. The blood supply of 75% of pulmonary sequestrations is derived from the thoracic or abdominal aorta. The remaining 25% of sequestrations receive their blood flow from the subclavian, intercostal, pulmonary, pericardiophrenic, innominate, internal mammary, celiac, splenic, or renal arteries.

3. Diaphragmatic hernia.

4. Intrapulmonary sequestration is usually diagnosed later in childhood or adolescence.

5. Embolization techniques for pulmonary sequestration are expanding, and may be a safe alternative method to surgery, especially for infants with extralobar pulmonary sequestration who present with congestive heart failure.

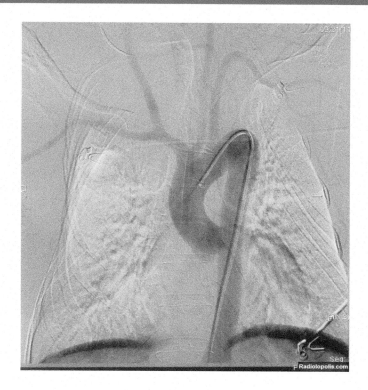

1. What is the diagnosis?

2. Which are aortic arch variants?

3. Where can the thyroidea ima artery arise from?

4. Where does the aortic arch terminate?

5. What is an aortic ductus diverticulum?

Case ranking/difficulty:

Answers

1. There is a bovine aortic arch and the patient has underlying necrotizing fasciitis (NF).

2. The aortic arch has numerous variations.

3. The thyroidea ima artery is an uncommon variant of the blood supply and can arise from all of the above locations.

4. The arch of the aorta is the direct continuation of the ascending aorta. Its origin is defined as a sternomanubrial joint. It terminates at the lower border of T4, when it becomes the descending aorta.

5. An aortic ductus diverticulum is a developmental outpouching of the aorta, usually seen at the anteromedial aspect of the aorta at site of the previous ductus arteriosus. This is also the site of 90% of traumatic aortic injuries, and differentiation of ductus arteriosus from a pseudoaneurysm is important. An aortic pseudoaneurysm usually forms sharp margins with the aorta, whereas the ductus diverticulum usually appears as a smooth focal bulge with gentle obtuse angles with the aortic wall.

Pearls

- The most common aortic arch branching pattern has separate origins for the innominate, left common carotid, and left subclavian arteries.
- The second most common pattern has a common origin for the innominate and left common carotid arteries. This pattern has erroneously been referred to as a bovine arch. A true bovine aortic arch bears no resemblance to any of the common human aortic arch variations. In cattle, a single great vessel originates from the aortic arch. This large brachiocephalic trunk gives rise to both subclavian arteries and a bicarotid trunk.

Suggested Reading

Jakanani GC, Adair W. Frequency of variations in aortic arch anatomy depicted on multidetector CT. *Clin Radiol.* 2010;65(6):481-487.

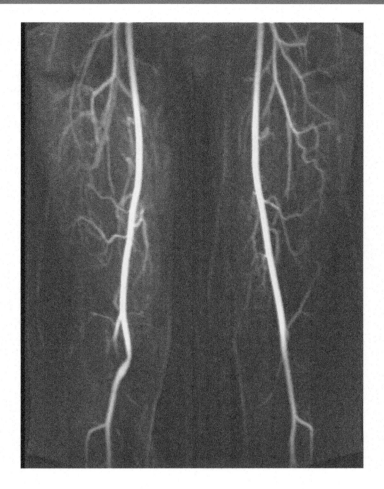

1. What is the diagnosis?

2. Which imaging modality can make the diagnosis and demonstrate the underlying anatomic abnormality?

3. What are the treatment options?

4. What is the key demographic?

5. What is island popliteal artery?

Case ranking/difficulty:

Category: Arterial system

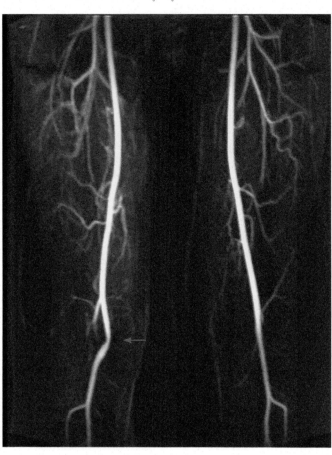

MRA of the proximal thigh and upper calf.

Answers

1. There is medial deviation of the popliteal artery consistent with popliteal entrapment syndrome.

2. The abnormal muscle or fibrous band can be seen on T1-weighted magnetic resonance (MR) images.

   Dynamic testing with plantar flexion (which can be combined with ultrasonography or angiography) does not demonstrate the underlying anatomical abnormality. Also, these dynamic tests can produce arterial compression in normal subjects.

   Magnetic resonance angiography (MRA) alone does not provide the high-resolution axial T1 images that are needed to look for the fibromuscular abnormalities.

3. Surgical treatment depends on the precise anatomic abnormality (as defined by the Delaney classification). The underlying artery may be damaged and so endarterectomy and bypass may also be required. There is no role for endovascular therapy.

4. It tends to affect young athletic men.

5. There is a variant branch from the popliteal artery to the proximal tibioperoneal trunk that gives the visual appearance of an "island."

Pearls

- The popliteal artery is entrapped as a result of an anomalous relationship with the surrounding musculotendinous structures. This is commonly caused by an abnormal attachment of the medial head of gastrocnemius but there are a range of underlying abnormalities.
- Repetitive arterial microtrauma leads to stenosis, thrombosis, occlusion, and pseudoaneurysm formation. Dynamic ultrasonographic testing is useful, but plantarflexion-induced arterial compression is a finding in normal subjects. MRI can image the arterial as well as identify the underlying anatomical cause. Treatment is surgical with musculotendinous release.

Suggested Reading

Macedo TA, Johnson CM, Hallett JW, Breen JF. Popliteal artery entrapment syndrome: role of imaging in the diagnosis. *AJR Am J Roentgenol*. 2003;181(5):1259-1265.

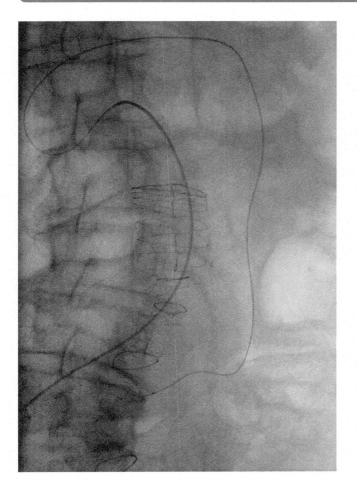 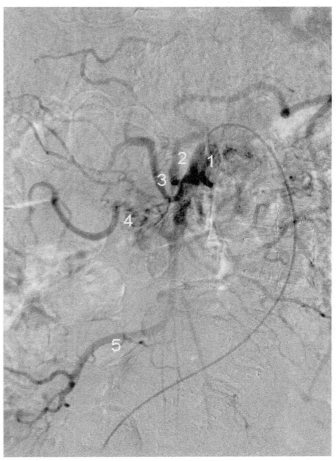

1. Regarding image on the left: what device is present, where is the catheter?

2. Regarding image on the right: name the annotated vessels.

3. State the classification of endoleaks.

4. What is the potential risk of a type 2 endoleak?

5. How should type 2 endoleaks be managed?

Case ranking/difficulty: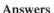

Category: Arterial system

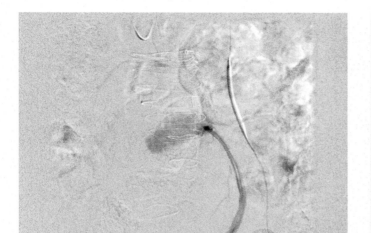

Advanced catheter position at the origin of the inferior mesenteric artery (IMA) with filling of the sac.

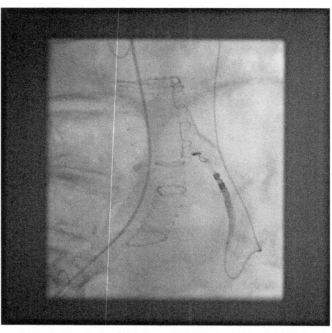

Endpoint showing coil embolization of the IMA and no filling of the sac.

Answers

1. The spot fluoroscopic image shows the presence of an EVAR and a host catheter that has selected the superior mesenteric artery and a microcatheter placed coaxially through this catheter, which passes from the superior mesenteric artery (SMA), through the middle colic, left colic, and back up the IMA to the sac.

2. (1) SMA trunk, (2) middle colic, (3) inferior pancreaticoduodenal artery, (4) right colic, and (5) ileocolic.

3. See discussion.

4. Delayed rupture has been reported. It is likely that an unrecognized type 2 endoleak can cause sac enlargement, which can then lead to graft migration and a high-pressure leak.

5. There should be regular surveillance, and intervention should occur if there is sac enlargement.

Pearls

- Type I endoleaks occur at the proximal and distal attachment sites. Type II endoleaks occur due to retrograde flow in arteries that feed the sac, such as lumbar arteries or the IMA. Type III endoleak occurs when there is stent graft fracture, holes in the fabric, or separation of the modular components. Type IV is thought to be due to graft porosity and may be device-specific. Type V is called "endotension," where there is expansion of the sac without standard imaging evidence of an endoleak.

- Type II endoleaks may occur in up to 20% of patients but can often be managed conservatively. Serial CT surveillance often demonstrates sac size reduction or sac stability. Increasing sac size with a type II endoleak is an indication for treatment.

- Embolization of the lumbar or IMAs can be performed with coils. Onyx embolization of the sac is an alternative. Percutaneous sac puncture can also be a useful technique.

Suggested Reading

Tolia AJ, Landis R, Lamparello P, Rosen R, Macari M. Type II endoleaks after endovascular repair of abdominal aortic aneurysms: natural history. *Radiology*. 2005;235(2):683-686.

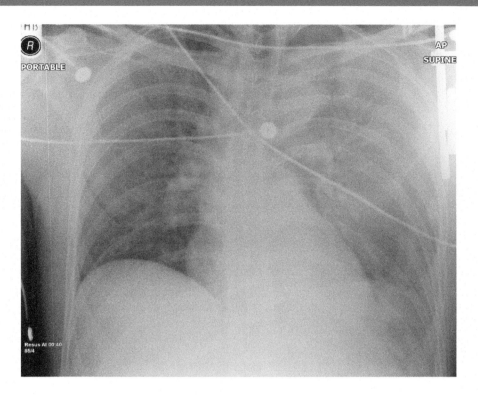

1. Review the chest radiograph—what is the major abnormality?

2. What chest radiograph signs are associated with aortic transection?

3. What percentage of patients with blunt aortic injury die at the scene?

4. What are the advantages of stent-grafting over open surgery?

5. What may be needed if the left subclavian artery is covered—either planned or inadvertently?

Case ranking/difficulty:

Category: Arterial system

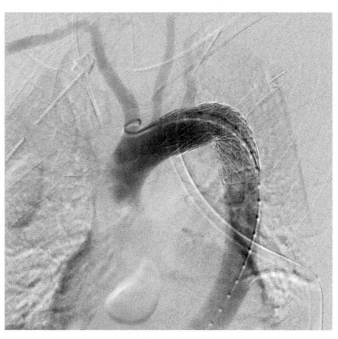

Post stent graft angiogram.

Pearls

- Traumatic aortic injuries can be managed with endovascular stent graft placement.
- Advantages over open surgery include that the potentially multiply injured patient can be managed in the supine position (compared to being turned for thoracotomy), without the need for one-lung ventilation, prolonged systemic heparinization, cardiopulmonary bypass, or aortic cross-clamping.

Suggested Readings

Marotta R, Franchetto AA. The CT appearance of aortic transection. *AJR Am J Roentgenol*. 1996;166(3):647-651.

Orford VP, Atkinson NR, Thomson K, et al. Blunt traumatic aortic transection: the endovascular experience. *Ann Thorac Surg*. 2003;75(1):106-111; discussion 111-112.

Answers

1. The aortic knuckle is abnormal and appearances are suspicious for an aortic injury.

2. Mediastinal width of >8 cm is concerning. Any sign of major intrathoracic injury should raise suspicion.

3. Eighty-five percent will die at the scene. Of those that arrive to hospital, around 20% will die.

4. Advantages of stent grafting include being able to manage the patient in a supine position, no requirement for one-lung ventilation, bypass, cross-clamping, or prolonged systemic heparinization.

5. A left subclavian-carotid bypass may be required.

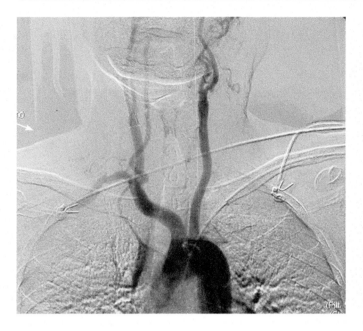 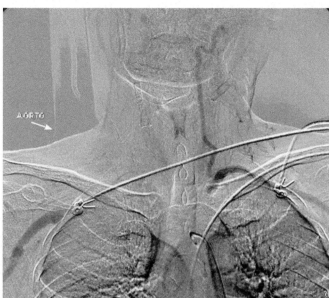

1. Review the 2 images—what is your diagnosis?

2. What is the most common clinical symptom of this condition?

3. Which clinical symptoms indicate vertebrobasilar insufficiency?

4. What causes this condition?

5. You identify reversed flow (away from the brain) during systole and antegrade flow during diastole in the Doppler ultrasonographic examination of the left vertebral artery of a 53-year-old man presenting with left arm claudication and dizziness. What is the most likely diagnosis?

Case ranking/difficulty:

Category: Arterial system

Answers

1. Subclavian steal syndrome.

2. The term *subclavian steal phenomenon* is reserved for asymptomatic patients. It indicates retrograde vertebral artery flow causing transient neurologic symptoms.

3. These symptoms may be related to vertebrobasilar insufficiency, an indication for treatment.

4. Subclavian steal syndrome results from occlusion or severe stenosis of subclavian artery or innominate artery proximal to origin of vertebral artery.

5. Partial subclavian steal syndrome—there is partial reversal of flow in the vertebral artery during systole. Full steal shows revered flow in vertebral artery throughout the cardiac cycle. The term subclavian steal phenomenon is reserved for asymptomatic patients.

Pearls

- Subclavian steal syndrome results from occlusion or severe stenosis of subclavian artery or innominate artery proximal to origin of vertebral artery. In this disorder, the arm obtains its blood supply by reverse flow down the ipsilateral vertebral artery from the opposite vertebral artery or from the circle of Willis.

Suggested Reading

Song L, Zhang J, Li J, et al. Endovascular stenting vs. extrathoracic surgical bypass for symptomatic subclavian steal syndrome. *J Endovasc Ther.* 2012;19(1):44-51.

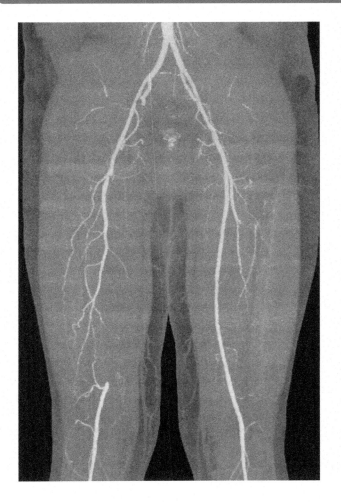
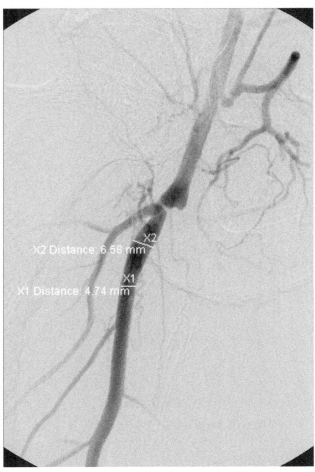

1. The profunda is easily accessed from the ipsilateral common femoral artery—true or false?

2. Revascularization of the profunda will treat major arterial ulceration—true or false?

3. What is the 3-year patency rate for profundaplasty?

4. Endovascular therapy is better than surgery in the profunda—true or false?

5. The medial circumflex femoral artery always arises from the main profundal trunk—true or false?

Category: Arterial system

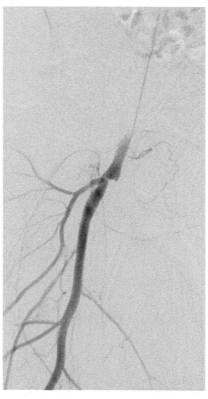

Post profundoplasty.

3. Small series have reported 3- and even 8-year patency rates of more than 80%.

4. Surgical endarterectomy and open surgical repair is the gold standard for patients with critical limb ischemia and profunda atherosclerosis.

5. The medial circumflex femoral artery arises from the profunda in 60%, and the lateral circumflex arises from the profunda in 80%.

Pearls

- The profunda femoris has variable anatomy with a profunda trunk and medial and lateral circumflex branches. The main trunk commonly comes off the common femoral laterally with a separate medial circumflex. The main trunk can arise medially or even anteriorly and the bifurcation can be high. Attenuation should always be paid to this anatomy when accessing the common femoral artery.
- Profunda is accessed from the contralateral common femoral artery with a crossover.
- Revascularization of the profunda is useful in selected patients with critical limb ischemia with rest pain or minor tissue loss.

Answers

1. A high puncture would be required and this would be in the setting of atherosclerosis or a postoperative groin and so the profunda is best accessed from the contralateral common femoral artery with a crossover.

2. PFA revascularization has a role where there is rest pain or minor tissue loss but will not have good results with major tissue loss where distal revascularization will probably be required. The profunda is the main collateral pathway when the SFA is occluded.

Suggested Readings

Donas KP, Pitoulias GA, Schwindt A, et al. Endovascular treatment of profunda femoris artery obstructive disease: nonsense or useful tool in selected cases? *Eur J Vasc Endovasc Surg.* 2010;39(3):308-313.

Karnabatidis D, Spiliopoulos S, Pastromas G, Katsanos K, Siablis D. Endovascular management of the arteria profunda fmoralis: long-term angiographic and clinical outcomes. *Cardiovasc Intervent Radiol.* 2012;35(5): 1016-1022.

75-year-old man with a thoracoabdominal aneurysm

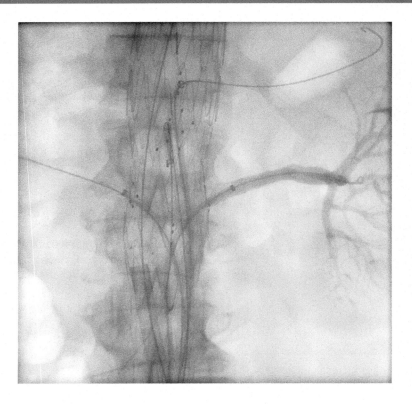

1. Is endovascular repair the standard of care for all aneurysms?

2. What year was first endovascular aneurysm repair (EVAR) was performed in?

3. What percentage of aortic aneurysms are abdominal?

4. What percentage of abdominal aortic aneurysms (AAAs) are infrarenal?

5. Which of the following conditions predispose to aneurysm formation?

Case ranking/difficulty:

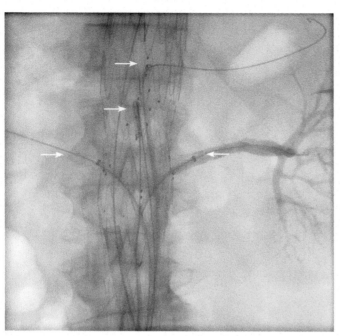

Fluoroscopic image of a fenestrated EVAR repair in progress. The right and left renal fenestrations have been completed.

Answers

1. No. This is probably true for infrarenal aneurysms. However, juxta- and suprarenal/thoracoabdominal aneurysms can be treated endovascularly but this should be done in centers of excellence. These centers can also treat aneurysms that involve the great vessels and arch. Intermediate-term outcome data suggest that advanced aneurysm repair is associated with good outcomes.

2. The first report by Parodi et al entitled "Transfemoral Intraluminal Gaft Implantation for Abdominal Aortic Aneurysm" was published in 1991.

3. About 75% of all aortic aneurysms are abdominal, and 25% of aortic aneurysms are thoracic or thoracoabdominal.

4. Ninety-five percent of AAAs are infrarenal. The other 5% are juxtarenal or thoracoabdominal.

5. Connective tissue diseases and vasculitides are associated with aneurysm formation.

Pearls

- Fenestrated aortic stent graft placement is a complex procedure.
- Complex aneurysm repairs for thoracoabdominal and juxtarenal aortic aneurysms are possible. Stent graft design allows exclusion of the aneurysm and the visceral vessels are preserved by placing balloon-expandable stent grafts through the reinforced "fenestrated" branches.
- Here, the device is in place and the right and left renal arteries have been stented. Sheaths and access wires are in place to complete the procedure by stenting the origins of the superior mesenteric artery and celiac trunk.

Suggested Readings

Greenberg R, Eagleton M, Mastracci T. Branched endografts for thoracoabdominal aneurysms. *J Thorac Cardiovasc Surg.* 2010;140(6 Suppl):S171-S178.

Parodi JC, Palmaz JC, Barone HD. Transfemoral intraluminal graft implantation for abdominal aortic aneurysms. *Ann Vasc Surg.* 1991;5(6):491-499.

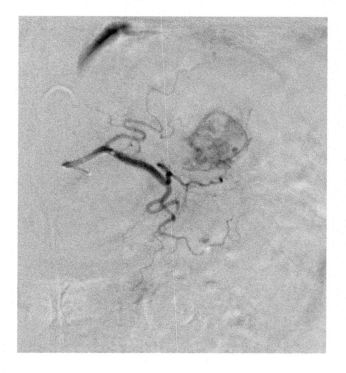
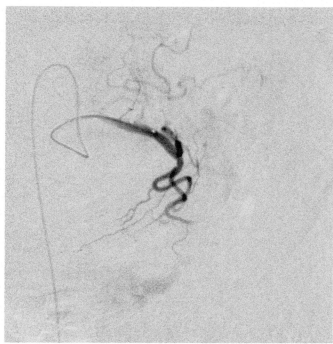

1. Review the pre- and postembolization angiographic images. What catheters do you see? What is the arterial territory?

2. What treatment strategies are available for gastrointestinal stromal tumor liver metastases?

3. What is the difference between PVA and trisacryl particles?

4. What is post-embolization syndrome?

5. How can bowel gas artefact be reduced in angiography?

Case ranking/difficulty: **Category:** Arterial system

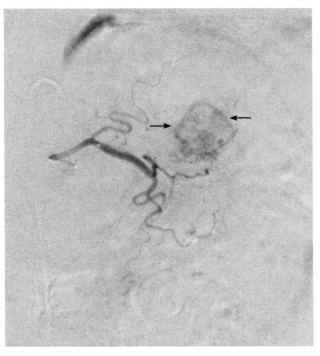

Preembolization angiogram.

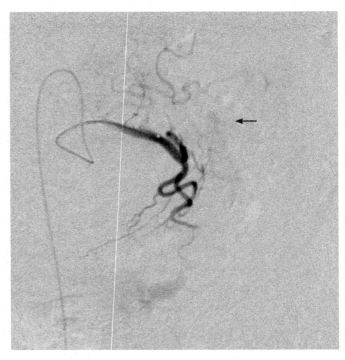

Postembolization angiogram.

Answers

1. There is a Simmonds catheter in the celiac trunk and a microcatheter in the left gastric artery. Angiogram demonstrates a hypervascular lesion consistent with the known GIST tumor. Post-embolization angiogram demonstrates stasis and nonvisualization of the tumor and otherwise preserved branches of the left gastric artery.

2. Tyrosine kinase inhibitor chemotherapy and transarterial chemoembolization (TACE) are efficacious.

3. PVA particles vary in size and are irregular, as opposed to trisacryl gelatin microspheres, which are homogenous in size and shape. The irregular nature of PVA particles is thought to lead to clumping or aggregation of particles, which may cause catheter obstruction or occlude larger vessels, and therefore may be a less effective embolic agent than the trisacryl particles.

4. Post-embolization syndrome is felt to be a response to tissue ischemia and inflammation. It tends to be a self-limiting illness that presents with flu-like symptoms between 2 and 14 days. However, attention must be paid to not miss a true septic complication such as abscess formation.

5. Buscopan and glucagon are commonly used. Buscopan and glucagon can be given intravenously.

Pearls

• GIST tumors are mesenchymal neoplasms. Liver and peritoneum are common metastatic sites. Tumors can respond to tyrosine kinase inhibitor chemotherapy. Liver metastases can respond to transarterial chemoembolization. Gastric GISTs frequently present with upper gastrointestinal bleeding, which can be controlled with embolization.

Suggested Reading

Kobayashi K, Gupta S, Trent JC, et al. Hepatic artery chemoembolization for 110 gastrointestinal stromal tumors: response, survival, and prognostic factors. *Cancer.* 2006;107(12):2833-2841.

22-year-old lady with right upper quadrant pain

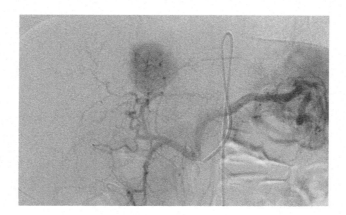

1. What do the images show?

2. What is the differential diagnosis?

3. What is the effect of oral contraceptives on FNH?

4. What is the best diagnostic sign of FNH?

5. What is the value of using superparamagnetic iron oxide (SPIO) as a contrast agent?

Case ranking/difficulty:

Category: Arterial system

Answers

1. There is a hypervascular tumor seen on the angiogram with a dense blush in the capillary phase.

2. Hepatic adenoma, cavernous hemangioma, fibrolamellar carcinoma, hepatocellular carcinoma, hypervascular metastasis and focal nodular hyperplasia are all possibilities.

3. Oral contraceptives do not cause FNH but have trophic effect on growth.

4. Best diagnostic clue for FNH: brightly and homogeneously enhancing mass in arterial phase computed tomography (CT) or magnetic resonance imaging (MRI) with delayed enhancement of central scar.

5. SPIO is taken up by Kupffer cells, which are present in FNH, and so there is decreased signal on T2W images.

Pearls

• The diagnosis of FNH is based on the demonstration of a central scar but this may not be visible in as many as 20% of patients.

• Angiographic signs show a hypervascular mass with a central arterial supply, a 'spoke wheel' pattern of enhancement with an intense capillary blush. The classical 'spoke wheel' appearance is said to be seen in up to a third of cases.

Suggested Readings

Huang D, Chen Y, Zeng Q, et al. Transarterial embolization using pingyangmycin lipiodol emulsion and polyvinyl alcohol for the treatment of focal nodular hyperplasia of the liver. *Hepatogastroenterology.* 2011;58 (110-111):1736-1741.

Fowler KJ, Brown JJ, Narra VR. Magnetic resonance imaging of focal liver lesions: approach to imaging diagnosis. *Hepatology.* 2011;54(6):2227-2237.

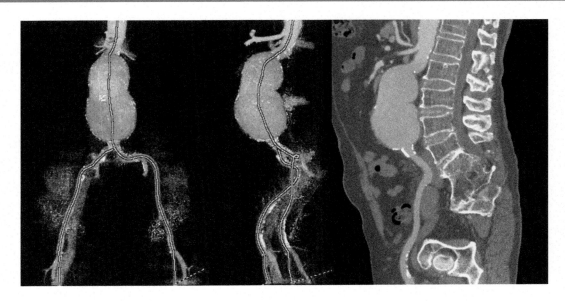

1. Is this aneurysm suitable for standard EVAR?

2. What feature is most challenging?

3. AUI is a proven strategy for emergency EVAR—true or false or unknown?

4. What is the 4-year patency of femoral–femoral cross-over grafts post EVAR?

5. Would you yourself have an open repair or an EVAR?

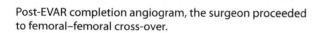

Category: Arterial system

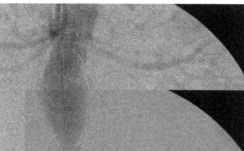

3. Emergency EVAR can be performed with bifurcated system, though an AUI graft take less planning and are more straight forward. Outcome data from prospective randomized trials such as the IMPROVE trial will give further insight.

4. One large series has found patency rates of over 90% at 4 years.

5. Despite whatever the evidence-base might be, any decision-making process should be patient-centered. There are short-term gains with EVAR, but there is the 'late equivalence' effect, and the need for close follow-up and secondary interventions is not needed with open repair and this should be discussed with the patient.

> ## Pearls
>
> - AUI grafts facilitate endovascular repair of aortic aneurysms in the setting of complex iliac anatomy.
> - They may be an option for emergency EVAR.
> - Femoral–femoral cross-over grafts are required, and their initial patency rates are high, but very long-term data is not available.

Post-EVAR completion angiogram, the surgeon proceeded to femoral–femoral cross-over.

Suggested Reading

Schanzer A, Greenberg RK, Hevelone N, et al. Predictors of abdominal aortic aneurysm sac enlargement after endovascular repair. *Circulation.* 2011;123(24):2848-2855.

Answers

1. No, a uni-iliac stent graft is required.

2. The aortic bifurcation is narrowed, and will not accept 2 limbs, and so an aorto-uni-iliac (AUI) graft with subsequent femoral–femoral cross-over grafting must be performed. Appropriate tube angulation is required to see the true length of neck.

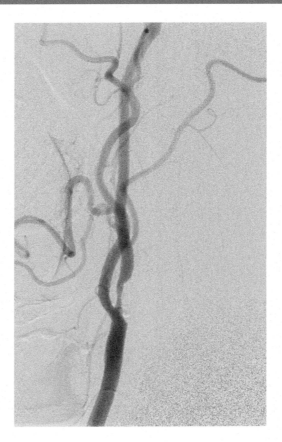

1. What are the indications for carotid artery stenting?

2. What are contraindications?

3. What is the evidence for embolic protection devices?

4. What is the management of anticoagulation status around stenting?

5. What medications may be useful during carotid stenting?

Case ranking/difficulty:

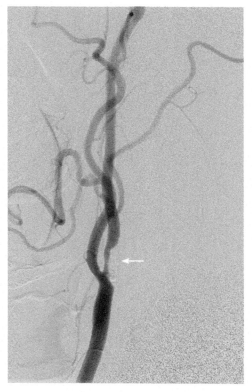

Carotid angiogram.

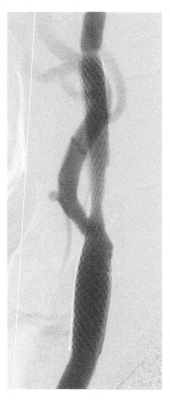

S/p stent.

Answers

1. CAS is indicated for symptomatic >70% stenosis where surgery is challenging because of anatomy, previous insults to the neck, or patient factors.

2. Total occlusions and hanging thrombus are contraindications to CAS. Surgery would allow control of the vessel distally, whereas endovascular approaches risk disrupting intraluminal thrombus. Quality of life is not improved in the setting of cognitive impairment. Benefits may not outweigh risks in patients with short life expectancy, but being an octogenarian is only a relative contraindication.

3. There is currently no randomized controlled trial evidence comparing CAS with and without EPDs. Several EPDs are available and operator experience is important to avoid complications.

4. Ideally, 5 days of pretreatment would be required and dual use of aspirin and clopidogrel is widespread.

5. Atropine may be used for bradycardia. Medications for anaphylaxis should always be at hand. Heparinization is important. Blood pressure monitoring and control is also important.

Pearls

- Carotid endarterectomy (CEA) and CAS have important roles in stroke prevention.
- Evidence is based upon several randomized controlled trials, but there is no consensus. CEA is associated with more MI, severe hematomas and cranial nerve injuries, CAS with more minor strokes.
- CAS may be beneficial in patients with significant operative risk, hostile gross anatomy of the neck (eg, previous surgery or radiotherapy) and is operator dependent. Existing guidelines suggest that case selection should be a multidisciplinary decision, and that operators have appropriate training and perform a high volume of complex endovascular procedures given the significant risk of stroke.

Suggested Reading

Macdonald S. Carotid artery stenting trials: conduct, results, critique, and current recommendations. *Cardiovasc Intervent Radiol.* 2012;35(1):15-29.

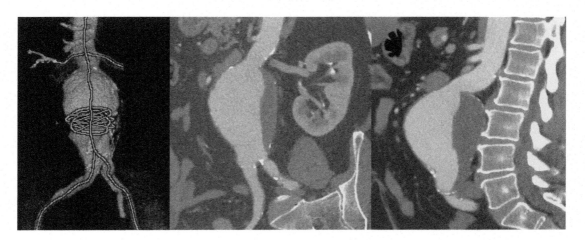

1. Does this aortic aneurysm look suitable for EVAR?

2. Which features at the neck would preclude EVAR?

3. Which features of iliac anatomy preclude EVAR?

4. High-quality computed tomographic (CT) angiography is mandatory for EVAR planning—true or false?

5. Vessel analysis programs can be used instead of manually reading the CT angiogram—true or false?

Case ranking/difficulty:

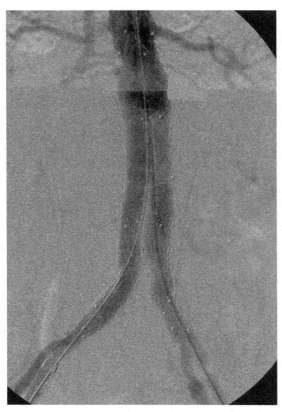

Post-EVAR completion angiogram.

Answers

1. Yes, there are single renal arteries on both sides, with a regular neck, which though angulated anteriorly is suitable for EVAR. There are no critical issues pertaining to the aortic bifurcation or iliac vessels.

2. Short, conical, and angulated necks preclude standard EVAR. Heavy calcification and circumferential thrombus are also hostile neck features.

3. Extreme tortuosity can be overcome by selecting a graft with flexible limbs. Low-profile devices allow placement

of EVAR in a 7 mm external iliac artery, but 5 mm is too small. Internal iliac artery aneurysm can be embolized and stent graft can be extended to "land" in the external iliac artery. Stent graft components can cater for large ectatic common iliac arteries, but an alternative is to sacrifice the internal iliac artery and again, land in the external iliac artery.

4. High-quality CT angiography should be obtained prior to EVAR. Catheter angiography or MR has been used, but CT is accepted practice.

5. Vessel analysis tools can aid EVAR planning, but should not be used as a substitute for closely reviewing the base data of the CT angiogram.

Pearls

- Suitability for endovascular aortic aneurysm repair involves the assessment of multiple factors—both patient factors and aneurysm factors.
- There is a wide range of aortic stent grafts available, each with particular advantages and disadvantages. Familiarity with multiple devices is useful, as there are differing indications and contraindications.
- The neck of the aneurysm must be assessed—its size, length, angulation, and the presence of thrombus and calcification taken into account. Length of the aneurysm and space in the sac and at the bifurcation is important to allow cannulation and 2 limbs. The iliac vessels must also be assessed—for aneurysmal change, caliber and tortuosity.

Suggested Reading

Schanzer A, Greenberg RK, Hevelone N, et al. Predictors of abdominal aortic aneurysm sac enlargement after endovascular repair. *Circulation*. 2011;123(24): 2848-2855.

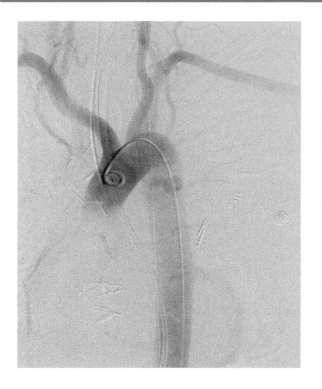

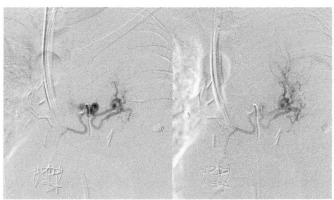

1. What is the definition of massive hemoptysis?

2. What are causes of massive hemoptysis?

3. What is the usual origin of the bronchial arteries?

4. What is the minimum particle size for bronchial artery embolization?

5. What is the role of CT before bronchoscopy or angiography?

Case ranking/difficulty:

Answers

1. Various accepted definitions are in the literature, but urgent interventional management is required where there is a large volume of blood in life-threatening situations.

2. Tuberculosis, cystic fibrosis, and lung cancer are common causes. With an aortobronchial fistula, the source of hemorrhage is aortic, and with a Rasmussen aneurysm, the source of hemorrhage is the pulmonary circulation.

3. Aortic origins are at T5 or T6. Care must be taken to identify radicular or anterior medullary arteries, as there is always a potential risk of spinal cord ischemia as a result of bronchial artery embolization.

4. Access can be challenging and a wide range of diagnostic catheters as well as microcatheters should be available. Particles smaller than 325 μm may pass through any bronchopulmonary anastomoses and into the lung. Recurrent hemorrhage can occur in up to 50% of patients.

5. Computed tomography (CT) can be useful, as angiography to identify and search for all potentially relevant branches can be time consuming.

Pearls

- Massive hemoptysis is a medical emergency. Patients die from asphyxiation or exsanguination. Principles of management are to maintain airway patency and oxygenation, localize the source of bleeding, and control hemorrhage.
- Bronchial artery anatomy is variable, but the arteries originate from the descending thoracic aorta at T5 or T6—with multiple or single trunk origins, and differing numbers of right and left arteries, each of which can be shared with an intercostal artery as an intercostal bronchial trunk.
- Anomalous bronchial arteries can arise from the internal thoracic, subclavian, costocervical, and thyrocervical trunks and even the abdominal aorta.

Suggested Reading

Yoon W, Kim JK, Kim YH, Chung TW, Kang HK. Bronchial and nonbronchial systemic artery embolization for life-threatening hemoptysis: a comprehensive review. *Radiographics.* 2002;22(6):1395-1409.

45-year-old man with clinical deterioration and cholestasis 5 months after liver transplantation

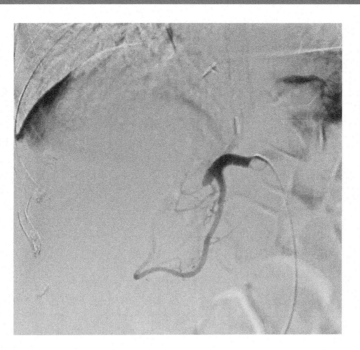

1. What is the diagnosis?

2. What is the most frequent vascular complication after liver transplant?

3. How does this condition present?

4. What are the common causes?

5. What are risk factors for this condition?

Case ranking/difficulty:

Category: Arterial system

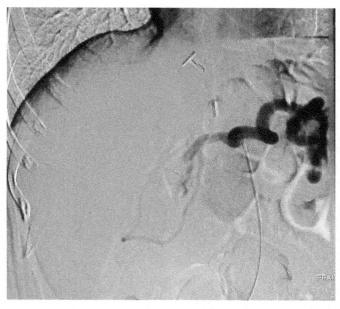

Celiac angiogram shows hepatic artery thrombosis in a liver transplant recipient.

Answers

1. Hepatic artery thrombosis after liver transplant.

2. The most frequent vascular complication after liver transplant is hepatic artery thrombosis, which occurs in 3% to 5% of cases, and more frequently in children.

3. Patients often show signs of fulminant liver failure, biliary leak, or sepsis.

4. The common causes are operative errors, progressive hepatic artery stenosis, rejection, and arterial kinking.

5. Donor age more than 60 years, extended cold ischemia time, lack of ABO compatibility, cigarette smoking, hypercoagulability, preservation damage to the endothelium, and a donor positive for CMV in a recipient who is CMV-negative are risk factors.

Pearls

- In the classic orthotopic liver transplant procedure, the hepatic arterial anastomosis is formed between the donor celiac axis or common hepatic artery and the recipient common hepatic artery. Knowledge of the anatomy of the surgical anastomosis (eg, end to end) is important prior to angiography.
- Because the biliary tree is exclusively supplied by the hepatic artery, bile duct ischemia occurs frequently without treatment, resulting in strictures, bilomas, or mucosal sloughing (ischemic cholangiopathy).
- Endovascular thrombolysis, angioplasty, and stent placement may allow graft salvage, and they require immediate revascularization to avoid the need for retransplantation.

Suggested Reading

Silva MA, Jambulingam PS, Gunson BK, et al. Hepatic artery thrombosis following orthotopic liver transplantation: a 10-year experience from a single centre in the United Kingdom. *Liver Transpl.* 2006;12:146-151.

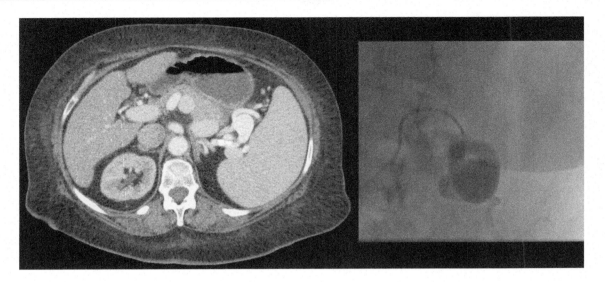

1. Elective repair is indicated at what size?

2. What is the mortality of (a) elective surgical repair (b) ruptured splenic artery aneurysm?

3. What endovascular agents or devices can be used?

4. What complications can result from endovascular treatment?

5. What other treatment should be considered if a large volume of the spleen infarcts?

Category: Arterial system

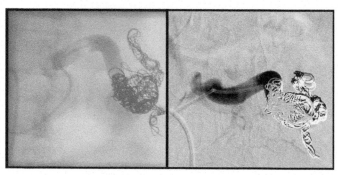

Postembolization fluoroscopic image and angiogram.

Answers

1. Elective repair can be considered when the aneurysm is larger than 2 cm. The average size of a ruptured splenic artery aneurysm is 3 cm.

2. Elective repair mortality is reported at 5%, and that of ruptured splenic artery aneurysm repair at 10% to 25%.

3. Coils can be used to close the front and back door, as can AVPs. Stent graft placement across the aneurysm can be performed, but may be precluded by tortuous anatomy. Liquid agents such as ethylene-vinyl alcohol (Onyx) can also be used, particularly when aneurysms are wide-necked or patency of the parent vessel is required.

4. Rupture can occur during the procedure. Splenic infarction or abscess formation can occur.

5. Vaccination against the meningococcus, pneumococcus, and haemophilus influenza is given.

Pearls

- Splenic artery aneurysms are the most common site of visceral aneurysms, accounting for 60% of them.
- The mean diameter of ruptured aneurysms is over 3 cm.
- General principles of aneurysm treatment apply—the aneurysm must be excluded from the circulation, and so "front-door" and "back-door" techniques are used to occlude the inflow and outflow vessels, or alternatively the aneurysm can be filled with other embolic agents such as Onyx.
- Stent grafts can be placed across the aneurysm. The MARS ("multilayer aneurysm repair system") may also be useful—stents are placed across the aneurysm, which modulates flow and encourages thrombosis within the aneurysm sac.

Suggested Reading

Belli AM, Markose G, Morgan R. The role of interventional radiology in the management of abdominal visceral artery aneurysms. *Cardiovasc Intervent Radiol.* 2012;35(2): 234-243.

84-year-old man patient with hepatocellular carcinoma (HCC) presenting for transarterial chemoembolization (TACE)

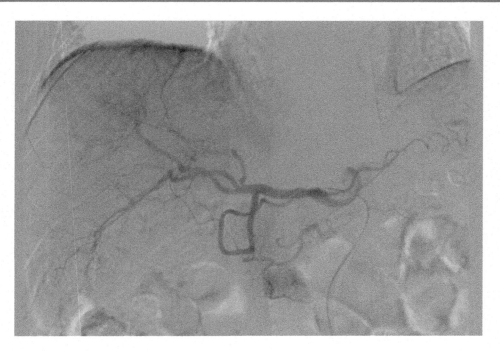

1. Review the angiogram and identify 3 relevant points.

2. What agents make up the embolization mixture in TACE?

3. What are absolute contraindications to TACE?

4. What are the quoted 1-, 2-, and 3-year survival rates post TACE for HCC?

5. What is the incidence of infective complications after TACE?

Case ranking/difficulty: **Category:** Arterial system

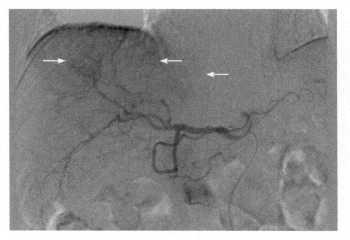

Angiogram with catheter in common hepatic artery.

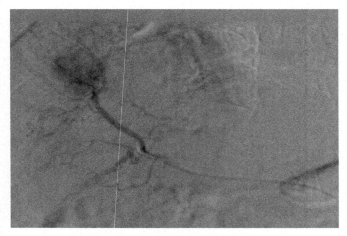

Selective angiogram in right hepatic branch.

Answers

1. 1. Hypervascular lesion in the right lobe.
   2. Nonvisualization of the left hepatic branches due to a replaced left hepatic artery off the left gastric.
   3. Although masked, lipiodol staining can be seen indicative of a previous treatment. All of these features are important, as the previous lesion may need treatment if it were to be fed from the left hepatic branches, which would require selective catheterization of the left gastric artery also.

2. Doxorubicin, cisplatin, and mitomycin C can be used as intraarterial chemotherapeutic agents. Lipiodol and particles are commonly added. Sorafenib is an oral chemotherapeutic, also effective in treating HCC.

3. If there are curative options such as ablation, surgery, or transplantation, TACE is not usually required. TACE can downstage tumors to turn a patient into a candidate for one of the above. Severe liver disease, as indicated by a high bilirubin, is also a contraindication because of the risk of treatment-induced liver failure. Portal vein thrombosis and AV shunting within the tumor are only relative contraindications, as are general poor health (as indicated by poor oncology performance scores). Each management decision should be made on a patient-by-patient basis by a multidisciplinary team.

4. One randomized study demonstrated 1-, 2-, and 3-year survival rates at 57%, 31%, and 26%, respectively.

5. Postembolization is common and generally self-limiting. Liver abscess formation is seen in up to 2% of patients.

Pearls

- Hepatocellular carcinoma can be treated with transplantation, resection, ablation (eg, radiofrequency ablation, ethanol), chemotherapy (eg, sorafenib, a tyrosine kinase inhibitor), and embolizations that include TACE, Y90, and bland embolization.
- The Milan criteria are used to stage HCC. Patients are transplant candidates if they have 1 lesion <5 cm, 3 lesions <3 cm, no vascular invasion, and no distant metastases.

Suggested Reading

Lencioni R. Loco-regional treatment of hepatocellular carcinoma. *Hepatology*. 2010;52(2):762-773.

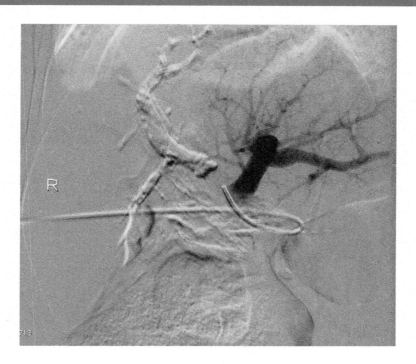

1. What are the indications for portal vein embolization?

2. What are the contraindications of portal vein embolization?

3. Which liver segments are supplied by the right portal vein branch?

4. What are the potential complications of portal vein embolization?

5. How can portal vein embolization be performed if the conventional transhepatic technique is impossible?

Case ranking/difficulty:

Category: Venous system

Answers

1. It can be performed prior to hepatic resection for any lesion when future liver remnant is expected to be less than 25%-40%.

2. Contraindications are related to the transhepatic access and the ability to access the portal vein. It can be performed after decompression of the biliary tree.

3. Right portal vein branch supplies segments 5 to 8. Left portal vein branch supplies segments 2 to 4. Multiple small branches for the caudate lobe come from the right and left portal veins.

4. Pneumothorax, subcapsular hematoma, arterial pseudoaneurysm after inadvertent arterial puncture, and portal vein thrombosis may occur.

5. A transjugular approach has been successfully used when performing the conventional transhepatic technique was impossible. Similarly, transjugular biliary accesses have been obtained where transhepatic puncture was not possible and yet a percutaneous biliary access was needed (a "TIBS").

Pearls

- Portal vein embolization is a safe and effective method that can induce hepatic hypertrophy prior to planned resection.
- It is frequently performed prior to hemihepatectomy for colorectal liver metastases.

Suggested Reading

Denys A, Prior J, Bize P, et al. Portal vein embolization: what do we know? *Cardiovasc Intervent Radiol.* 2012;35(5):999-1008.

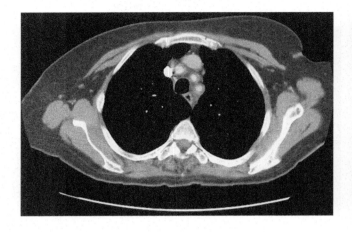 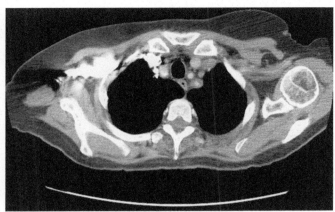

1. What do the images show?

2. What is the differential diagnosis?

3. What biopsy might be helpful?

4. True or false—given the cold arm and axillary lesion, urgent angioplasty should be performed.

5. Coronary arteries are also particularly at risk here—true or false?

Case ranking/difficulty:

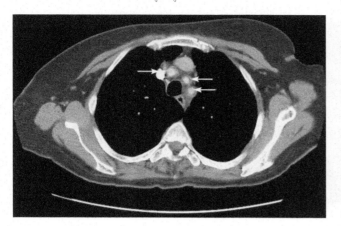

Mural thickening is seen in the origins of the great vessels.

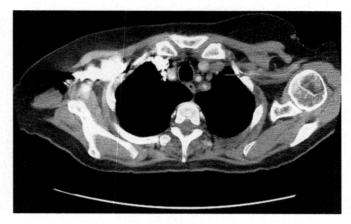

Further thickening is seen in the left axillary artery.

Answers

1. There is vessel wall thickening, which affects the arch, great vessels, and axillary arteries.

2. Differential of large vessel vasculitis includes giant cell arteritis (GCA) and Takayasu arteritis (TA).

3. A temporal artery biopsy may be helpful.

4. False. These conditions may be steroid responsive.

5. False. Kawasaki disease is associated with coronary artery lesions. TA is infrequently associated with coronary lesions.

Pearls

- Large-vessel vasculitis is due to GCA or TA.
- GCA is characterized by granulomatous infiltrates in large and medium-sized arterial walls. It commonly presents with headache, affects women older than 50, and inflammatory markers such as ESR are significantly raised at 40 to 140 mm/hr. Vessel wall thickening of more than 1.5 mm is typical in GCA. T2-weighted MR demonstrates high signal in the aortic wall as a result of edema and positron emission tomographic scan also shows increased ^{18}F-fluorodeoxyglucose (^{18}F-FDG) uptake in inflammatory segments. Diagnosis can be established with temporal artery biopsy. GCA does not involve the common carotid artery, affecting mainly medium-sized branches such as the subclavian and axillary arteries.

- TA is a granulomatous arteritis that affects the arch and great vessels. Coronary and pulmonary arteries can also be affected. Skip lesions are characteristic. Tapering of extracranial aortic branches such as subclavian and axillary arteries is seen. This condition usually affects those younger than 50 years old and is the only vasculitis that causes stenosis or occlusion of the aorta itself. There is a strong female and Oriental predominance. TA can involve the left subclavian artery (<50%), common carotid artery (20%), pulmonary arteries (>50%), as well as the renal, superior mesenteric (SMA), and celiac arteries. It infrequently involves the axillary, brachial, and coronaries. ESR is mildly raised at over 20 mm/hr.

Suggested Reading

Spira D, Kötter I, Ernemann U, et al. Imaging of primary and secondary inflammatory diseases involving large and medium-sized vessels and their potential mimics: a multitechnique approach. *AJR Am J Roentgenol.* 2010;194(3):848-856.

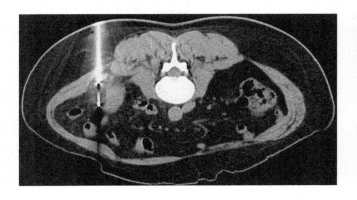 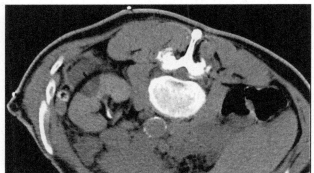

1. Is cryoablation indicated in younger patient with a large central tumor?

2. What are contraindications to cryoablation?

3. What are technical considerations in a cryoablation circuit?

4. What are relative advantages and disadvantages of partial nephrectomy, radiofrequency ablation, and cryoablation as treatments for renal tumors?

5. What are potential complications?

Answers

1. Larger central lesions are more challenging, and partial nephrectomy may still be the gold standard, particularly in younger patients.

2. Large tumors may have a higher risk of local recurrence and hemorrhage. Long-term data on recurrence are awaited and so younger patients may be more suitable for laparoscopic partial nephrectomy.

3. Cell death occurs at −20°C and the probe can reach a temperature as low as −190°C. Probes can be cooled by argon gas. Two freeze-thaw cycles improve outcomes and the ice ball should extend 5 mm beyond the lesion.

4. Partial nephrectomy may be more expensive but long-term data are clear. RFA and cryoablation can be performed without general anesthesia. RFA may be more painful than cryoablation. There is a higher risk of hemorrhage with cryoablation than RFA.

5. Complications can occur from needle placement and from collateral damage from the ice ball or ablation zone. Tumor seeding in the tract is extremely rare.

Pearls

- Case selection, planning, intraprocedural imaging guidance, and monitoring as well as surveillance for disease progression are important components of an ablation service.
- Cryoablation and radiofrequency ablation are both options for renal lesions with different advantages and disadvantages. Complications of cryoablation include probe site pain, hemorrhage, incomplete ablation, and tumor recurrence.

Suggested Reading

Allen BC, Remer EM. Percutaneous cryoablation of renal tumors: patient selection, technique, and postprocedural imaging. *Radiographics*. 2011;30(4):887-900.

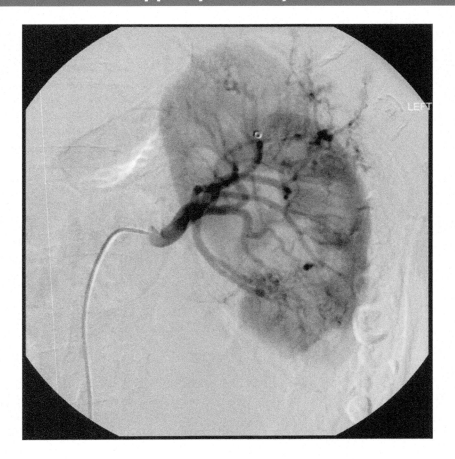

1. What is the diagnosis?

2. What is the preferred embolic strategy?

3. What are potential complications?

4. At what size should treatment be considered?

5. What is the significance of this lesion in pregnancy?

Case ranking/difficulty:

Category: Arterial system

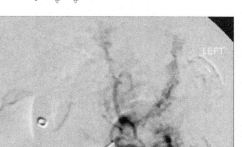

Superselective left renal angiogram.

Answers

1. The angiogram demonstrates multiple areas of abnormality with long tortuous vessels extending outside the nephrogram, and appearances are diagnostic of angiomyolipoma.

2. The use of polyvinyl alcohol particles (PVA) alone has been reported to be associated with a higher risk of post-procedure hemorrhage, and so PVA and coils are a recommended strategy.

3. Postembolization syndrome occurs frequently, and abscess formation, pleural effusion, and post embolization hemorrhage are also reported.

4. Most centers would treat any AML once it was 4 cm in size.

5. The influence of pregnancy on AML is not fully known, but there is a suggestion that rapid growth can occur, largely based on case reports of very large AMLs undergoing hemorrhage. Close ultrasonographic surveillance is generally recommended.

Pearls

- Angiographic signs of abnormal vasculature include long, dilated tortuous vessels that are clearly different from the normal renal vasculature, extending outside the nephrogram.
- The "light bulb" sign has been described, where the light bulb is a region with no vessels representing acute hematoma and may help to localize the abnormal vessel.

Suggested Reading

Lenton J, Kessel D, Watkinson AF. Embolization of renal angiomyolipoma: immediate complications and long-term outcomes. *Clin Radiol*. 2008;63(8):864-870.

78-year-old man presents for evaluation for endovascular aneurysm repair (EVAR)

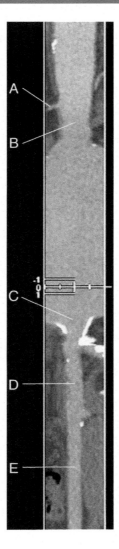

1. What is A? Why is this important?

2. What is B? What features would you consider?

3. What is C? What features would you analyze?

4. What is D? Is the length of D important?

5. What is E? What anatomic considerations are important here?

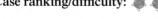

Case ranking/difficulty:

Answers

1. A could represent either renal artery, but typically this would be the lowest renal artery. This landmark is important, as it is used to judge where the neck starts, and also is the landmark used to measure device length against.

2. Structure B is the infrarenal aorta and represents the neck of the aneurysm. Neck length and diameter, and the presence and degree of tortuosity, calcification, and mural thrombus are important.

3. Normally around 20 mm of space at the bifurcation is needed to allow both limbs to sit unconstrained, but this differs according to different devices. Similarly, more than 10 mm is needed for uni-iliac devices.

4. D represents the common iliac artery, and the length is important, as there must be sufficient length of landing zone, which, again, is device dependent.

5. E is the external iliac artery. Note that the origin of the internal can also be appreciated. The internal iliac artery origin is important, as the aim is to preserve these arteries. The external iliac artery must be of sufficient caliber to allow insertion of the device.

Pearls

- Software and reconstructions can aid visualization and the decision-making process, and a centerline analysis is presented in this case.
- The aneurysm must be seen as a 3D structure, and judgment must be exercised even when doing something as simple as measuring the size—which ought to be perpendicular to its long axis, and therefore not necessarily a transverse measurement.
- Postprocessing techniques are invaluable.

Suggested Reading

Schanzer A, Greenberg RK, Hevelone N, et al. Predictors of abdominal aortic aneurysm sac enlargement after endovascular repair. *Circulation.* 2011;123(24): 2848-2855.

73-year-old with a type 2 endoleak after inferior mesenteric artery (IMA) embolization

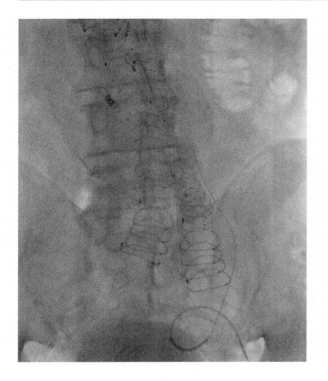 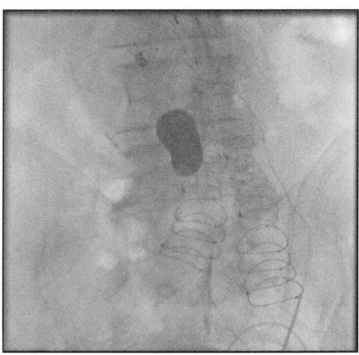

1. Where is the tip of the catheter?

2. What embolization agent was used?

3. Where is this agent most commonly used?

4. What is the rate of type 2 endoleak after endovascular aneurysm repair (EVAR)?

5. List some possible management options.

Case ranking/difficulty:

Category: Arterial system

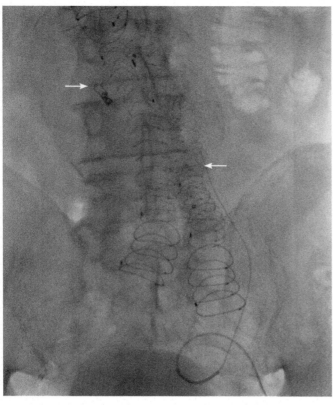

Pretreatment.

3. Brain arteriovenous malformations.

4. An endoleak rate of up to 22% has been reported.

5. Surveillance, transcatheter embolization of the IMA, lumbar or deep circumflex iliacs, and percutaneous translumbar embolization are the reported treatment strategies.

Pearls

• Endoleaks occur in up to 20% of EVAR. Conservative management with surveillance of sac size is required. If the sac is enlarging, treatment options include embolization of the feeding arteries (commonly the IMA and lumbars) or direct percutaneous sac puncture.

Suggested Reading

Nevala T, Biancari F, Manninen H, et al. Type II endoleak after endovascular repair of abdominal aortic aneurysm: effectiveness of embolization. *Cardiovasc Intervent Radiol.* 2010;33(2):278-284.

Answers

1. The tip of the catheter is in the aneurysm sac.

2. Onyx. Onyx is a liquid embolization system and is composed of ethylene vinyl alcohol (EVOH) copolymer, which is dissolved in dimethyl sulfoxide (DMSO), and suspended micronized tantalum powder, which provides contrast allowing visualization under fluoroscopy. It is available in different viscosities, for example, Onyx 18 and Onyx 34.

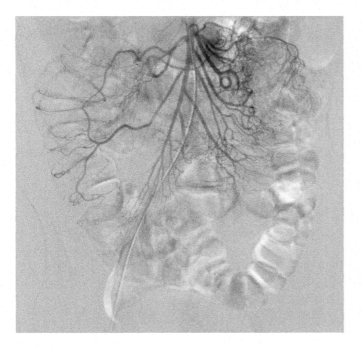
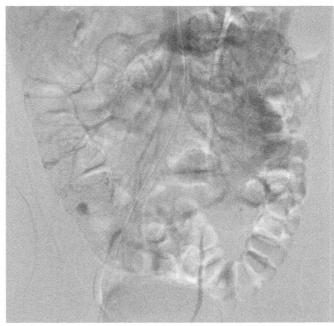

1. Review the early- and late-phase images—
   where is the abnormality?

2. What vessel is the culprit?

3. Where would you embolize from?

4. What would you do if there was spasm in the
   ileocolic artery, which stopped you selecting
   the bleeding vessel?

5. How can you make sure you do not miss a
   bleeding point?

Case ranking/difficulty:

Category: Arterial system

Answers

1. Bleeding point is seen in the cecum.

2. A branch of the right colic artery.

3. This should occur distal to the marginal artery, from the bleeding vasa recta.

4. Administer glyceral trinitrate (GTN). The branch could potentially be approached from another colic branch via the marginal artery—in this case the right colic artery, for example.

5. Images should be closely reviewed both with and without digital subtraction. Images should be taken with breath-holding. Antiperistaltic agents such as buscopan or glucagon should be used. Multiple projections and magnified views may be required. Contrast medium should be sufficiently dense and injected at appropriate rates. Imaging should continue through the portal venous phase.

Pearls

- Arterial embolization for gastrointestinal hemorrhage is a commonly requested procedure.
- Preprocedure imaging and endoscopy can help to narrow down the arterial territory. Computed tomographic angiography can identify the bleeding point and exclude other causes of bleeding, which may require surgery, such as a tumor.
- Good angiographic technique and use of microcatheters are important to identify, and then treat the source of hemorrhage.

Suggested Reading

Walker TG. Acute gastrointestinal hemorrhage. *Tech Vasc Interv Radiol.* 2009;12(2):80-91.

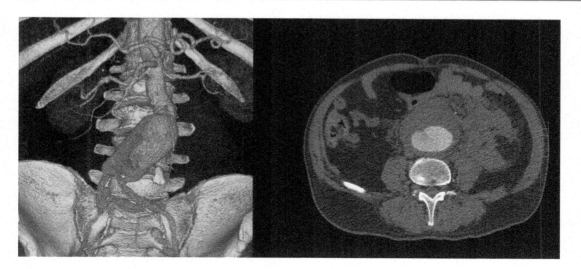

1. What percentage of those with ruptured abdominal aortic aneurysms (AAAs) die in the community?

2. What is the 30-day mortality of open repair of a ruptured AAA?

3. What is the reported 30-day mortality of ruptured AAAs treated with endovascular aneurysm repair (EVAR)?

4. What factors influence the outcome for ruptured EVARs?

5. What complication is not associated with open surgery but is specific to EVAR in this setting?

Case ranking/difficulty: 　　　　　　　　　　Category: Arterial system

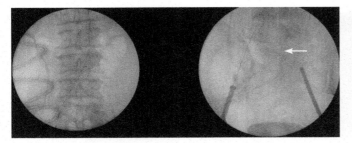

AUI and left-sided iliac occluder (annotated).

Answers

1. Fifty percent die in the community.

2. The 30-day mortality for open repair of a ruptured abdominal aortic aneurysm is 50%.

3. The 30-day mortality for ruptured aneurysms treated with EVAR is 25%.

4. Timing of heparin and use of occlusion balloons is not yet standardized. Supraceliac occlusion balloon can cause renal and splanchnic ischemia and distal embolization. Prompt endograft deployment may be favorable.

5. Abdominal compartment syndrome can occur where there is massive retroperitoneal hemorrhage and hematoma formation in a closed abdomen.

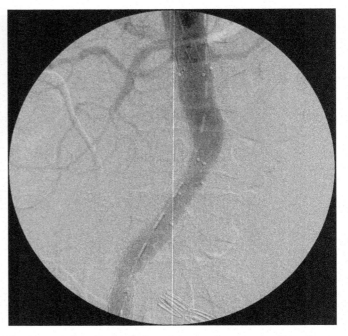

Angiogram showing exclusion of the aortic aneurysm. Vascular surgeons then proceeded to perform a femoral–femoral cross-over graft.

Suggested Reading

Alsac JM, Kobeiter H, Becquemin JP, Desgranges P. Endovascular repair for ruptured AAA: a literature review. *Acta Chir Belg*. 2005;105(2):134-139.

Pearls

- Open repair has a 30-day mortality in the order of 50%. Some selected series have shown a 30-day mortality of 25%.
- Bifurcated EVAR or AUI are options for REVAR. Timing and use of heparin and occlusion balloons must be considered. Teamwork between anesthetists, ED, vascular surgeons, and interventional radiology is key to providing a streamlined emergency EVAR service.

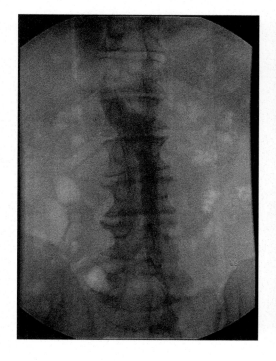
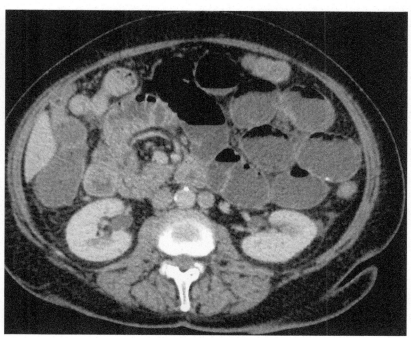

1. What do you notice?

2. How would you ensure the patient is protected from pulmonary embolism (PE)?

3. What percentage of patients have caval anomalies?

4. Name 4 other caval abnormalities.

5. What is the definition of a megacava?

Case ranking/difficulty:

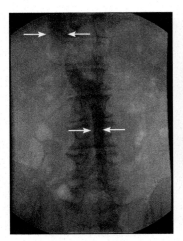

Left transfemoral cavagram.

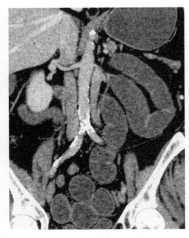

Coronal computed tomography (CT)—showing double IVCs.

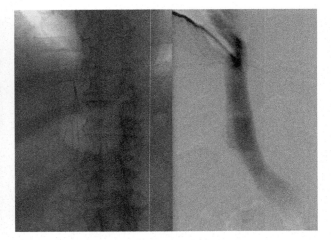

Suprarenal filter placement.

Answers

1. Note the vertical left-sided IVC and also the caliber change, which is suggestive of dual IVC. CT shows bilateral cavas either side of the aorta.

2. Options include placing 1 suprarenal filter, or studying both limbs and placing 2 IVC filters. The decision is based on the balance of risks—there would be low risk of renal vein thrombosis due to a suprarenal filter, and placing 2 filters in relatively small cava of 1 to 1.5 cm would not be without risk—a second access, potential problems with retrieval and a constrained filter in a small vessel may increase the risk of caval thrombosis.

3. Caval abnormalities occur in around 3% of cases.

4. Megacava, left-sided IVC, azygous continuation of the IVC, absent IVC.

5. Megacava is >28 mm.

Pearls

- In double IVC, IVC filters have been placed in both cavas, but a suprarenal filter also suffices.
- The risks of either need to be balanced—there is a low risk of renal vein thrombosis and suprarenal filters are not associated with added risk of complications. Placing and retrieving, or leaving 2 filters in small undersized vessels, could be problematic.

Suggested Readings

Hashmi ZA, Smaroff GG. Dual inferior vena cava: two inferior vena cava filters. *Ann Thorac Surg.* 2007;84(2):661-663.

Kalva SP, Chlapoutaki C, Wicky S, Greenfield AJ, Waltman AC, Athanasoulis CA. Suprarenal inferior vena cava filters: a 20-year single-center experience. *J Vasc Interv Radiol.* 2008;19(7):1041-1047.

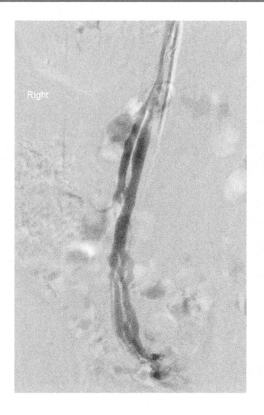 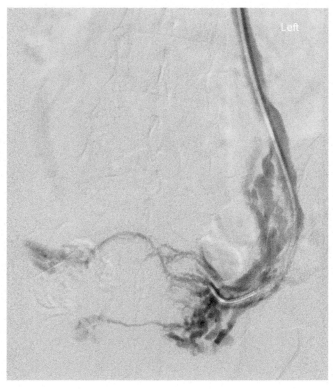

1. What is the incidence of pelvic varicosities?

2. List some risk factors.

3. Where is the origin of the right ovarian vein?

4. Where is the origin of the left ovarian vein?

5. What other vessels may supply pelvic varicosities?

Case ranking/difficulty: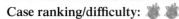

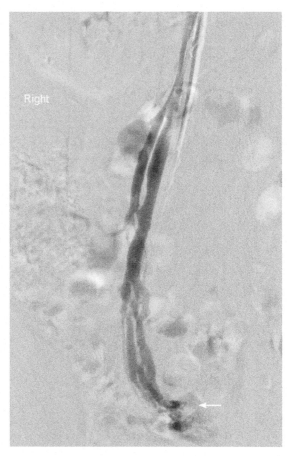

Right ovarian venogram.

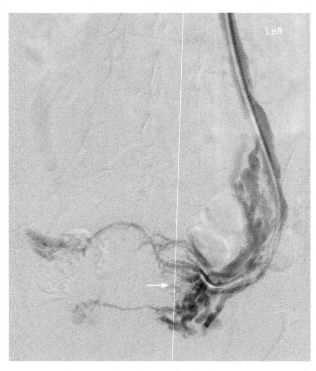

Left ovarian venogram.

Answers

1. Up to 15% of females may have pelvic varicosities, and about 50% of these may be symptomatic. However, there is a broad differential diagnosis for chronic pelvic pain.

2. Age between 20 and 50, previous pregnancy, polycystic kidneys, and hormonal dysfunction.

3. The right ovarian vein originates from the anterolateral aspect of the cava, below the right renal vein.

4. The left ovarian vein originates from the left renal vein.

5. Internal iliac veins can contribute to pelvic varicosities. These varicosities can also be in continuity with superficial vein, particularly in the case of vulval varices.

Pearls

- Pelvic congestion syndrome is caused by retrograde flow through incompetent ovarian veins.
- Ovarian varices are present in 10% of the population, and 50% of patients may be symptomatic.
- Bilateral selective ovarian vein and internal iliac vein embolization is effective in reducing symptoms in this condition resulting from ovarian and pelvic varices.

Suggested Readings

Ganeshan A, Upponi S, Hon L-Q, Uthappa MC, Warakaulle DR, Uberoi R. Chronic pelvic pain due to pelvic congestion syndrome: the role of diagnostic and interventional radiology. *Cardiovasc Intervent Radiol.* 2007;30(6):1105-1111.

Kim HS, Malhotra AD, Rowe PC, Lee JM, Venbrux AC. Embolotherapy for pelvic congestion syndrome: long-term results. *J Vasc Interv Radiol.* 2006;17(2 Pt 1): 289-297.

44-year-old woman who has a right thigh loop arteriovenous (AV) graft for dialysis. Ultrasonography detects stenosis

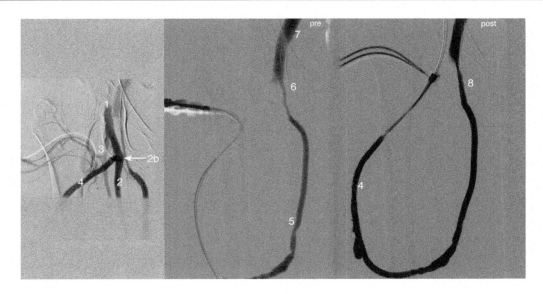

1. Review the images and name the structures 1 through 7.

2. The patient chose this dialysis access, as she did not want to have an arm fistula for cosmesis issues. True or false?

3. What are the 1- and 2-year patency rates?

4. What is the main reason for graft failure at this site?

5. Name some other fistula accesses in the lower limb.

Case ranking/difficulty:

Answers

1. 1. Common femoral artery. 2. Superficial femoral artery. 2b. Arterial anastomosis. 3. Profunda femoris artery. 4. Arterial limb. 5. Venous limb. 6. Great saphenous vein. 7. Common femoral vein.

2. The thigh loop graft is generally reserved for when all upper limb accesses have been exhausted.

3. Based on a series of 46 mid-thigh loop AV grafts, 1- and 2-year primary patency rates were found to be 68% and 43%, respectively.

4. Infection is a common reason for graft failure at this site.

5. The thigh loop AV graft, the mid-thigh loop AV graft, and femoral vein transposition AV fistula can be made. The loop AV grafts do have a high risk of infection, but the femoral vein transpositions have been reported to be associated with ischemic lower limb complications due to steal.

Pearls

- Thigh loop AV grafts are yet another access point for fistula formation, commonly created after failures of the bilateral arm venous accesses.
- Radiocephalic, brachiocephalic, brachiobasilic, brachioaxillary graft, and forearm loop grafts can be fashioned in the upper limb.
- Other dialysis routes include axillary–axillary necklace grafts. Even more desperate dialysis access routes include translumbar and transhepatic dialysis lines after the major upper body and lower body venous accesses have become exhausted.

Suggested Reading

Scott JD, Cull DL, Kalbaugh CA, et al. The mid-thigh loop arteriovenous graft: patient selection, technique, and results. *Am Surg.* 2006;72(9):825-828.

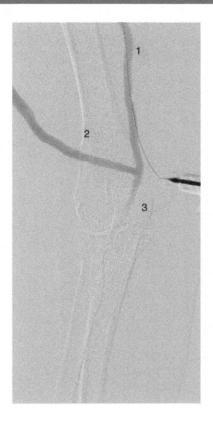

1. How was this image obtained? Name the structures.

2. How does steal present?

3. How common is steal?

4. Retrograde flow in the artery distal to the anastomosis is indicative of steal—true or false?

5. The diagnosis is clinical—true or false?

Case ranking/difficulty: 🐾 🐾

Category: Arterial system

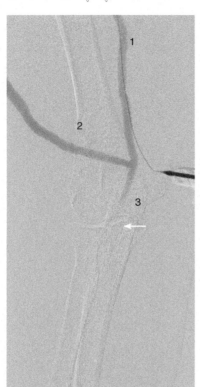

Brachial arteriogram.

Answers

1. This is a brachial angiogram, performed using a micropuncture access needle that is then exchanged over the wire for the inner 3-Fr component of the micropuncture set. (1) Brachial artery. (2) Outflow brachioaxillary graft. (3). Distal brachial artery with preferential flow into the arteriovenous (AV) graft indicating steal.

2. Steal can present with ischemic pain during dialysis, ischemic and neurologic symptoms in the distal limb (this can affect both hand, forearm, and leg depending on the fistula site), and tissue loss.

3. Steal is rare, but some fistulas may be at higher risk of steal, such as the transposed femoral AV fistula. Other risk factors include diabetes and atherosclerosis.

4. False: Retrograde flow in the artery distal to anastomosis can be a normal finding. For example, up to 20% of the inflow to a radiocephalic fistula can be from retrograde flow (ulna inflow, via palmar arch to the distal radial artery back into the fistula).

5. The diagnosis of steal syndrome is clinical, though noninvasive measurements of pulse volume recordings can be useful. Ultrasonography, vascular imaging, and invasive fistulograms can be important to aid the planning of any surgical treatment.

Pearls

- Steal can occur with any fistula. It can range in severity, some patients may get problematic symptoms during dialysis only. Others can have tissue loss.
- DRIL is a procedure that can salvage the fistula and maintain distal arterial flow. This is the "distal revascularization-interval ligation" procedure. It involves the creation of a short surgical bypass, connected above and below the arterial anastomosis of the fistula. The inflow then bypasses the fistula's inflow, and distal blood flow is maintained.
- Alternatives include refashioning of the anastomosis, or ligation and placement of a new fistula.

Suggested Reading

Knox RC, Berman SS, Hughes JD, Gentile AT, Mills JL. Distal revascularization-interval ligation: a durable and effective treatment for ischemic steal syndrome after hemodialysis access. *J Vasc Surg.* 2002;36(2):250-255; discussion 256.

56-year-old man who is 7 days status post orthotopic liver transplant has elevated liver function tests and increased resistive index on hepatic arterial Duplex examination

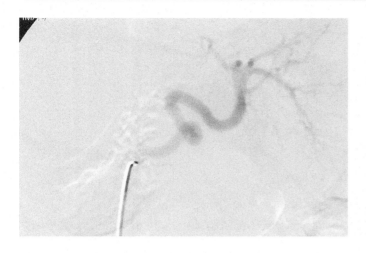 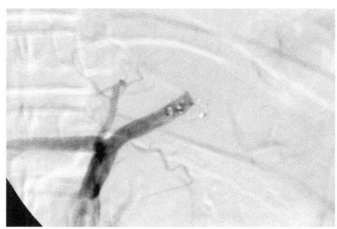

1. What is your diagnosis based on the clinical information and angiogram?

2. What are indications for splenic artery embolization?

3. What is the best technique for treating this condition?

4. How many named branches does the splenic artery have?

5. What are arterial complications after liver transplant?

Case ranking/difficulty:

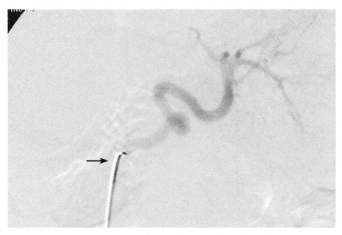

Celiac arteriography shows minimal flow to the common hepatic artery. Majority of the flow goes to the splenic artery.

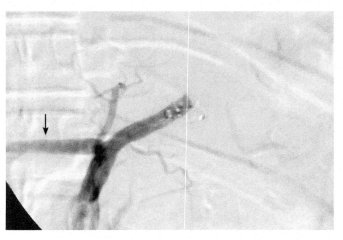

After deploying 2 Amplatzer vascular plugs (AVPs) at the proximal trunk of the splenic artery, the splenic arterial flow was stopped, and the common hepatic artery is well visualized (*arrow*) along with the left gastric artery.

Answers

1. The diagnosis is splenic artery steal syndrome.

2. Trauma, aneurysms, hypersplenism, and portal hypertension are other indications for splenic artery embolization.

3. Studies have shown that although proximal embolization with AVP or coils or both is a good technique, Gelfoam-assisted AVP embolization is best in the setting of splenic arery steal syndrome (SASS) where this is a hyperdynamic circulation.

4. The dorsal pancreatic, pancreatic magna, left gastroepiploic artery, and short gastric arteries arise from the splenic artery.

5. Thrombosis, stenosis, fistula, and pseudo- or true aneurysm formation can occur.

Pearls

- Early transplant rejection can be caused by hepatic artery complications, which include hepatic artery thrombosis and splenic artery steal syndrome. SASS may affect up to 7% of OLT recipients.
- Diagnostic angiography can demonstrate shift in blood flow into the splenic or gastroduodenal arteries. Hepatic arterial flow improves after embolization of the proximal splenic artery.

Suggested Reading

Zhu X, Tam MD, Pierce G, et al. Utility of the Amplatzer vascular plug in splenic artery embolization: a comparison study with conventional coil technique. *Cardiovasc Intervent Radiol*. 2011;34(3):522-531.

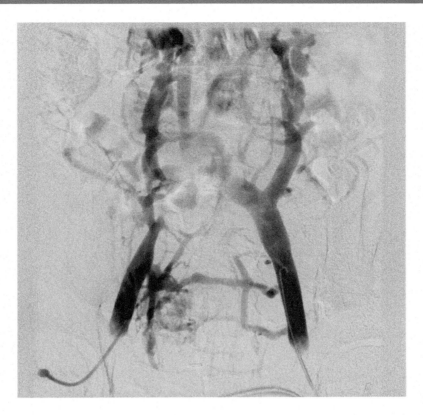

1. List 5 causes of iliac vein obstruction.

2. If you could not pass the occlusion from the femoral access, what would you do?

3. If you could cross the lesion with a wire, but the stent does not track, what would you do?

4. Should this patient be anticoagulated?

5. What are the main collateral pathways for venous drainage if the cava is occluded?

Case ranking/difficulty:

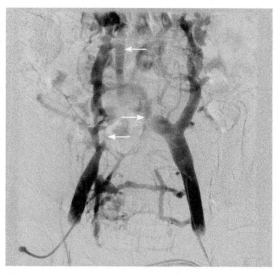

Bilateral iliac venogram. Note the massive paralumbar collateral veins. (Arrows indicate the sites of obstruction and filling of a diminutive cava.)

Answers

1. Venous thrombosis, postthrombotic, malignancy, retroperitoneal fibrosis, May-Thurner syndrome.

2. If an occlusion cannot be crossed from one direction, there is often another access route—with venous obstruction, this may be the popliteal, brachial, jugular, or subclavian route, for example.

3. In this case, predilatation of the right-sided tract was required to facilitate passage of the stent device. Through-and-through access can be obtained by creating a jugular access and snaring the transfemoral wire—having control of both ends of the guidewire facilitates passage of a device—which can be both pushed and pulled using the through-and-through ("flossing") wire.

4. The venous obstruction has occurred often in the setting of thrombosis, but also with fibrotic lumen and slow-flow states, all of which predispose to venous thrombosis, and so anticoagulation or antiplatelet therapy after venous stenting is generally recommended.

5. The paralumbar venous plexuses ascend in the posterior abdominal wall and drain into the cava or continue cephalad and drain into the azygous and hemiazygous systems. Drainage can collateralize through the pelvis into gonadal veins and back into the upper cava/renal veins. Anterior abdominal pathways also exist.

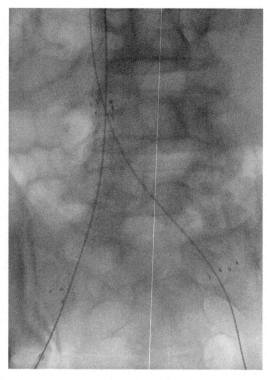

Spot fluoroscopic image after stent placement. Post stent venograms demonstrated improved flow through the iliac veins and cava, and reduction of filling of the collaterals.

Pearls

- Iliocaval occlusion can occur due to extensive venous thrombosis, as a postthrombotic complication, be caused by malignancy, or happen in compression syndromes such as May-Thurner syndrome. Retroperitoneal fibrosis is another cause.

Suggested Readings

Nazarian GK, Bjarnason H, Dietz CA, Bernadas CA, Hunter DW. Iliofemoral venous stenoses: effectiveness of treatment with metallic endovascular stents. *Radiology*. 1996;200(1):193-199.

Razavi MK, Hansch EC, Kee ST, Sze DY, Semba CP, Dake MD. Chronically occluded inferior venae cavae: endovascular treatment. *Radiology*. 2000;214(1):133-138.

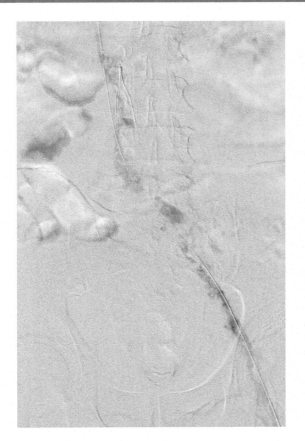 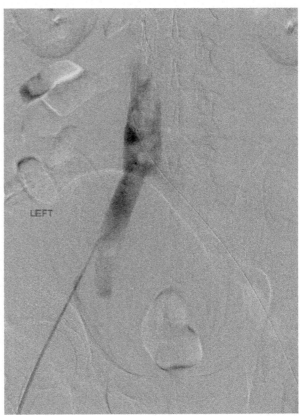

1. How might patients with caval thrombosis present?

2. What is phlegmasia cerulea dolens?

3. What is the role of venous thrombolysis for acute deep vein thrombosis (DVT)?

4. List 5 risk factors for caval thrombosis.

5. List 4 congenital anomalies of the inferior vena cava (IVC).

Case ranking/difficulty:

Category: Venous system

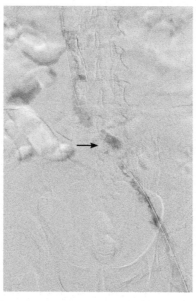

Left popliteal venogram. Arrow indicates filling defect in the common iliac vein.

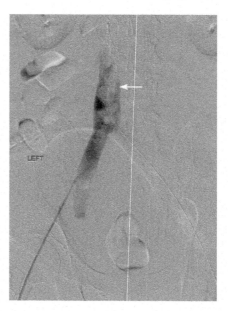

Right femoral venogram. Arrow demonstrates caval thrombosis.

Answers

1. Patients present with lower body edema, and often with visible dilated abdominal wall veins. Pain is common.

2. Phlegmasia cerulea dolens means "painful blue edema" and occurs with extensive DVT, which extends into collateral veins, which leads to massive edema. Further extension of thrombosis into the capillary bed leads to irreversible venous ischemia and gangrene. This is associated with a pulmonary embolism (PE) rate of 30%, mortality rate up to 40%, and amputation rate up to 50%. Phlegmasia alba dolens describes massive fulminant venous thrombosis without ischemia.

3. The vast majority of patients with acute DVT are anticoagulated—this stops clot propagation and embolization, but it does not remove the clot burden. Many patients have postphlebitic symptoms, so the role for lysis of acute DVT may lead to better long-term outcomes as the treatment aims to remove all clot in the acute phase.

4. Renal cell carcinoma is associated with tumor and bland thrombosis of the IVC. Extrinsic compression from any retroperitoneal disease, underlying malignancy, and inherited thrombophilias are risk factors. Extensive iliofemoral DVT can progress, and femoral catheters and IVC filters are other risk factors.

5. Absent IVC, dual IVC, left-sided IVC, and azygous continuation of the IVC are anomalies.

Pearls

- Caval thrombosis and extensive iliofemoral thrombosis can cause significant symptoms.
- Lysis procedures include mechanical, infusional, pulse-spray rheolytic techniques.
- There is debate as to whether IVC filters are pro-thrombotic. Some filter designs are thought to lead to disruption of laminar flow, particularly in the setting of thrombus. Thrombus in a filter may act as a nidus for further thrombosis. Filter placement (if one is not present) during lysis is a controversial issue. The argument for filter placement is to protect the patient from PE (eg, a filter could be placed above the thrombosis from a jugular access).

Suggested Reading

O'Sullivan GS. The role of interventional radiology in the management of deep venous thrombosis: advanced therapy. *Cardiovasc Intervent Radiol.* 2011;34(3): 445-461.

24-year-old man with flank pain and macroscopic hematuria after competing in a triathlon

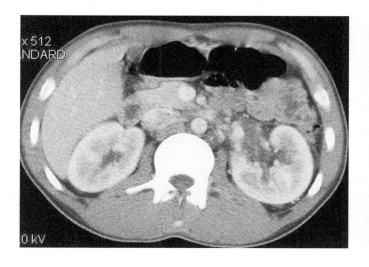 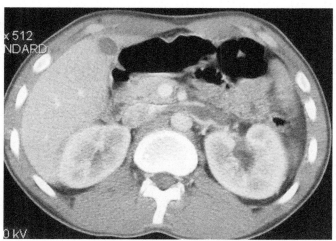

1. What is the diagnosis?

2. What are the causes of this condition?

3. What is the most common cause in adults?

4. What is the standard treatment?

5. What are CT signs?

Case ranking/difficulty:

Answers

1. Renal vein thrombosis.

2. Nephrotic syndrome and extension of inferior vena cava (IVC) thrombosis are also causes.

3. Nephrotic syndrome is the commonest cause in adults.

4. The standard treatment for acute renal vein thrombosis is anticoagulation.

5. CT findings include an enlarged kidney, with an enlarged renal vein with low attenuation filling defect/thrombus, capsular venous collaterals, thickening of the Gerota fascia, and pericapsular stranding also seen. Abnormal enhancement is seen that can be delayed and persistent.

Pearls

- Renal vein thrombosis has multiple causes including nephrotic syndrome, glomerulonephritis, and dehydration. It can result from extension of caval thrombus, affect transplant kidneys, or occur in hypercoagulable states such as with antiphospholipid syndrome.
- Anticoagulation is the mainstay of treatment. Catheter-directed thrombectomy or thrombolysis has been reported in limited series with evidence of rapid restoration of flow in native renal veins and salvage of renal transplants.

Suggested Reading

Urban BA, Ratner LE, Fishman EK. Three-dimensional volume-rendered CT angiography of the renal arteries and veins: normal anatomy, variants, and clinical applications. *Radiographics.* 2009;21(2):373-386; questionnaire 549-555.

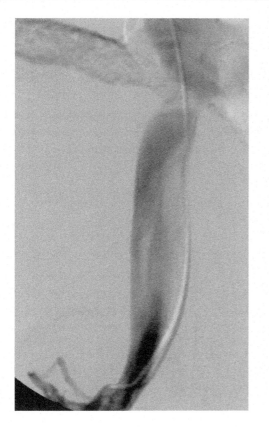 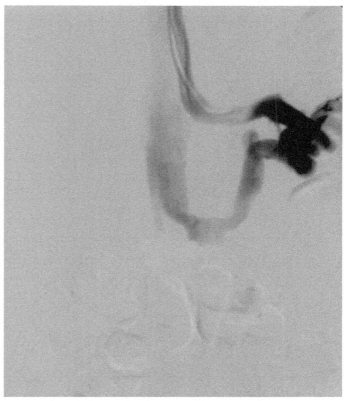

1. List some scenarios where knowledge of the presence of a circumaortic renal vein would be of value.

2. Selective renal venography should be performed at IVC filter placement; discuss.

3. Optimum filter placement should be above both renal veins—true or false?

4. Computed tomography (CT) is more sensitive than cavagram for diagnosing a circumaortic renal vein—true or false?

5. Which of the following are associated with circumaortic renal veins?

Case ranking/difficulty: 🐢🐢

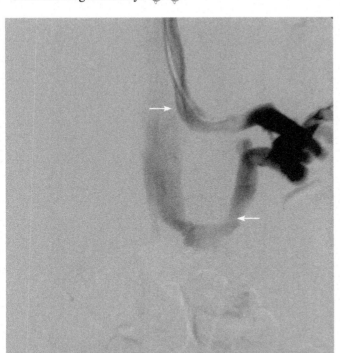

Selective left renal venogram.

Answers

1. Aneurysm, renal and retroperitoneal surgery, IVC filter placement, varicocele embolization, and adrenal vein sampling.

2. Most operators perform a cavagram. Some operators favor a jugular approach and selective catheterization of the renal veins and both iliac veins. Evidence does suggest that more IVC and venous anomalies are found by performing selective venograms—11% in cavagrams, 37% with selective venography, finding 20/108 significant variants not seen on the initial standard cavagram.

3. IVC filter placement should be below both renal veins. Placement of a filter in between the renal veins is not advised, as the circumaortic conduit is a route for potential emboli. If there was no space for a filter in the infrarenal cava, or thrombus, then a suprarenal filter would be preferred.

4. True. One study reported finding 19 retroaortic or circumaortic renal veins on CT scans of their patients (12.8%) undergoing filter placement, none of which were detected by the cavagram performed at time of placement.

5. There are no reported associations of the circumaortic renal vein.

Pearls

- Circumaortic renal vein is a common venous anomaly. The superior left renal vein is preaortic, and the inferior left renal vein is retroaortic.
- IVC filter placement between the 2 veins may not be sufficient, as there is often significant hilar connection between the 2 renal veins, which would be a potential route for emboli.

Suggested Readings

Jaskolka JD, Kwok RPW, Gray SH, Mojibian HR. The value of preprocedure computed tomography for planning insertion of inferior vena cava filters. *Can Assoc Radiol J.* 2010;61(4):223-229.

Tay K-H, Martin ML, Mayer AL, Machan LS. Selective spermatic venography and varicocele embolization in men with circumaortic left renal veins. *J Vasc Interv Radiol.* 2002;13(7):739-742.

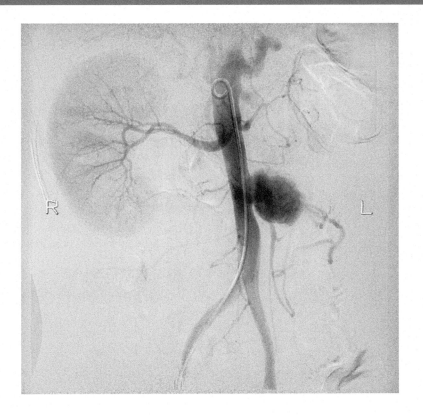

1. What is your diagnosis?

2. Most posttraumatic abdominal aortic pseudoaneurysm are caused by penetrating injury of the upper abdomen—true or false?

3. The mortality rate from abdominal aortic injury is higher for suprarenal injuries—true or false?

4. What are the possible clinical presentations of posttraumatic abdominal aortic pseudoaneurysms?

5. How late has delayed presentation of this lesion been reported?

Case ranking/difficulty:

Answers

1. There is pseudoaneurysm of the infrarenal aorta.

2. True, most posttraumatic abdominal aortic pseudoaneurysms are caused by penetrating injury.

3. The mortality rate from abdominal aortic injury is greater than 75% and is higher for suprarenal injuries.

4. Clinical presentation may be dramatic. Spontaneous rupture induces hypovolemic shock. Symptoms of unruptured PAAPs are variable, with pain, local compression, distal thromboembolism, or even sepsis having been reported.

5. Time of delayed presentation from initial injury to symptomatic presentation has ranged from 4 days to 32 years!

Pearls

- Posttraumatic abdominal aortic pseudoaneurysms (PAAPs) are rare.
- Most PAAPs are caused by penetrating injury of the upper abdomen, such as a gunshot wound or stabbing.
- Treatment can be surgical with open repair, or endovascular with stent graft placement.

Suggested Reading

Hussain Q, Maleux G, Heye S, Fourneau I. Endovascular repair of an actively hemorrhaging stab wound injury to the abdominal aorta. *Cardiovasc Intervent Radiol.* 2008;31(5):1023-1025.

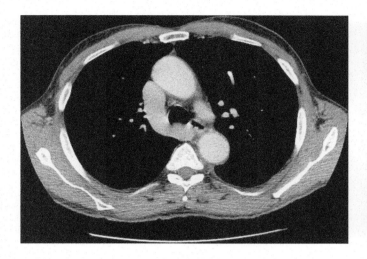
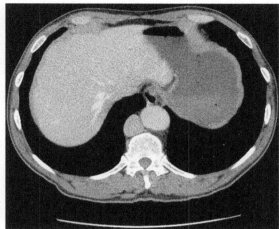

1. Review the CT images and describe the anatomy of the venous drainage pathways.

2. What is the incidence of this condition?

3. This is commonly associated with polysplenia—true or false?

4. This is commonly associated with asplenia—true or false?

5. This is commonly associated with a left-sided superior vena cava (SVC)—true or false?

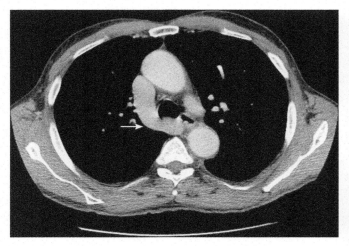
Category: Venous system

CT thorax.

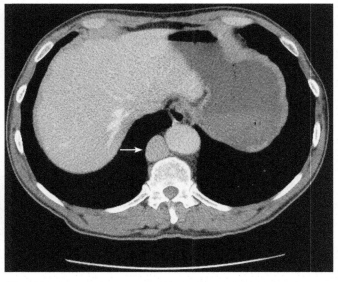

CT abdomen.

Answers

1. There is azygous continuation of the IVC.

2. 0.6%.

3. True.

4. False, this is rarely associated with asplenia.

5. True.

> **Pearls**
>
> - Azygous continuation of the IVC occurs because of absence of the IVC between the right atrium and renal veins as a result of embryologic abnormality. The right subcardinal vein does not anastomose with the hepatic veins. The right subcardinal vein atrophies. The retrocrural azygous vein persists from an anastomosis between the subcardinal and cranial portion of the supracardinal vein. IVC interruption can occur with azygous or hemiazygous continuation.
> - The hepatic veins are directly connected to the right atrium.

Suggested Reading

Fulcher AS, Turner MA. Abdominal manifestations of situs anomalies in adults. *Radiographics*. 2002;22(6): 1439-1456.

Interventional radiology is consulted about a 55-year-old woman who is short of breath and hypotensive with known large pulmonary emboli

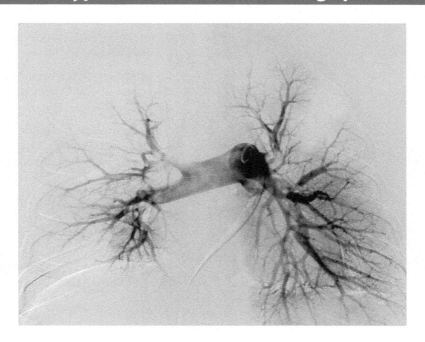

1. List 5 indications for pulmonary angiography.

2. How can pulmonary angiography be performed, and what are contraindications?

3. List the clinical features associated with massive pulmonary embolism (PE).

4. List some techniques that may be used in the setting of acute PE in the interventional suite.

5. What is the evidence base for intervention in PE?

Case ranking/difficulty:

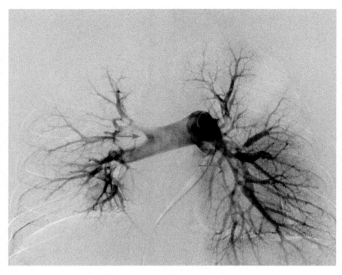

Pulmonary angiogram.

3. Dyspnea, tachycardia, hypoxia, hypotension, and a feeling of impending doom are experienced by the patient with massive life-threatening PE.

4. Catheter-directed fragmentation, aspiration thrombectomy, and thrombolysis can be used. Rheolytic therapy is avoided due to the risk of cardiac dysrhythmia.

5. Catheter-directed intervention has been reported to be successful but there is no large evidence base for its efficacy and is often provided on a case-by-case merit.

Pearls

- Catheter-directed intervention in acute PE can be life-saving. Techniques include catheter-directed embolectomy and fragmentation, catheter-directed infusion, and rheolytic thrombolysis.

Answers

1. Diagnostic indications include evaluation of congenital heart disease and mapping for pre-pulmonary endarterectomy. Pulmonary angiography is also a precursor for treatment of massive PE and pulmonary AVMs.

2. Jugular or femoral access can be used. Left bundle branch block is a relative contraindication as catheter-induced right bundle block can lead to complete heart block. The risk of procedure-related mortality is increased in severe pulmonary hypertension.

Suggested Reading

Kuo WT, van den Bosch MAAJ, Hofmann LV, Louie JD, Kothary N, Sze DY. Catheter-directed embolectomy, fragmentation, and thrombolysis for the treatment of massive pulmonary embolism after failure of systemic thrombolysis. *Chest*. 2008;134(2):250-254.

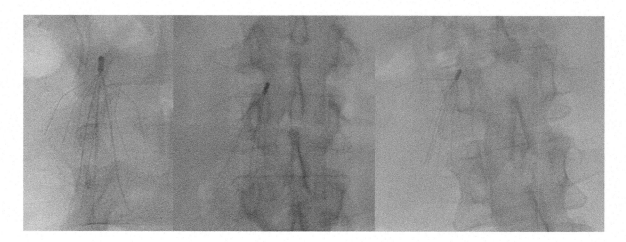

1. Think of 5 generic device-related complications.

2. Would you remove a broken filter?

3. Filters have been deployed into which of the following sites by mistake—the aorta, spinal canal, paralumbar collateral veins, and the right ventricle?

4. Filters deployed in the IVC can migrate into the right side of the heart, true or false?

5. What can lead to improved rates of filter retrieval?

Case ranking/difficulty:

Answers

1. Any device can be misplaced, migrate, break, occlude, act as a nidus for thrombosis or infection, or cause damage at its target site. Devices/tubes/drains should therefore be removed when their job is done! All device complications can be reported back to manufacturers or to national databases.

2. There are pros and cons to removing broken filters. A broken filter may expose the patient to a higher risk of pulmonary embolism (PE) as there are larger gaps through which a deep vein thrombosis (DVT) could pass. However, a broken filter itself may have risks of distal embolization with significant complications.

3. Yes, unbelievably, a filter has been deployed in the spinal canal. Good technique will avoid such complications. Presumably, a lumbar collateral was put up without appropriate imaging and checking of position. There are also reports of aortic placement. These misplacements have been reported in the vascular surgery literature. There are no reports about intracardiac placement, though several filters have migrated into the heart after placement, possibly due to unrecognized mega-cava. Filters can be placed in iliac veins in the setting of double IVC or indeed megacava with 2 large iliac veins, so this is not necessarily a misplacement! Upside down placement is also possible—if so, this should be retrieved, as most filters have hooks or designs that prevent migration.

4. Almost 100 cases are reported in the literature. Intracardiac filters can cause tamponade, arrhythmias, and intracardiac thrombus. Patients have survived for several years with filters or wall stents or other migrated material in the right atrium, so a conservative approach can be possible! Intracardiac migration can occur due to unrecognized trauma, or operator error. They can be removed with endovascular snaring techniques or by open surgery.

5. An agreed management plan prior to insertion, multidisciplinary work-up, follow-up clinics, patient communication, and dedicated IR staff to contact patients can drive up retrieval rates.

Pearls

- IVC filters can also migrate en bloc into the heart, where they have caused death, been removed at open-heart surgery, or also removed using multiple-access endovascular techniques.

Suggested Readings

Owens CA, Bui JT, Knuttinen MG, et al. Intracardiac migration of inferior vena cava filters: review of published data. *Chest.* 2009;136(3):877-887.

Tam MD, Spain J, Lieber M, Geisinger M, Sands MJ, Wang W. Fracture and distant migration of the Bard Recovery filter: a retrospective review of 363 implantations for potentially life-threatening complications. *J Vasc Interv Radiol.* 2012;23(2):199-205.

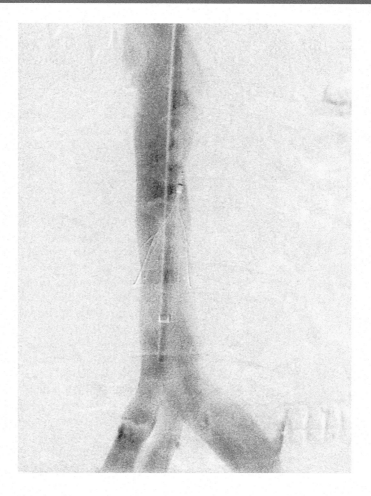

1. Under what conditions might you not proceed to attempt filter retrieval?

2. What filter can be removed from a femoral access?

3. Which filters must be removed before 3 months?

4. What factors explain why IVC retrieval rate is low?

5. What percentage of retrievable filters are removed in the United States?

Case ranking/difficulty:

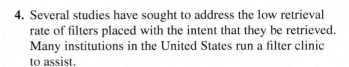

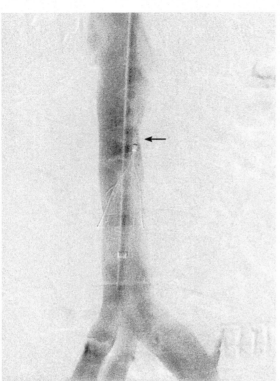

PA projection of cavagram with tilted filter and with the retrieval hook seen to be embedded to the caval wall (indentation).

4. Several studies have sought to address the low retrieval rate of filters placed with the intent that they be retrieved. Many institutions in the United States run a filter clinic to assist.

5. Large series show low retrieval rates, but there are many ventures underway to improve this figure. Success of filter retrieval is greater than 90%.

Pearls

- It is known that long-term implantation of IVC filters can lead to complications such as fracture, migration, and caval occlusion. The aim should be to retrieve filters as soon as is clinically possible. A good management plan made prior to insertion in conjunction with the radiologist, primary service, and hematology is important.
- Filter retrieval rates can be maximized by good communication between physicians and between the physicians and patient, as well as having dedicated follow-up clinics.
- More than 90% of filters can be removed; tilted or embedded filters can also be removed using advanced techniques, self-made wire loops, and even biopsy forceps and laser-assisted procedures.

Answers

1. Large thrombus in the filter, severely tilted filters, filters embedded in the caval wall, fractured filters, and migrated filters pose relative challenges and risks with attempted retrieval.

2. The OptEase filter is retrieved via a femoral approach.

3. The OptEase filter has a short retrieval period of 23 days, but studies report successful retrieval up to 60 days post placement.

Suggested Readings

Kuo WT, Tong RT, Hwang GL, et al. High-risk retrieval of adherent and chronically implanted IVC filters: techniques for removal and management of thrombotic complications. *J Vasc Interv Radiol.* 2009;20(12): 1548-1556.

Zhou D, Spain J, Moon E, McLennan G, Sands MJ, Wang W. Retrospective review of 120 select inferior vena cava filter retrievals: experience at a single institution. *J Vasc Interv Radiol.* 2012;23(12):1557-1563.

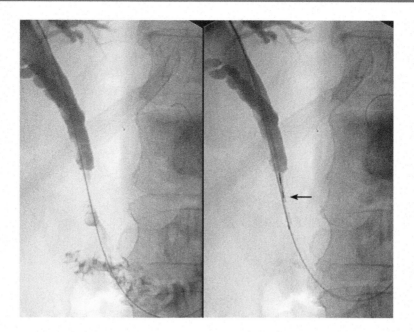

1. What can you see? What is the device labeled with an arrow?

2. What is the sensitivity of bile aspiration cytology?

3. What is the sensitivity of biliary brush biopsy?

4. What is the sensitivity of a pinch forceps biopsy?

5. What is the average life expectancy after diagnosis of cholangiocarcinoma?

Case ranking/difficulty:

Answers

1. There is a distal common bile duct (CBD) stricture. The device is a brush biopsy kit.

2. Less than 1/3.

3. 30% to 60%.

4. 40% to 80%.

5. 6 months.

Pearls

• Biliary strictures can be benign (eg, postpancreatitis) or malignant. Cytology of bile aspirate has a low diagnostic yield. Brush biopsy has a sensitivity of 30% to 60% for malignant strictures. Pinch biopsy with forceps has a sensitivity of around 40% to 80%.

Suggested Reading

Weber A, Schmid RM, Prinz C. Diagnostic approaches for cholangiocarcinoma. *World J Gastroenterol.* 2008;14(26):4131-4136.

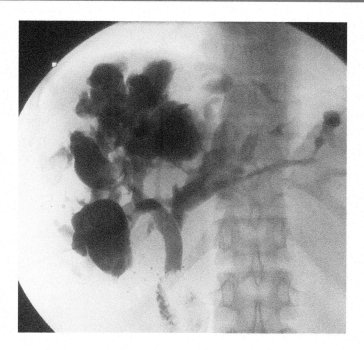

1. What is the diagnosis?

2. What are the differences between the disease and the syndrome?

3. What are the complications of Caroli disease?

4. What considerations should be paid to PTC in children?

5. Pediatric PTC can be performed safely under local anesthesia in what conditions?

Case ranking/difficulty:

Category: Gastrointestinal system

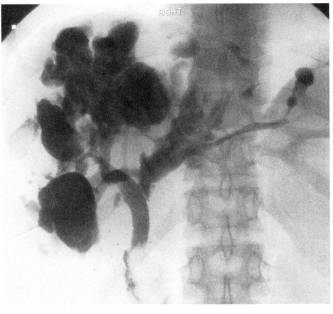

Percutaneous transhepatic cholangiogram shows diffuse saccular dilatation of intrahepatic bile duct.

4. Although much of the equipment and techniques are the same, specific exposure to pediatric interventional radiology during training is required—both technical and nontechnical skills including child protection and communication skills. Pediatric interventions should be performed in high-volume well-staffed centers.

5. The vast majority of pediatric IR is performed under general anesthesia by dedicated skilled teams.

Pearls

• Caroli disease is diagnosed by imaging studies showing nonobstructive, saccular, or fusiform dilatations of the intrahepatic bile ducts.
• Periportal Caroli disease (known as Caroli syndrome) is inherited and associated with congenital hepatic fibrosis.
• Cholangiocarcinoma develops in approximately 7% of cases. Intrahepatic duct stones, cholangitis, and abscesses are also potential complications.

Answers

1. The appearances are consistent with Caroli disease.

2. All of the above apply. The term Caroli disease is applied if the disease is limited to ectasia or segmental dilatation of the larger intrahepatic ducts. This form is less common than Caroli syndrome, in which malformations of small bile ducts and congenital hepatic fibrosis are also present.

3. Complications include stone formation, cholangitis, abscess formation, cirrhosis, and a risk of cholangiocarcinoma.

Suggested Reading

Lefere M, Thijs M, De Hertogh G, et al. Caroli disease: review of eight cases with emphasis on magnetic resonance imaging features. *Eur J Gastroenterol Hepatol.* 2011;23(7):578-585.

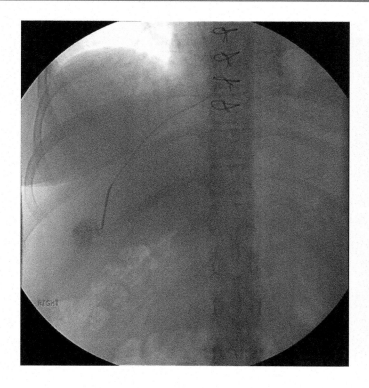 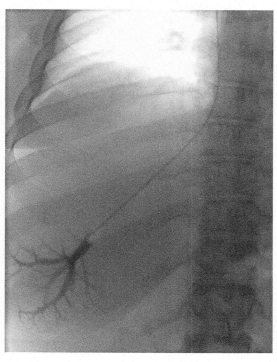

1. What is the normal hepatic venous pressure gradient and how is it calculated?

2. What are the hepatic sinusoids? What are their functions?

3. If there is azygous continuation of the inferior vena cava (IVC), where do the hepatic veins drain?

4. Name some indications for hepatic venography.

5. What level of hepatic venous pressure gradient is associated with risk of variceal hemorrhage?

Case ranking/difficulty:

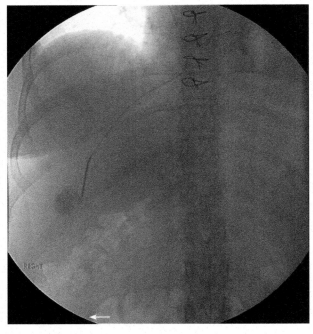

Catheter tip in a wedged position.

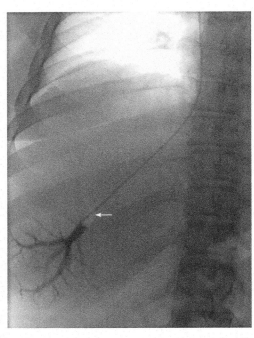

Fogarty balloon catheter also demonstrating a wedged position.

Answers

1. The pressure gradient is equal to the wedged hepatic venous pressure minus the free hepatic venous pressure and is between 1 and 5 mmHg.

2. The hepatic sinusoids are vessels that surround the hepatocytes. The hepatocytes and the sinusoids are separated by the space of Disse.

   They are low-pressure vessels that receive blood from both the terminal branches of the hepatic artery and portal vein in the periphery of lobules and deliver it into central veins. They are also highly fenestrated, which allows plasma exchange between the portal venous blood from the intestine and hepatocytes and the formation of lymph. The sinusoids also contain specialized macrophages, the Kupffer cells.

3. In this situation, they drain into the coronary sinus.

4. Transjugular biopsy, pressure measurements, investigation of Budd Chiari, assessment of the posttransplant anastomosis, a prelude to transjugular intrahepatic portosystemic shunt (TIPS) formation, and for venous sampling during arterial stimulation tests performed for localizing tumors such as insulinomas.

5. Although 10 mmHg is accepted as a sign of significant portal hypertension, a gradient of 12 mmHg is associated with increased risk of variceal hemorrhage.

Note, however, that most literature pertain to variceal hemorrhage reports on the portoatrial gradient, which requires direct measurement of the portal pressure.

Pearls

- Hepatic wedge pressure is a reflection of the sinusoidal pressure. The catheter tip or catheter balloon results in stasis of flow and the generation of a static column of blood, which then can transmit pressure from the proximal vascular bed (in this case, the hepatic sinusoids) to the catheter. The principle is the same for that of a wedged pulmonary artery pressure.
- The hepatic venous pressure gradient = wedged hepatic venous pressure – free hepatic venous pressure. This is normally between 1 and 5 mmHg. A gradient of >10 mmHg is taken to be indicative of significant portal hypertension.

Suggested Reading

Kumar A, Sharma P, Sarin SK. Hepatic venous pressure gradient measurement: time to learn! *Indian J Gastroenterol.* 2008;27(2):74-80.

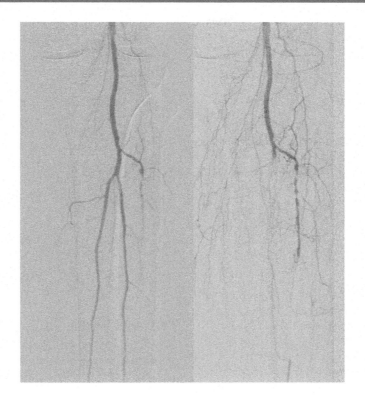

1. Why are appearances worse after femoral angioplasty?

2. What would you do next?

3. What do you need to perform aspiration thrombectomy?

4. What are disadvantages of aspiration thrombectomy?

5. What are advantages and disadvantages of infusional thrombolysis?

Case ranking/difficulty:  **Category:** Arterial system

Answers

1. There has been distal thromboembolism that has resulted in occlusion of the peroneal and posterior tibial arteries.

2. Aspiration thrombectomy should be considered.

3. A larger sheath is required, and a guiding catheter or aspiration catheter is passed down the artery into the proximal thrombus. Suction is then performed with a 20-mL syringe, which is then maintained as the guiding catheter is withdrawn.

4. Aspiration thrombectomy catheters can be guided rapidly into any of the 3 crural vessels, which is a key advantage compared to the use of Fogarty balloon catheters used at surgical embolectomy. (8-Fr sheaths may be required.)

5. It is labor-intensive requiring close monitoring in critical care and multiple trips to the angiography suite, and clearance can take more than 24 hours. There can be severe hemorrhagic complications. It can also be painful and uncomfortable. However, it can be performed relatively easily, can clear thrombus in small vessels, and has good outcomes.

Pearls

- Surgical embolectomy is performed for acute arterial embolus. This can result in rapid and effective clearing when there is embolic thrombi in normal arteries. Success of surgical embolectomy decreases in the presence of underlying chronic atherosclerotic disease.

- Catheter-directed thrombolysis can be performed for acute thromboembolism. It is minimally invasive, can be performed without GA, does not directly damage the endothelium, and can clear thrombus in small vessels. Treatment is not rapid, there are associated hemorrhagic risks and it requires multiple visits and close monitoring in a critical care environment.

- Aspiration thrombectomy is another technique that can remove acute thromboembolic disease. AT can treat patients with acute or early chronic thromboembolism. AT has advantages over surgical embolectomy as the direction of the Fogarty balloon catheters cannot be controlled. AT catheters can be guided into any of the 3 crural vessels. Disadvantages include need for large sheaths and risk of dissection and vessel perforation.

Suggested Reading

Oğuzkurt L, Ozkan U, Gümüş B, Coşkun I, Koca N, Gülcan O. Percutaneous aspiration thrombectomy in the treatment of lower extremity thromboembolic occlusions. *Diagn Interv Radiol.* 2010;16(1):79-83.

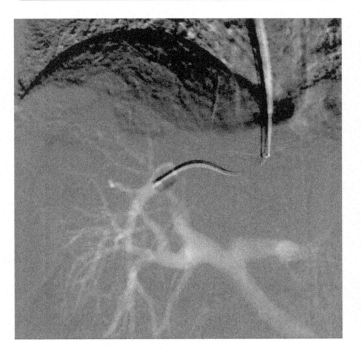 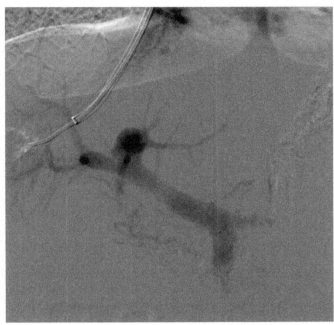

1. List some potential advantages of using carbon dioxide as a contrast agent.

2. List 10 methods of imaging the portal vein.

3. List some potential hazards associated with carbon dioxide angiography.

4. Should the CO_2 cannister remain connected to the delivery system during case, and if so, why?

5. Why is large 50-ml delivery syringe recommended to inject the CO_2?

Category: Venous system

Answers

1. CO_2 is nonallergenic, nonnephrotoxic, has a low viscosity, and is inexpensive.

2. Ultrasonography (US), computed tomography (CT), magnetic resonance (MR), CO_2 portogram, superior mesenteric artery (SMA) angiogram, transsplenic portogram, direct portal venogram via transhepatic/transjugular/direct percutaneous variceal puncture/cut-down of mesenteric branch.

3. As CO_2 is invisible, there is a risk of contamination and injection of air. Attention must therefore be paid to purging any air from the delivery system. CO_2 is buoyant and will displace rather than mix with blood, and so it rises to an anterior position with a risk of CO_2 trapping in anterior sites, and as such ischemia may result from this "vapor lock" that could occur, for example, in the SMA origin. This can be dealt with by waiting between injections, watching with fluoroscopy, aspirating, or ultimately changing the patient's position. Arterial injections of CO_2 above the diaphragm should be avoided.

4. The delivery system should be disconnected from the cylinder to avoid risk of inadvertent injection of large volumes of gas. The tubing system can be used to purge air from the system.

5. A larger delivery syringe reduces compression of the CO_2 at injection; it is not related to the volume of injection required.

Pearls

- The portal vein can be imaged in many ways.
- Noninvasive imaging with US, CT, or MRI can be performed.
- Indirect invasive imaging can be performed from a wedged position in the hepatic vein with reflux of contrast medium (normally CO_2) through the hepatic sinusoids. Capsular laceration has been reported, and so some operators prefer injecting behind a balloon catheter rather than through a wedged catheter tip. Indirect portogram can also be obtained via angiography; portal venous phase imaging from a superior mesenteric artery (SMA) angiogram also fills the portal system.
- Direct portal vein imaging can be performed via a transhepatic direct access, via a transjugular route during a TIPS procedure, via a collateral at cut-down or percutaneous puncture of a varix (eg, caput medusa or stomal varix). Historically, transsplenic portography was performed, which was associated with a small risk of splenic rupture.

Suggested Reading

Hidajat N, Stobbe H, Griesshaber V, Felix R, Schroder RJ. Imaging and radiological interventions of portal vein thrombosis. *Acta Radiol.* 2005;46(4):336-343.

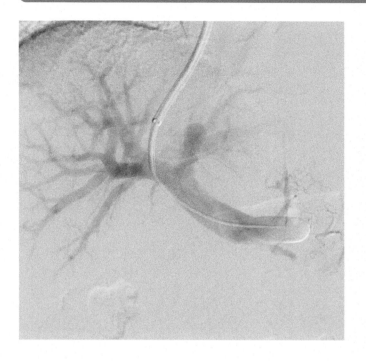 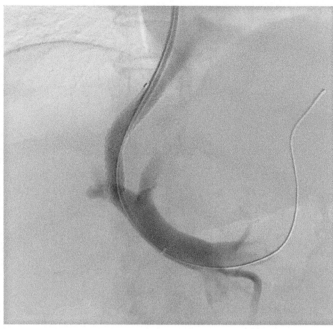

1. What is a TIPS?

2. What are the indications for TIPS?

3. What is the portoatrial gradient?

4. What is the target portoatrial gradient for a TIPS for variceal bleeding?

5. List some contraindications for TIPS.

Case ranking/difficulty: **Category:** Gastrointestinal system

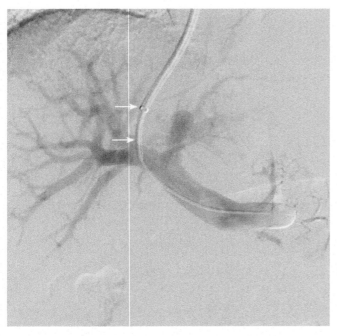

Portal venogram pre-TIPS. Arrows indicate the tract between the hepatic vein and portal vein.

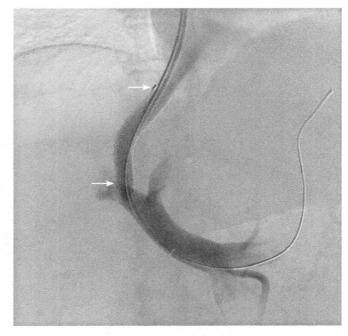

Portal venogram post-TIPS. Arrows indicate the covered portion of the stent graft.

Answers

1. This is a transjugular intrahepatic portosystemic shunt.

2. TIPS is used to treat the sequelae of portal hypertension, most commonly for variceal bleeding, but also for refractory ascites and hepatic hydrothorax.

3. This is the direct portal pressure minus the right atrial pressure.

4. The portoatrial gradient should be reduced below 11 mmHg if the TIPS is performed to stop variceal bleeding.

5. A right heart pressure of >25 mmHg is an absolute contraindication. Liver failure and coagulopathy are relative contraindications. Portal vein thrombosis and cavernous transformation of the portal vein are not contraindications to TIPS formation.

- A Colapinto or Rosch-Uchida needle is passed from hepatic vein to portal vein. A guidewire is then inserted through the needle, this tract dilated and then stented.
- Some operators use CO_2 portograms for guidance. Some experienced operators use no guidance. Transhepatic wires and snares and advanced techniques such as "gun sight" TIPSs or direct intrahepatic portacaval stent (DIPS) may be required, particularly in cases performed for Budd-Chiari syndrome.
- Polytetrafluoroethylene (PTFE)-covered stents (eg, VIATORR stent graft) have better patency than self-expanding metal stents (eg, Wallstent).
- Reduction of the portoatrial gradient to less than 11 mmHg is required for TIPS performed for variceal bleeding; reduction of this gradient to less than 5 mmHg is required for ascites.

Pearls

- Transjugular intrahepatic portosystemic shunt can be performed for variceal bleeding and other complications of portal hypertension.
- A shunt is created by placing a stent across a tract that is created between the portal vein and hepatic vein.

Suggested Reading

Boyer TD, Haskal ZJ, Haskal ZJ. The role of transjugular intrahepatic portosystemic shunt (TIPS) in the management of portal hypertension: update 2009. *Hepatology.* 2010;51(1):306.

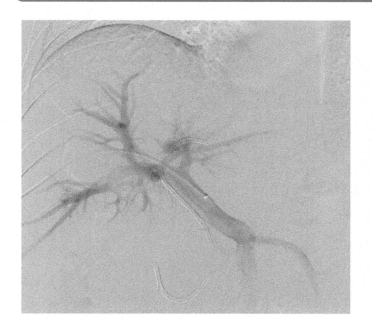
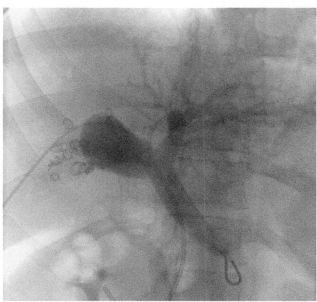

1. What access has been obtained? What has been done?

2. How much liver can be resected?

3. What is a trisegmentectomy?

4. Describe the normal portal venous anatomy.

5. How much liver can be resected if there is underlying parenchymal disease?

Case ranking/difficulty:

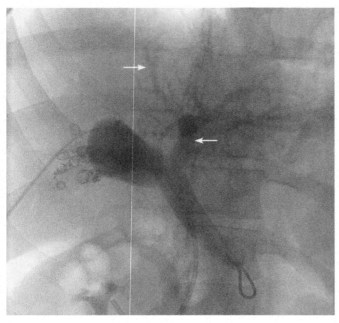

Postembolization portal venogram. Arrows indicate patency of the left-sided portal veins; the right side has been occluded.

Answers

1. A right-sided transhepatic portal vein access is obtained, and the right portal branches have been embolized.

2. Patients with no underlying background liver disease can tolerate 60 to 70% of their liver being resected.

3. A trisegmentectomy is an extended right hepatectomy, which involves removal of all of the true right lobe but also the medial aspect of the lateral segments.

4. The portal bifurcation is extrahepatic in 50%. On the right, there are normally 2 major branches—anterior and posterior sectoral branches. The main left portal vein has 2 parts, an extrahepatic horizontal part and an intrahepatic vertical or umbilical part. The sectoral branches divide into segmental branches. Segments may receive more than 1 segmental branch. Variations occur in 15%. The commonest variation is the portal trifurcation where the main portal vein divides into 2 right and 1 left branch. The right anterior portal vein can arise from the left, and similarly the left can arise from the right anterior portal vein.

5. The future liver remnant (FLR) to total estimated liver volume (TELV) ratio should be above 25% for normal livers and 40% for diseased livers. Portal vein embolization can push people above this threshold and make them into operative candidates.

Suggested Reading

Madoff DC, Hicks ME, Vauthey J-N, et al. Transhepatic portal vein embolization: anatomy, indications, and technical considerations. *Radiographics.* 2002;22(5):1063-1076.

74-year-old man with hydronephrosis due to malignant lower ureteric obstruction

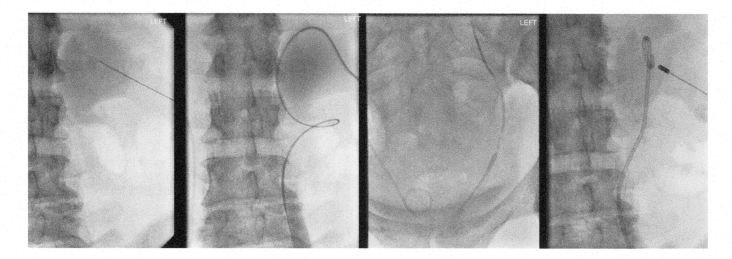

1. Review the first panel; what is the optimal access for antegrade stenting?

2. Regarding the second panel, what is the issue here?

3. Regarding the third panel, what is the issue?

4. Regarding the fourth panel—how do you deploy the top end of a JJ stent?

5. What are the roles of the pusher?

Case ranking/difficulty:

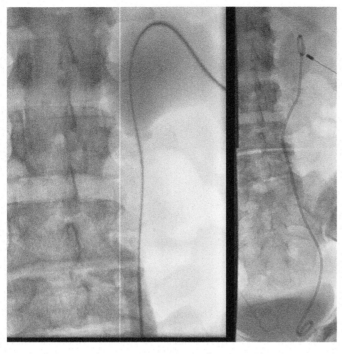

Reduction of the ureteric loop and final stent position.

Answers

1. Lower pole caliceal access may result in an unforgiving bend that makes it difficult to push the stent through the renal pelvis and down the ureter. Upper pole access may result in a higher complication rate. Therefore, a midpole calyx is probably better overall, but antegrade JJ stenting can be completed with any access.

2. There is a loop in the upper ureter, but this will tend to straighten. Various wire and catheter moves can facilitate this straightening if it does not occur automatically.

3. There is a distal stricture. The JJ stent may not freely pass without balloon dilatation, which should be considered here.

4. The top end is deployed by coordinating a number of factors. The wire is pulled back through the stent, which allows the loop to form. The thread that allows countertraction must be cut and pulled. The pusher allows the thread to be pulled without pulling the stent out of the collecting system by providing counter traction against the stent. The pusher should also be controlled so that access to the collecting system is not lost.

5. The pusher gives countertraction, allowing the thread to be pulled. The pusher also allows access to the collecting system to be retained to facilitate placement of a safety catheter should one be required.

Pearls

- Antegrade JJ stent placement is performed by accessing the renal system, passing a wire into the bladder, and then advancing the JJ stent over the wire, forming the distal loop in the bladder, and then releasing the top end of the catheter in the renal pelvis.
- It can be performed safely as a primary procedure without the need of a safety catheter. Nevertheless, a safety catheter should be considered if there is a high-grade obstruction.
- In the setting of obstructing ureteric calculi, a retrograde approach may be more comfortable for the patient.

Suggested Reading

Chitale S, Raja V, Hussain N, et al. One-stage tubeless antegrade ureteric stenting: a safe and cost-effective option? *Ann R Coll Surg Engl.* 2010;92(3):218-224.

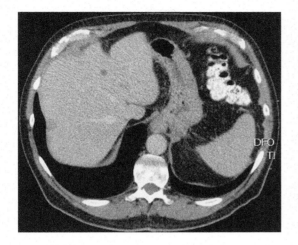
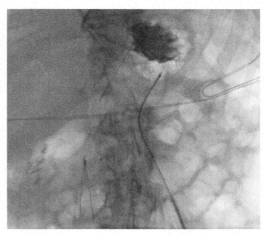
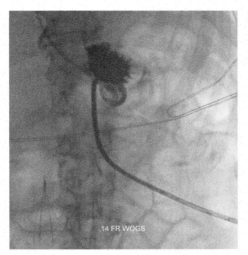

1. What are the contraindications to radiologically inserted gastrostomy tube (RIG) placement?

2. What strategies can be used to identify and avoid the transverse colon?

3. Can a RIG be inserted from the mouth?

4. Which patients benefit from gastrojejunostomy placement rather than RIGs?

5. Is it easy to covert a G tube to a GJ tube?

Case ranking/difficulty:

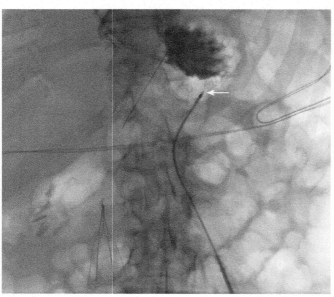

Gastric access.

Answers

1. Coagulopathy is a contraindication for RIG because of the risk of uncontrollable hemorrhage. The other selections are not absolute contraindications but make the procedure challenging. Particular care should be taken to note the position of the transverse colon. Ascites can be drained at time of RIG placement to decrease the risk of leak.

2. Lateral screening, GI contrast medium prior to procedure, ultrasound, CT, and pullback tractogram are all techniques to locate, identify, and check the position of the transverse colon, techniques that can be important in difficult cases.

3. Gastrostomy can be performed with radiologic guidance only and still be placed via the mouth. Orogastric access

and percutaneous access is obtained and connected via a snare. In fact, the gastric access can be directed to the gastroesophageal junction and a wire passed from stomach and out of the mouth. Once a through-and-through wire is obtained, the tube can be passed orally and passed via the mouth and out the abdominal wall. Some manufacturers make so-called PUSH and PULL tubes.

4. Patients who have a higher risk of aspiration may benefit from GJ placement over a G tube.

5. G to GJ conversion may be complicated by the fact that the existing access for a G tube is usually directed to the fundus whereas for a primary GJ tube, access is directed toward the pylorus. This difference in direction can lead to wire looping, which makes negotiation around the duodenum and passing the ligament of Treitz challenging. This process is usually assisted by curved or rigid sheaths and metallic trocars.

Pearls

• RIG can be performed with a high or intrathoracic gastric position. It can also be performed where there is a hiatus hernia. If there is no subcostal window, then the stay sutures and access can be made intercostally and may be performed with computed tomographic guidance.

Suggested Reading

Lyon SM, Pascoe DM. Percutaneous gastrostomy and gastrojejunostomy. *Semin Intervent Radiol.* 2004;21(3):181-189.

40-year-old woman who is known to have mild left hydronephrosis secondary to cervical cancer presents with sudden onset of left flank pain

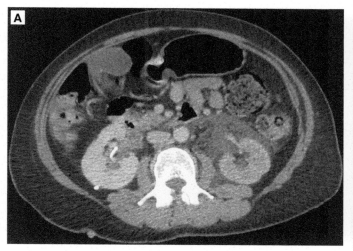 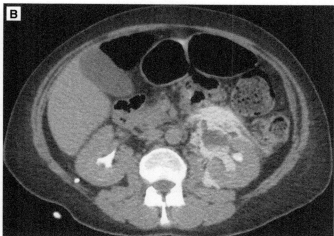

1. Describe the phases and findings of the images.

2. What should be done next?

3. How can non-dilated systems be accessed?

4. Name some indications for nephrostomy tube placement into a non-dilated system.

5. Can obstruction and non-dilatation exist, and if so, why?

Case ranking/difficulty:

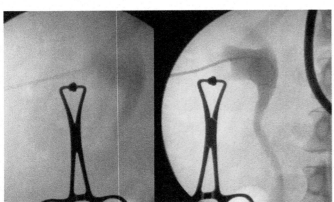

Nephrostomy placement.

Answers

1. Image A is portal venous phase, and image B is a delayed phase. The images demonstrate contrast extravasation around the left kidney due to a ruptured renal collecting system.

2. Urine diversion is necessary to prevent a urine leak into the retroperitoneum and subsequent urinoma development. Urgent nephrostomy placement is preferable but stenting may be feasible.

3. Opacifying the system aids placement. If renal function is normal, then a contrast bolus can opacify the system. A fluid challenge may also open the calices. A two-puncture technique can be used: the first needle finds and opacifies the system, and a second definitive access is found to insert the tube.

4. Renal collecting system rupture, ureteric leak, sepsis with stone disease, acute renal failure, and access for PCNL are indications.

5. It may account for up to 5% of obstructions. Dilatation may not be seen because diagnostic imaging is performed too early. Also, dilatation may not occur as a result of low flow, resistance of the renal tissues to dilate, or resistance due to fibrosis of perirenal tissues such as in retroperitoneal fibrosis.

Pearls

- Spontaneous rupture of the renal pelvis can occur due to ureteric obstruction. Nephrostomy placement is required to divert the urine, and further management is dependent upon the primary cause.
- In a nondilated collecting system, several techniques can assist in gaining access and they include opacification of the collecting system with an intravenous bolus of contrast medium (not possible with renal dysfunction), ultrasound guidance, or a 2-needle technique with initial access into the renal pelvis allowing the system to be distended followed by a second definitive access.

Suggested Reading

Patel U, Hussain FF. Percutaneous nephrostomy of nondilated renal collecting systems with fluoroscopic guidance: technique and results. *Radiology.* 2004;233(1):226-233.

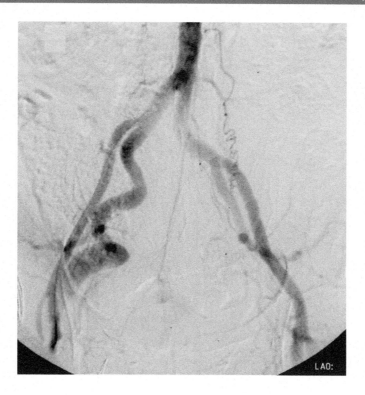

1. What is the diagnosis?

2. What is the commonest site of aneurysm formation in this condition?

3. What are potential complications?

4. When do complications present?

5. What is the incidence of distal arterial occlusion?

Case ranking/difficulty:

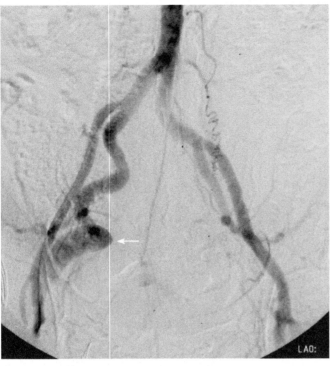

Left anterior oblique (LAO) aortic angiogram.

Answers

1. The apparently hypertrophied right internal iliac artery is a persistent sciatic artery.

2. Aneurysm formation tends to occur between piriformis and the greater trochanter, the site where the artery is S-shaped. The mechanism for aneurysm formation is, however, poorly understood.

3. Aneurysm formation, thrombosis, mass effect, and distal arterial occlusive disease occur. Failure to recognize the underlying anatomy during angiography or embolization for other reasons can also lead to significant complications.

4. Complicated PSA presents in the 40s and 50s.

5. Around 8% of patients with PSA will have distal arterial occlusions.

Pearls

- The persistent sciatic artery is a rare but important anatomic variant. It arises from an enlarged internal iliac artery and can be the dominant supply to the lower extremity. The SFA can be hypoplastic, absent, or normal.
- Complications occur due to aneurysm formation, thrombosis, and distal embolization. Localized pressure effects can cause sciatic neuropathy.

Suggested Readings

Mousa A, Rapp Parker A, Emmett MK, AbuRahma A. Endovascular treatment of symptomatic persistent sciatic artery aneurysm: a case report and review of literature. *Vasc Endovascular Surg.* 2010;44(4):312-314.

van Hooft IM, Zeebregts CJ, van Sterkenburg SM, de Vries WR, Reijnen MM. The persistent sciatic artery. *Eur J Vasc Endovasc Surg.* 2009;37(5):585-591.

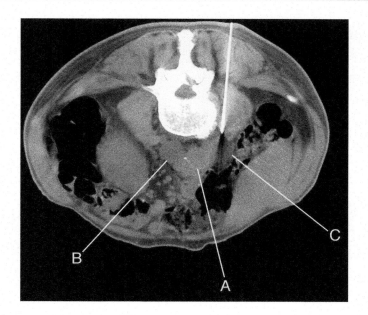

1. Name the structure labelled A.

2. The needle has been inserted by the staff radiologist and you attend midway through the case. The staff asks you to take the biopsy. Will you proceed?

3. Name the structures labelled B and C.

4. Would you perform a fine-needle aspiration (FNA) or cutting biopsy?

5. What is the incidence of a left-sided inferior vena cava (IVC)?

Case ranking/difficulty:

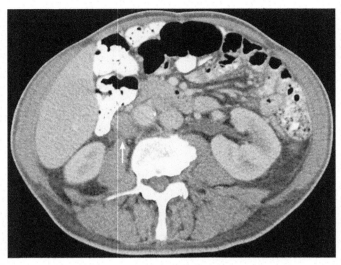

Note the paraaortic lymph node and the left-sided IVC (arrow), the aorta with its focus of mural calcification, and the left-sided IVC.

Answers

1. A is the aorta. Note the calcification.

2. Preprocedure planning includes review of all relevant diagnostic studies as well as informed consent and so it may not be appropriate to perform the biopsy. Also, are you concerned about where the needle is?

3. This patient has a left-sided vena cava.

4. Cutting biopsy is most likely to give useful information in this setting.

5. The incidence is quoted to be between 0.2% and 0.5%.

Pearls

- Review all imaging before performing procedures.
- A preprocedure safety checklist is important.
- Understanding normal anatomy and anatomic variants is of critical importance.
- There are several safety checklists available—for example, those from the World Health Organization or those from specific radiology and interventional radiology societies.

Suggested Reading

Tomozawa Y, Inaba Y, Yamaura H, et al. Clinical value of CT-guided needle biopsy for retroperitoneal lesions. *Korean J Radiol.* 2011;12(3):351-357.

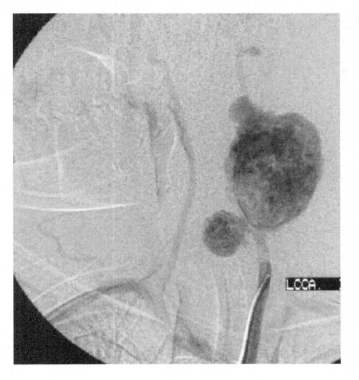 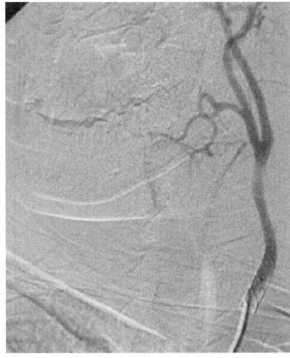

1. What is the most common cause
   of a pseudoaneurysm?

2. What is the principal imaging modality
   for head and neck trauma?

3. What are the indications of catheter
   angiography in head and neck trauma?

4. Name some important variations of the internal
   carotid artery.

5. What are the complications of stent graft
   placement?

Case ranking/difficulty:

Category: Arterial system

Answers

1. They are most commonly associated with blunt or penetrating trauma.

2. Computed tomographic (CT) angiography is the principal imaging modality for head and neck trauma. It provides excellent images of the bony structures, including the face, cranium, and spine, and can readily delineate arterial injuries.

3. Catheter angiography is usually reserved for patients who are clinically unstable and have a high clinical suspicion for an arterial injury, for difficulty with diagnosis, or as a prerequisite to intervention. In evaluating the trauma patient, complete, "4 vessel" angiography is recommended and this includes both carotids and both vertebral arteries.

4. Persistent trigeminal and persistent hypoglossal arteries as well as the proatlantal intersegmental arteries are important carotid-basilar arterial anastomoses.

5. Possible complications of stent grafts include microembolism or vascular rupture.

Pearls

- Common carotid artery (CCA) pseudoaneurysms are rare and potentially lethal, and adequate treatment is warranted in order to prevent rupture or neurologic sequelae. The causes of CCA pseudoaneurysm include trauma, infection, vasculitis, and iatrogenic causes.
- Surgery has been the standard treatment for pseudoaneurysms. However, endovascular surgical approaches such as stent graft placement or coiling have become effective alternatives, with minimal morbidity and high success rates.

Suggested Readings

Cox MW, Whittaker DR, Martinez C, Fox CJ, Feuerstein IM, Gillespie DL. Traumatic pseudoaneurysms of the head and neck: early endovascular intervention. *J Vasc Surg.* 2007;46(6):1227-1233.

Defillo A, Zelensky A, Pulivarthi S, et al. Noninfected carotid artery pseudoaneurysm 29 years after endarterectomy, endovascular management with covered stent. *J Neurosurg Sci.* 2012;56(2):145-150.

Golarz SR, Gable D. Use of a Viabahn stent for repair of a common carotid artery pseudoaneurysm and dissection. *Ann Vasc Surg.* 2010;24(4):550.e11-e13.

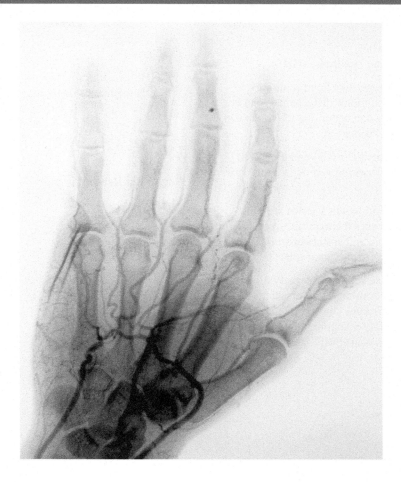

1. What is the diagnosis?

2. What are key clinical features?

3. Describe Allen's test and its role in this condition.

4. What are the angiographic findings in this syndrome?

5. What is the epidemiology of the condition?

Case ranking/difficulty:

Category: Arterial system

Answers

1. This is hypothenar hammer syndrome (HHS).

2. Occupational history of repetitive hand trauma is present. Pain, sensory, and motor disturbances can be present. Digitial ischemia can occur due to vasospasm, thrombosis, or aneurysm formation.

3. Allen's test involves sequential radial and then ulna artery occlusion. It is not specific and negative in 17% of patients with HHS.

4. Common angiographic findings in a series are ulna artery occlusions as it crosses the hamate, occlusion of digital arteries, aneurysms, and spiral deformation or "corkscrew configuration" of the ulnar artery.

5. HHS is an uncommon disease, which largely affects men, with a 9:1 male predominance, and typically involves the right hand. Studies showed that HHS can occur in persons with preexisting palmar ulnar artery fibromuscular dysplasia (FMD) and a history of repetitive palmar trauma.

Pearls

- HHS is caused by repetitive microtrauma to the hand over the hook of hamate, which can cause thrombosis of the superficial palmar arch of the ulnar artery. This leads to vascular insufficiency of the ulnar side of the hand. Treatment can involve surgical bypass.

Suggested Reading

Molvar CA, Funaki BS. AJR teaching file: carpenter with cold, numb fingers. *AJR Am J Roentgenol.* 2009;193(3 Suppl):S46-S48.

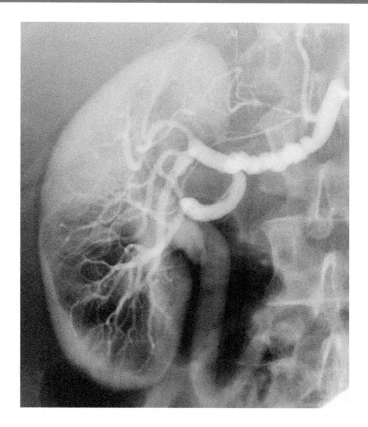

1. What is the most common cause of spontaneous renal artery dissection?

2. What are the complications of fibromuscular dysplasia?

3. What is the gold-standard treatment of spontaneous renal artery dissection?

4. What is the best imaging modality for diagnosing spontaneous renal artery dissection?

5. Spontaneous renal artery dissection can occur at which sites?

Case ranking/difficulty:

Answers

1. Fibromuscular dysplasia is the most commonly reported cause of isolated spontaneous renal artery dissection in the literature.

2. Complications include hypertension, renal infarction, renal artery dissection, and aneurysm formation and rupture.

3. Spontaneous renal artery dissection is a rare condition and often involves a small branch. There is no consensus regarding standard treatment.

4. Renal angiography is the preferred imaging modality for detecting renal artery pathology, especially in small arterial segments.

5. Dissection can occur in the main or segmental arteries, and can be single, multiple, or recurrent.

Pearls

• Spontaneous renal artery dissection is rare and is most commonly seen in fibromuscular dysplasia. Dissection can result in renal parenchymal loss and severe hypertension. The correct diagnosis is often delayed because of the rarity and nonspecific presentation of the disease. Furthermore, successful revascularization is often limited because of the involvement of small branches. Diagnostic workup includes computed tomographic and magnetic resonance angiography but renal angiography is a better imaging modality for detecting renal artery pathology, especially in smaller segmental branches. Management options for spontaneous dissection include surgical revascularization, endovascular intervention, or anticoagulation.

Suggested Reading

Ramamoorthy SL, Vasquez JC, Taft PM, McGinn RF, Hye RJ. Nonoperative management of acute spontaneous renal artery dissection. *Ann Vasc Surg.* 2002;16(2):157-162.

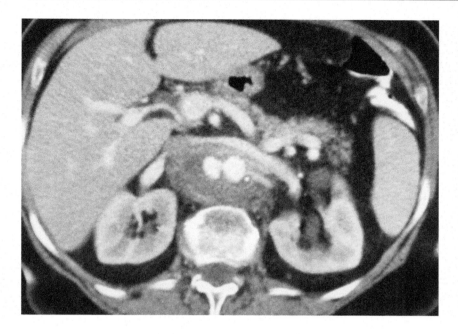

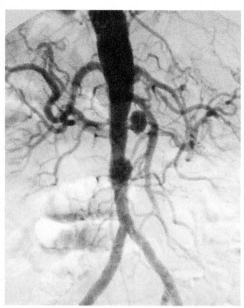

1. What is the diagnosis?

2. What would you include in the differential diagnosis?

3. What is the current gold-standard treatment?

4. What is the incidence of aneurysm wall infection in abdominal aortic aneurysms in autopsy specimens?

5. What are the most common pathogens responsible?

Category: Arterial system

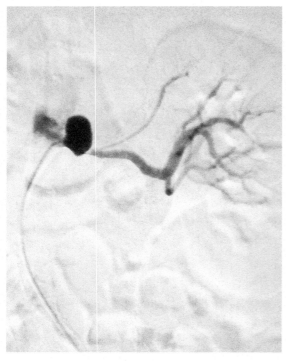

Selective left renal arteriogram shows a focal outpouching at the superior aspect of the proximal renal artery.

Answers

1. There are mycotic aneurysms.

2. Other aortic syndromes, such as penetrating ulcers, pseudoaneurysms, and saccular aneurysms, can have similar appearances.

3. Open surgery remains the gold standard.

4. Infected arterial aneurysms of the aorta are not common, comprising approximately 3% of abdominal aortic aneurysms (AAAs) in autopsy specimens.

5. The majority of cases are due to staphylococcus, with salmonella being the second most common.

Pearls

• Mycotic aneurysms occur when there is an infectious break in the wall of an artery with formation of a saccular outpouching that is contiguous with the arterial lumen. Conventional surgery for treatment of mycotic aortic aneurysm has rather high surgical morbidity and mortality rates. This requires debridement or infected tissue, removal of any infected prosthetic material, and arterial reconstruction. Endovascular repair provides rapid aneurysm exclusion, and stent graft placement can be performed and active infection managed medically.

Suggested Readings

Leon LR Jr, Mills JL Sr. Diagnosis and management of aortic mycotic aneurysms. *Vasc Endovascular Surg.* 2010;44(1):5-13.

Setacci C, de Donato G, Setacci F. Endografts for the treatment of aortic infection. *Semin Vasc Surg.* 2011;24(4):242-249.

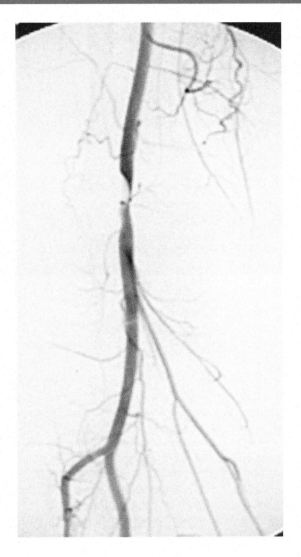 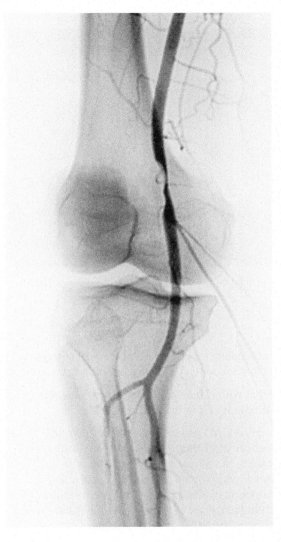

1. The patient is otherwise fit and healthy with no risk factors and no signs of atherosclerosis on the CT angiogram. What is the diagnosis?

2. What is the most common presenting symptom?

3. What is the proposed etiology of this condition?

4. How can this disease be managed?

5. What imaging signs favor this diagnosis?

Case ranking/difficulty:

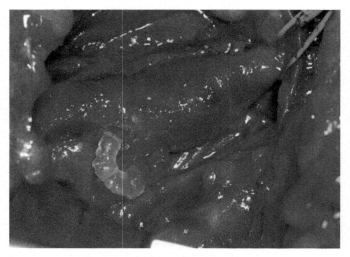

Intraoperative photograph shows the cysts around the popliteal artery.

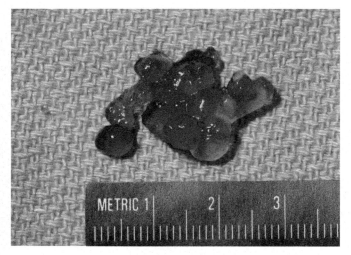

The specimen shows grapelike cysts filled with clear liquid.

Answers

1. There is an eccentric, extrinsic narrowing of the popliteal artery and this is due to cystic adventitial disease.

2. It can present with claudication, pain, local mass effect, or as a pulsatile lesion in the popliteal fossa.

3. The etiology of CAD remains debatable. Repetitive trauma may cause adventitial degeneration, leading to cyst formation. Mucin-secreting cells from adjacent joints may be incorporated into the popliteal artery during development. Others suggest that adventitial cysts develop from the adjoining joint synovium as the cysts have histologic similarities to ganglion cysts.

4. Spontaneous regression of the cysts can occur. The diseased segment of the popliteal artery can be excised and repaired, patched, or bypassed. Image-guided aspiration of the cyst may be a simple alternative. Recurrence has been reported after excision and aspiration. In patients with severely compressed artery, angioplasty or endograft placement may be necessary.

5. Classical descriptions report the presence of a "scimitar sign" (a curvilinear narrowing of the vessel) or an "hourglass" configuration. Other imaging techniques have the capacity to show not only the lumen but also the lesion within the vessel wall. Of course, ultrasound appearances are quite striking!

Pearls

- Cystic adventitial disease typically affects popliteal artery (up to 85% cases) and patients present with symptoms of claudication that is usually of short or sudden onset.
- It is a rare vascular disease that primarily affects the arteries. It was first reported in 1947 by Atkins and Key, who described a case of a myxomatous tumor arising from the external iliac artery. Since then, fewer than 400 cases have been published.
- Other sites of involvement include the external iliac, femoral, radial, ulnar, brachial, and axillary as well as the abdominal aorta.

Suggested Reading

Paravastu SC, Regi JM, Turner DR, Gaines PA. A contemporary review of cystic adventitial disease. *Vasc Endovascular Surg.* 2012;46(1):5-14.

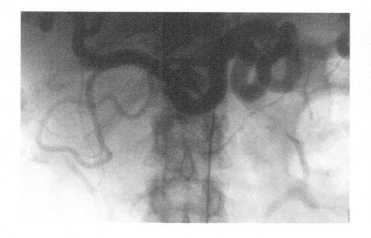 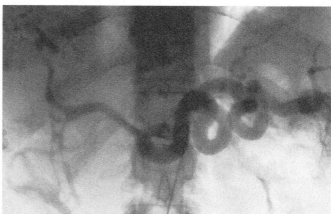

1. Review the 2 images, what has happened?

2. What are signs of arterial dissection?

3. If this occurs during a TACE procedure, what is your management strategy?

4. What are the principles of balloon fenestration technique?

5. What are complications from selective hepatic artery catheterization?

Case ranking/difficulty:

Category: Arterial system

Answers

1. There is a dissection of the common hepatic artery.

2. A double-lumen sign, eccentric extrinsic narrowing, decreased distal flow, loss of side branches, and slow flow in the false lumen are key angiographic signs of dissection.

3. When a celiac trunk or hepatic artery dissection develops, the procedure should be aborted and repeated after 1 month as there is a high rate of spontaneous recanalization as high as 60%. However, if the dissection causes a complete arterial occlusion as in this case, the chance of recanalization is believed to be low.

4. The entry tear in iatrogenic dissection of the celiac or hepatic artery is considered to be small because it is caused by a guidewire, catheter, or contrast injection. Even though it is small, the dissected false lumen does not have an outflow and behaves like a windsock. Inflow through the entry tear causes propagation of the dissection, and the resultant compromise of the true lumen.

   If a reentry tear larger than the entry tear can be made, the false lumen may collapse or shrink as a result of an increase in false lumen outflow capacity. In our case, balloon fenestration of the reentry tear immediately decompressed the false lumen and reopened the true lumen. The dissected artery was patent with mild residual stenosis.

5. Again, dissection, occlusion, pseudoaneurysm formation, or perforation can occur!

Pearls

- Iatrogenic arterial dissection can occur during any procedure. Celiac trunk or proper hepatic artery dissection can occur during transarterial chemoembolization procedures. Recognition of the complication is important to avoid further progression to complete occlusion. Iatrogenic arterial dissections can be managed by catheterization of the true lumen and balloon dilatation. A large percentage can resolve spontaneously, so conservative management may be considered in noncritical situations.

Suggested Reading

Yoon DY, Park JH, Chung JW, Han JK, Han MC. Iatrogenic dissection of the celiac artery and its branches during transcatheter arterial embolization for hepatocellular carcinoma: outcome in 40 patients. *Cardiovasc Intervent Radiol.* 1995;18(1):16-19.

83-year-old man with abdominal pain, radiating to the back, has a repeat computed tomography (CT) 3 days later because of increasing pain

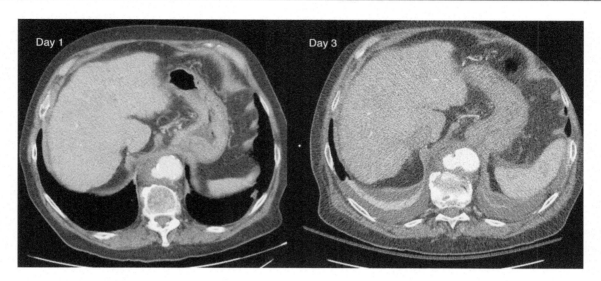

1. What are complications of penetrating aortic ulcers?

2. Name some acute aortic syndromes.

3. What is the most common form of acute aortic syndrome?

4. What is the pathophysiological basis of a penetrating ulcer?

5. What is your management strategy for this case?

Case ranking/difficulty: **Category:** Arterial system

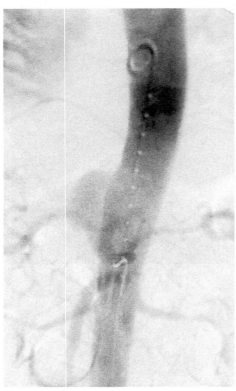

Abdominal aortogram shows a focal contrast collection at the right aspect of the aorta, just above the origin of the celiac artery.

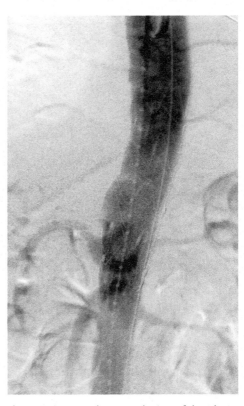

Postprocedure angiogram shows exclusion of the ulcer.

Answers

1. Complications include progression to overt aortic dissection, pseudoaneurysm formation after breaking through the adventitia, and, in as many as 40% of patients, rupture.

2. Acute aortic syndromes occur when either a tear or an ulcer allows blood to penetrate from the aortic lumen into the media, which can lead to aortic dilatation and rupture. These conditions include aortic dissection, intramural hematoma, and penetrating atherosclerotic ulcer and trauma that cause intimal tears.

3. Aortic dissection is most common.

4. Penetrating ulcers occur due to plaque rupture within an ulcerated atherosclerotic lesion that then erodes and penetrates the internal elastic lamina, which progresses into the media.

5. Conservative, endovascular, or surgical management is possible. If the lesion is enlarging, treatment may be indicated. Conventional stent grafting requires an adequate landing zone. Multilayered stents, which modulate flow encouraging thrombosis in the sacs outside the stent meshes, may also be indicated. In this case, a stent graft was deployed sacrificing the celiac trunk to give a landing zone.

Pearls

• Penetrating atherosclerotic ulcer describes an ulcerating atherosclerotic lesion that penetrates the elastic lamina and is associated with hematoma formation within the media of the aortic wall. The natural history of penetrating atherosclerotic ulcer is not clear, but many authors consider this to have a poorer prognosis than classic aortic dissection, particularly in patients with persistent pain due to rapid extension of the ulceration.

Suggested Reading

Stanson AW, Kazmier FJ, Hollier LH, et al. Penetrating atherosclerotic ulcers of the thoracic aorta: natural history and clinicopathologic correlations. *Ann Vasc Surg.* 1986;1(1):15-23.

72-year-old man who is status post endograft placement for an 8-cm rapidly expanding descending thoracic aortic aneurysm. The proximal end of the endograft was positioned at the left subclavian artery origin. Two overlapping extension cuffs were placed distally

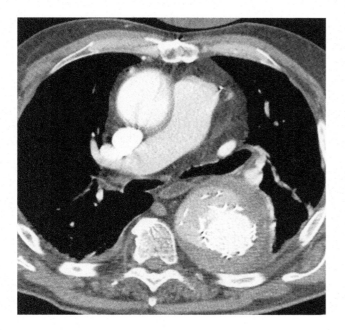
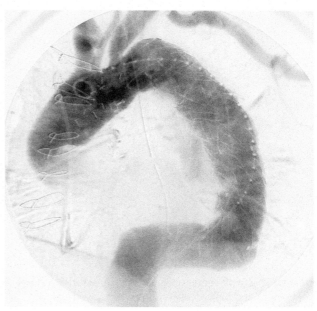

1. What is the diagnosis?

2. Why does this occur?

3. Will it resolve spontaneously? If not, what will you do?

4. What disadvantages does CT have in detecting and characterising endoleaks?

5. If you place another stent, would you oversize it and post-dilate it, or not?

Case ranking/difficulty:

Category: Arterial system

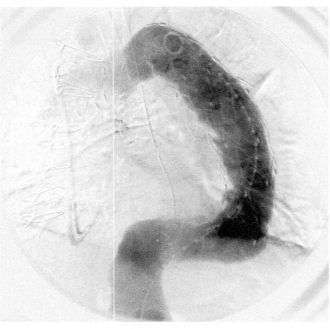

Posttreatment with placement of an additional extension at the level of the leak and balloon dilatation with resolved leak.

Answers

1. This is a type 3 endoleak.

2. Type 3 endoleaks result from gaps between modular components or fabric tears.

3. Type 3 endoleaks do not spontaneously resolve and usually require additional stent-graft components.

4. CT angiography has a limited ability to determine blood flow direction, which is critical for endoleak classification, although 4D time-solved CT angiography may have some useful applications.

5. Oversizing and dilation in TEVAR should be avoided in acute dissection due to the risk of causing a retrograde type A. In this case, oversizing and post-dilatation is indicated.

Pearls

- Type 3 endoleak occurs due to inadequate overlapping of graft components or tears in the graft fabric. Some endoleaks can require early treatment—such as type 1 and type 3 leaks, as there is high or pressurized flow in the aortic sac with potential risk of rupture.

Suggested Reading

Stavropoulos SW, Charagundla SR, Imaging techniques for detection and management of endoleaks after endovascular aortic aneurysm repair. *Radiology.* 2007;243(3):641-655.

54-year-old man with a history of alcohol abuse presents with massive gastrointestinal hemorrhage

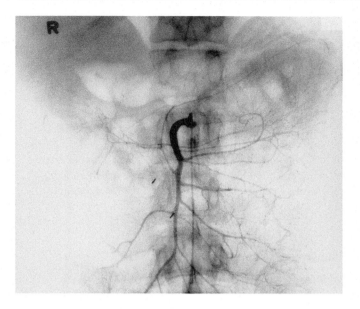 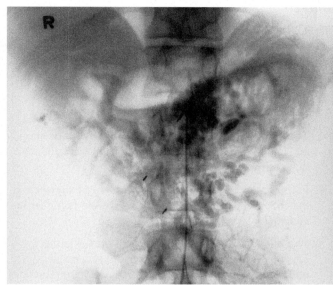

1. What procedure is this and what does it show?

2. What are the complications of what is seen?

3. What are possible management strategies?

4. What other sites can similar lesions be found?

5. Where are common sites of porto-systemic anastomoses?

Case ranking/difficulty:

Category: Venous system

Answers

1. This is a superior mesenteric angiogram with delayed portal venous phase imaging. Large duodenal varices can be seen.

2. Hemorrhage from dudodenal varices is rare but life-threatening. They may be underrecognized as compared to esophageal varices.

3. There is no accepted strategy but options include surgical and endoscopic ligation, TIPS, duodenal resection, and injection sclerotherapy.

4. Ectopic varices can be found in stomas and anywhere in the abdomen around the GI tract as well as being vesical and vaginal.

5. These include the gastro-esophageal plexus to the azygous system, hemorrhoidal plexus, recanalized umbilical vein, and pancreaticoduodenal venous arcade to the retroperitoneum with communication with the IVC and veins of Retzius.

Pearls

• Duodenal varices are a rare but devastating cause of gastrointestinal hemorrhage. The etiology of duodenal varices can be classified into hepatic (eg, cirrhosis) or extrahepatic (eg, portal, splenic, or superior mesenteric vein thrombosis). Endoscopic injection and variceal ligation are widely accepted as primary therapies for esophageal variceal bleeding, whereas bleeding gastric fundal varices are usually treated with cyanoacrylate injection or shunt procedures. However, there is no widely accepted treatment modality for duodenal varices.

Suggested Readings

Akazawa Y, Murata I, Yamao T, et al. Successful management of bleeding duodenal varices by endoscopic variceal ligation and balloon-occluded retrograde transvenous obliteration. *Gastrointest Endosc.* 2003;58(5): 794-797.

Hashizume M, Tanoue K, Ohta M, et al .Vascular anatomy of duodenal varices: angiographic and histopathological assessments. *Am J Gastroenterol.* 1993;88(11):1942-1945.

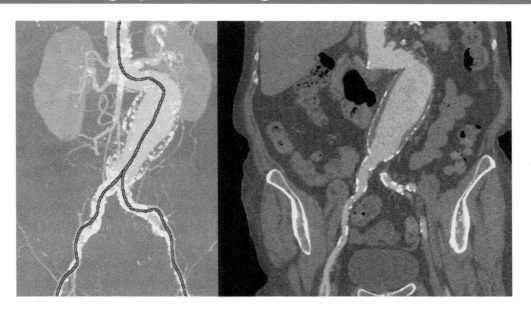

1. What defines "severe" neck angulation?

2. Severe aortic neck angulation >60 degrees
   is seen in what percentage of AAAs?

3. What is the effect of neck angulation
   on outcome?

4. What are treatment strategies for dealing
   with severe neck angulation?

5. What defines "severe" iliac tortuosity?

Case ranking/difficulty:

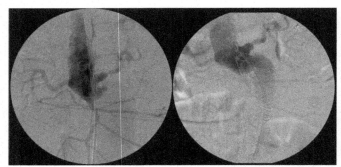

Endovascular aneurysm repair (EVAR) angiograms. Note the reduction in neck angulation with two stiff wires in position.

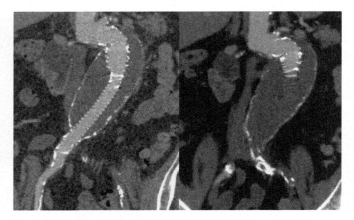

Postprocedure computed tomography demonstrating graft position at the neck and successful exclusion of the aneurysm.

Answers

1. A neck angle of 60 degrees between the neck and centerline of the aneurysm is deemed to represent severe angulation at this site. However, angulation is complex and can occur in 3 planes and also between the neck and suprarenal aorta (alpha angle) and the neck and the aneurysm sac proper (beta angle).

2. About 10% of AAAs have severe neck angulation.

3. Angled necks are associated with higher mortality, type 1 leaks, migration, and conversion, with studies reporting higher incidence of complications, particularly when some stent grafts are used off-label outside of manufacturer recommendations. Some grafts are available that can treat angulated necks of up to 90 degrees with good outcomes.

4. Severe neck angulation is seen in the region of the visceral vessels, so fenestrated grafts or chimney/snorkel techniques are probably not going to be helpful because although the proximal landing zone above the neck angulation could be used (as the visceral vessels preserved via fenestration or chimney/snorkel stents), the angulation will still be a significant problem. Hybrid repair in this situation would not confer any benefit over standard open repair.

5. Again, iliac tortuosity is complex and the CT volume should be reviewed in multiple planes. Passage of a stiff wire through the tortuosity can be a guide as to whether a device will pass. Tortuosity makes stent graft placement more challenging, and the device is harder to manipulate, as it is effectively gripped by the tortuosity of the access vessels.

Pearls

- Neck length, angulation, conicity, and diameter must be assessed to determine whether conventional EVAR is possible.
- Chimney/snorkel techniques or FEVAR may be performed if there is hostile neck anatomy.
- Though most devices recommend a neck angulation of 60 degrees, there are commercially available grafts specifically designed to treat highly angulated necks as seen in this case.

Suggested Reading

Balasubramaniam K, Hardman J, Horrocks M, Bulbulia R. The advantages of Aorfix for endovascular repair of abdominal aortic aneurysm. *J Cardiovasc Surg (Torino).* 2009;50(2):139-143.

32-year-old woman presents with sudden onset of right arm and leg weakness and global language disturbance

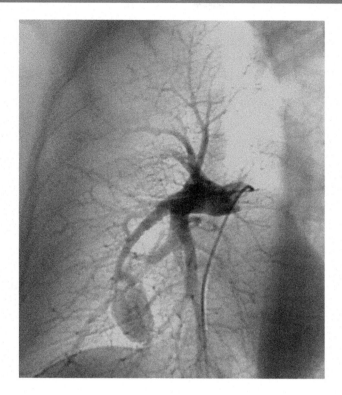

1. What is the biological basis of the underlying syndrome?

2. What 2 tests have improved outcomes in recent years?

3. What is a paradoxical embolus?

4. What are "complex" pulmonary AVMs?

5. What are indications for treatment?

Case ranking/difficulty:

Answers

1. HHT, also known as Osler-Weber-Rendu syndrome, is caused by mutations in at least 5, and perhaps 6, different genes. Patients are heterozygous for a mutation in one allele, so inheritance is autosomal-dominant. Knowing that each offspring of an affected person has a 50% risk of having inherited the condition.

2. A major advance in the past decade has been the development of genetic testing of at-risk relatives. Coupled with contrast-enhanced echocardiography, the diagnosis of HHT and PAVM has improved.

3. A PAVM bypasses the pulmonary capillary bed, providing a direct right-to-left shunt the diameter of the feeding artery. Patients may present due to paradoxical emboli with migraine, transient ischemic attack, stroke, or brain abscess. Other blood-borne infections such as osteomyelitis may result from PAVM via the same mechanism. Furthermore, paradoxical emboli can cause end-organ damage in other sensitive organs like the myocardium that are not typically recognized as PAVM-related.

4. A PAVM may be simple, with one or more feeding arteries arising from the same segmental artery, or complex, with multiple feeders from different segmental arteries. Complex PAVMs constitute approximately 10% of lesions, and a subset of these (approximately 5% of complex PAVMs) has recently been described as diffuse-type, with innumerable feeders and often lobar distribution. The diffuse-type PAVM introduces additional challenges to PAVM management, not only from an embolotherapy standpoint but also during follow-up.

5. In the 2 decades since the introduction of the "3-mm guideline," the HHT community has gradually come to the realize that PAVM with feeding arteries smaller than 3 mm also need to be treated. The 2009 HHT treatment guidelines now acknowledge that it is appropriate to treat PAVM with feeders smaller than 3 mm. The advances in technology since 1993 have dramatically improved our ability to detect and treat PAVM in this size range.

Pearls

- PAVMs are direct high-flow, low-resistance fistulous connections between pulmonary arteries and veins. The resulting right-to-left shunt can be clinically silent in small malformations, but often results in hypoxia or a variety of neurologic sequelae in larger malformations. PAVMs are most often associated with hereditary hemorrhagic telangiectasia. Patients commonly present as an incidental lung lesion. Untreated, they can present as stroke or brain abscess due to paradoxical embolization.

Suggested Reading

Trerotola SO, Pyeritz RE. PAVM embolization: an update. *AJR Am J Roentgenol.* 2010;195(4):837-845.

White RI Jr, Pollak JS, Wirth JA. Pulmonary arteriovenous malformations: diagnosis and transcatheter embolotherapy. *J Vasc Interv Radiol.* 1996;7:787-804.

15-year-old woman with history of tuberculosis presents with massive hemoptysis

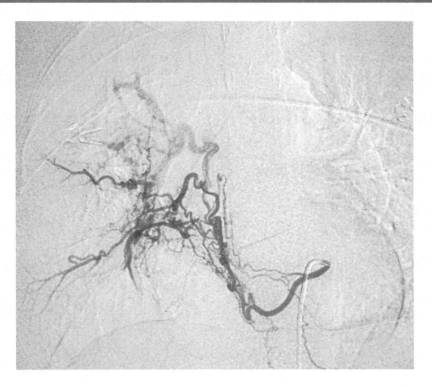

1. What is the diagnosis?

2. What embolic material can be used to treat this patient?

3. What is a Rasmussen aneurysm?

4. Where are multiple bronchial arteries more likely?

5. Where can anomalous bronchial arteries arise from?

Case ranking/difficulty:

Answers

1. Note the delayed filling of the pulmonary artery indicating a bronchial artery to pulmonary artery fistula.

2. Most operators select particle sizes ranging from 350 to 500 µm. Gelfoam is also a safe embolic agent.

3. Rasmussen aneurysm is a pulmonary artery aneurysm adjacent or within a tuberculous cavity. It occurs in up to 5% of patients with such lesions.

4. Multiple bronchial arteries are more likely on the left.

5. The internal thoracic and subclavian arteries are more common than the others.

Pearls

- Bronchial artery fistulas can form with the aorta, pulmonary circulation and have even occurred with the coronary arteries. Aortobronchial fistula usually results from primary aortic pathology. Bronchial artery to pulmonary artery fistula presents added challenges when performing embolization due to increased risk of lung infarction.
- A Rasmussen aneurysm is a pulmonary artery aneurysm.

Suggested Reading

Yon JR, Ravenel JG. Congenital bronchial artery-pulmonary artery fistula in an adult. *J Comput Assist Tomogr.* 2010;34(3):418-420.

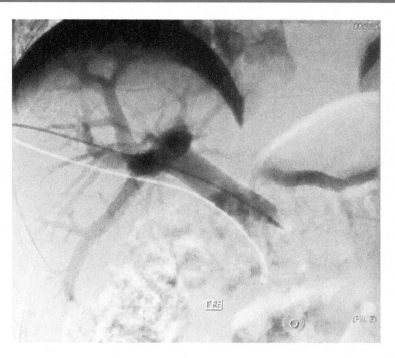

1. Islet cell transplantation is being performed. How would you perform this procedure?

2. What is the most likely complication?

3. Where should the catheter tip be positioned ideally?

4. What is the key investigation in a pre-transplant work-up?

5. Why is portal venous pressure (PVP) recorded during islets infusion?

Case ranking/difficulty:

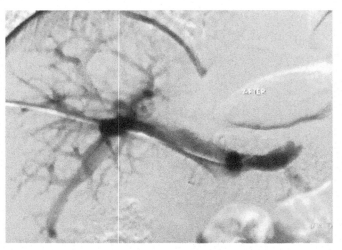

Portal venogram (frontal projection) shows a 4-F catheter tip positioned, proximal to the portal confluence.

Pearls

- Islet cell TP can treat IDDM patients with recurrent hypoglycemia/labile control/early complications despite optimal medical management.
- Purified islet cells are harvested from donor pancreas glands. The infusion is delivered into the portal vein via a transhepatic access. PVPs are recorded and heparin administered.
- The catheter and/or sheath is best sited just proximal to the confluence of the portal vein. PVP >20 mmHg is a contraindication for islet cell transplantation. If the PVP doubles or rises to 22 mmHg, the procedure should be terminated.
- There is a 3% risk of thrombosis. Focal hepatic steatosis can occur.

Answers

1. Portal vein is accessed, pressures measured, islets infused, and tract is plugged.

2. Hemorrhage due to the transhepatic access is the commonest complication.

3. The tip of the cannula is positioned within the main portal vein, just proximal to the confluence.

4. Ultrasonography is important to document the patency of the portal vein.

5. PVP is recorded intermittently. The infusion takes around 15 minutes, and there is around 7.5 mL of tissue in 250 mL of medium. The procedure is terminated if the pressure is more than 20 mmHg at the start, or doubles or rises to above 22 mmHg.

Suggested Reading

Gaba RC, Garcia-Roca R, Oberholzer J. Pancreatic islet cell transplantation: an update for interventional radiologists. *J Vasc Interv Radiol.* 2012;23(5):583-594.

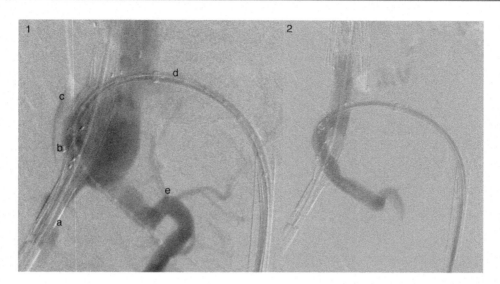

1. Review the image and name (a) to (e).

2. Which are advantages of branched iliac grafts?

3. What are important design features of vascular sheaths?

4. What are the complications of branched iliac repair?

5. What are the incidences of ischemic complications after internal iliac artery embolization?

Case ranking/difficulty: **Category:** Arterial system

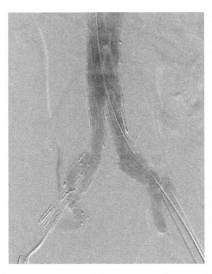

Completion angiogram showing exclusion of the aneurysm and patency of both internal iliac arteries.

Answers

1. A to E are as above. The use of the terms ipsilateral and contralateral are relative to the main device and are useful terms to aid communication when planning or during the case.

2. These grafts incur higher costs, suitability is limited, and planning can be complex.

3. Hemostatic valves are design features of a sheath; otherwise, it could be called a guiding catheter. French (Fr) size refers to the inner diameter of a sheath, so a 6-Fr sheath will accommodate a 6-Fr catheter. Long sheaths provide support, and sheaths can be used coaxially. A buddy wire alongside another catheter/wire, etc, will provide additional support. Sheaths can be reinforced or angled and have differing tapered introducers. Know your equipment and use the right tool for the right job!

4. Iliac branch repairs have similar complications to EVAR. The bridging stents can occlude and this may be related to tortuosity. Self-expanding and balloon-mounted stents can be used, or a combination of both can be used, should a stent appear kinked at deployment during the primary procedure.

5. Buttock claudication occurs in 20%, impotence is less likely, and bowel ischemia is very rare.

Pearls

- Branched iliac grafts preserve flow into the internal iliac artery. This reduces potential ischemic complications which include buttock claudication, bowel ischemia, and spinal ischemia.
- The ipsilateral bifurcation module has an indwelling catheter loaded through the side branch. This is used to cross over and the wire is snared. There is then a through-and-through access wire, which then allows a sheath to be placed from the contralateral side, over the bifurcation and into the side branch and then on into the internal iliac artery. A covered bridging stent is then deployed that forms a seal between the side branch and the native internal artery.

Suggested Reading

Paraskevas K, Möllendorf C, Fernandes E, Fernandes R, Tielliu I, Verhoeven E. EVAR for aortoiliac aneurysms, including iliac branched grafts. *J Cardiovasc Surg (Torino)*. 2012;53(1 Suppl 1):67-72.

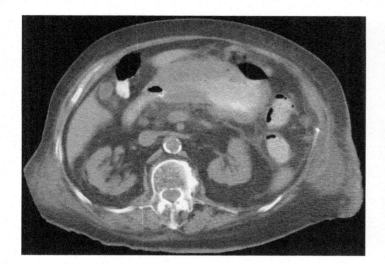

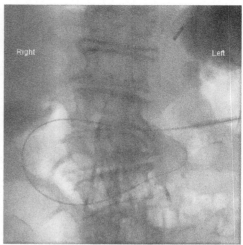

1. What is the goal of stenting in malignant gastric outlet obstruction?

2. What are potential complications?

3. What is mean survival after stenting in this situation?

4. How should the gastric access be obtained?

5. Describe the anatomy of the duodenum.

Case ranking/difficulty:

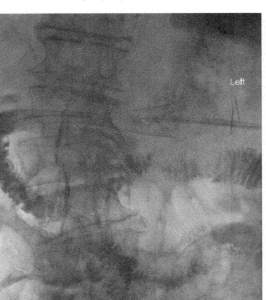

Stent placement.

Suggested Reading

Nadır I, Parlak E, Küçükay F, et al. Palliative treatment of malignant gastroduodenal obstruction: applications of self-expandable metal stent. *Turk J Gastroenterol.* 2011;22(1):6-9.

Answers

1. The aim of treatment is to improve quality of life.

2. Bleeding and perforation can complicate gastroduodenal stenting. Stent obstruction and stent migration can occur. Obstructed stents can be cleared with endoscopic techniques. Migration can occur in 10% and may require repeat stenting.

3. Patient survival is of the order of 90 days, as by time of presentation, they already have advanced upper gastrointestinal malignant disease.

4. Percutaneously and pointing toward the pylorus. Conventional access for RIG is directed at the fundus and this points away from the obstruction, and leads to looping and makes the procedure technically challenging.

5. The duodenum has 4 parts and is derived from the foregut and midgut, and is 25 to 38 cm in length. The major and minor papilla open onto the duodenal surface. Duodenal diverticulum is a relatively common variant.

57-year-old man with colorectal carcinoma and hepatic metastases who presents for portal vein embolization

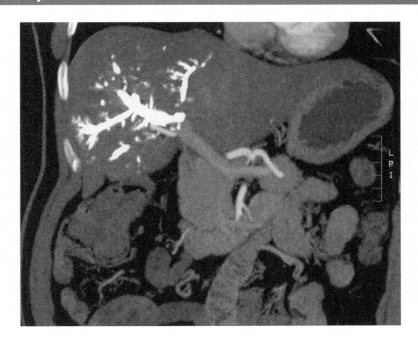

1. Which embolic agent has been used?

2. What are the advantages of this agent?

3. What are disadvantages of this agent?

4. Name other liquid agents?

5. What is effect of adding lipiodol?

Case ranking/difficulty:

Answers

1. Cyanoacrylate glue has been used. "Glue" commonly refers to the use of *n*-butyl-2-cyanoacrylate (*n*-BCA).

2. Glue is mixed with iodized oil and is relatively cheap.

3. Glue can stick to catheters and is not pre-mixed. Contact with normal saline and blood must be avoided until injection. Catheters are therefore flushed with D5W. Test angiograms with 0.1 to 0.6 mL of contrast can be performed to guide the volume required for embolization.

4. Onyx and ethanol are other liquid embolics. Sodium tetradecyl sulfate is also a liquid but is often used as a foam.

5. The ratio of n-BCA to lipiodol at 1:1 means the mixture will polymerize in around 1 second. A more dilute 1:4 mixture will polymerize in around 4 seconds. Lipiodol also makes the glue mixture radio-opaque.

Pearls

- Glue is another useful tool for the interventional radiologist.
- Liquid embolic agents have many advantages, but require some experience to use safely.
- Glue polymerizes on contact with ionic solutions and so contact with blood must be avoided and catheters should be flushed and handled with D5W. Glue is mixed with lipiodol in various ratios such as 1:1 and 1:4.

Suggested Reading

Pollak JS, White RI. The use of cyanoacrylate adhesives in peripheral embolization. *J Vasc Interv Radiol.* 2001;12(8):907-913.

16-year-old female adolescent presents for treatment of a venous malformation

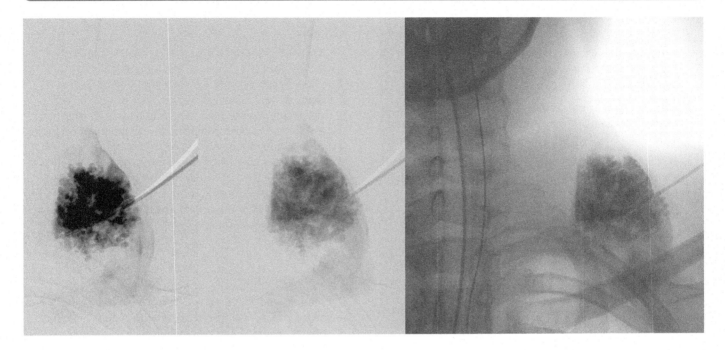

1. Where around the body are venous malformations found?

2. What are the relative roles of ultrasound and MRI and angiography?

3. How would you perform direct phlebography and what is seen?

4. How would you perform sclerotherapy?

5. What is the clinical outcome?

Case ranking/difficulty:

Category: Venous system

Answers

1. Venous malformations are the most common, and overlying skin can have a bluish tinge, or be normal. Forty percent occur in the head and neck, 40% in the extremities, and 20% in the trunk.

2. Ultrasonography can help with diagnosis, and MRI can aid with planning of intervention by showing the extent of lesions. Angiography is not usually required.

3. It is performed with a 20- or 21-G needle. Access can be facilitated with ultrasound guidance. Contrast medium can be injected when blood is aspirated. Common patterns seen are (a) cavitatory patterns with late venous drainage, (b) honeycombing pattern with late venous drainage, and (c) more rarely rapid drainage via dysmorphic veins.

4. Treatment decisions should be made in a multidisciplinary setting. Sodium tetradecyl sulfate is used as a sclerosant, and volume is determined by the intial phlebogram. Application of manual compression or a tourniquet can minimize distal passage of the sclerosant.

5. Lesions can become inflamed after and there is a risk of cutaneous necrosis. Treatment is frequently performed in stages.

Pearls

- Vascular malformations cover a broad spectrum of subtypes and can occur throughout the body. Classification systems are supported by clinical, imaging, and histologic factors. The Mulliken and Glowacki classification is helpful and divides lesions firstly into vascular tumors and vascular malformations. Another important classification is that made in 1992 by the International Society for the Study of Vascular Anomalies. This classifies malformations into low-flow subtypes (venous, capillary, lymphatic, and combinations of the above) and high-flow lesions like arteriovenous fistulas and arteriovenous malformations.

Suggested Reading

Dubois J, Soulez G, Oliva VL, Berthiaume MJ, Lapierre C, Therasse E. Soft-tissue venous malformations in adult patients: imaging and therapeutic issues. *Radiographics.* 2007;21(6):1519-1531.

39-year-old man who is hemodialysis dependent is known to have exhausted venous accesses with bilateral occluded upper and lower body central venous occlusions

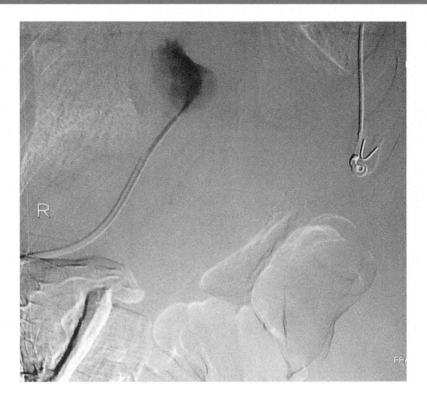

1. What procedure has been done?

2. When this procedure is indicated?

3. What are recognized complications?

4. What is the most common postprocedure complication specific to transhepatic placement?

5. When would this procedure be contraindicated?

Case ranking/difficulty:

Category: Venous system

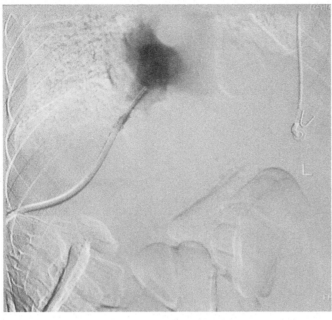

The transhepatic dialysis catheter has been placed with the tip positioned in the right atrium.

Answers

1. Transhepatic venous access for dialysis.

2. Transhepatic catheter access for hemodialysis is an alternative way in patients with limited options. Patients may have exhausted central venous accesses due to multiple past cannulations for temporary or permanent dialysis catheters.

3. Bleeding, infection, bacteremia, dysfunction, and occlusion.

4. Line dysfunction and infection remain significant complications. The hepatic venous system is a low-pressure system and so if a catheter is to be removed, it is simply pulled and access site pressure is sufficient.

5. The contraindications to placement are coagulopathy and ascites. Patent upper inferior cava and hepatic veins are required. The presence of liver lesions is only a relative contraindication.

Pearls

- Percutaneous transhepatic venous access for hemodialysis is an alternative route for patients with end-stage renal failure who have exhausted central venous accesses, particularly in the upper body.
- Early failure (≤7 days after placement) requires catheter exchange. Bleeding is the most common postprocedure complication, which we also noted in our case and it is the main cause of procedure-related death.

Suggested Readings

Smith TP, Ryan JM, Reddan DN. Transhepatic catheter access for hemodialysis. *Radiology.* 2004;232:246-251.

Stavropoulos SW, Pan JJ, Clark TWI, et al. Percutaneous transhepatic venous access for hemodialysis. *J Vasc Interv Radiol.* 2003;14:1187-1190.

69-year-old man with abnormal finding on a post–endovascular aneurysm repair (EVAR) surveillance computed tomography (CT)

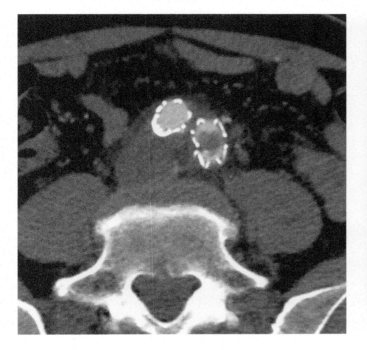 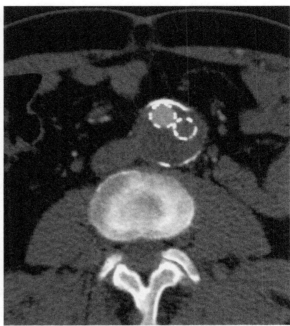

1. Review the images, what has happened and how can it present?

2. What is the rate of limb occlusion?

3. What are risk factors for limb occlusion?

4. What can be done to reduce the risk?

5. Is limb occlusion an early or late phenomenon?

Case ranking/difficulty: 🐢 🐢 🐢

Category: Arterial system

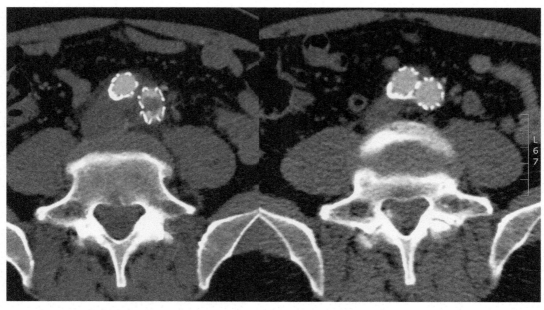

In fact, the thrombosis initially resolved after anticoagulation.

Answers

1. There is some thrombus in the limb that has progressed to frank occlusion. Limb occlusion can present with acute ischemia, rest pain, or buttock claudication but can be asymptomatic.

2. Large series report a limb occlusion rate of 3% to 5% and even up to 7% in older studies. This rate is around 1% to 3% in the common iliac artery (CIA) and up to 8% in the external iliac artery (EIA).

3. Kinked limbs, older stent graft generations, younger patients, and small-caliber grafts in external iliac arteries are associated with limb occlusion.

4. Device selection is key as some endografts are specifically designed and tailored to be placed through iliac tortuosity. Aorto-uni-iliac grafts may be beneficial when there is a narrow bifurcation that would put limbs at risk. Similarly, planning to have the main device up the ipsilateral or contralateral side and positioning of the gate can aid with the lie of the larger iliac limb. Adjunctive bare metal stenting may be required at points of angulation.

5. Limb occlusion can occur early or late but is increasingly seen as an early complication that occurs within a few months after the primary procedure. It is possible that this is due to unrecognized technical factors like kinking and placement of grafts through stenotic lesions or through a narrow aortic bifurcation.

Pearls

• Active graft surveillance is important in the management of post-EVAR patients. This tends to be performed with computed tomography or ultrasonography. Plain radiographs can complement an ultrasonographic surveillance programme. Stent graft limbs appear to have a higher rate of occlusion when extended into the EIA due to compression or kinking. Treatment options include conservative management, femoral–femoral crossover graft, axillofemoral bypass, thrombectomy, and stenting. In this case, thrombus was seen during routine surveillance and no limb kinking of stenosis was seen. The patient was anticoagulated and the thrombus cleared. Later, on routine ultrasonographic surveillance, the limb occluded despite anticoagulation!

Suggested Reading

Cochennec F, Becquemin JP, Desgranges P, Allaire E, Kobeiter H, Roudot-Thoraval F. Limb graft occlusion following EVAR: clinical pattern, outcomes and predictive factors of occurrence. *Eur J Vasc Endovasc Surg.* 2007;34(1):59-65.

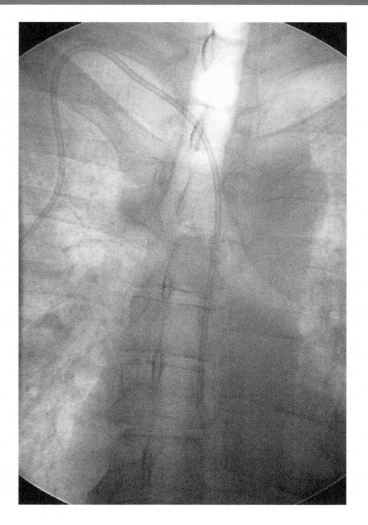

1. Where is the line?

2. What would you do?

3. What are risk factors for this complication?

4. What happens when central lines are placed into the pleural space?

5. List complications of arterial placement of large-bore central venous catheters.

Case ranking/difficulty: 🐾🐾🐾   **Category:** Venous system

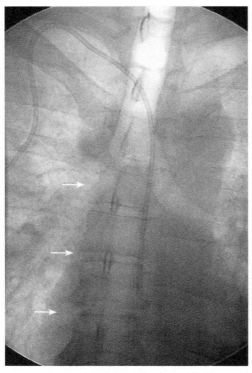

Spot fluoroscopic image after line placement. Arrows indicate the expected course of a central line.

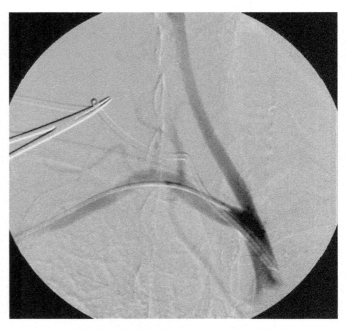

Angiogram demonstrates the line entering the subclavian artery.

Answers

1. The central line crosses the midline to lie on the left side of the vertebra, suggesting it is arterial.

2. Stop using the line immediately. Air or thrombus could potentially cause a stroke. A computed tomography would help delineate where the line is. The line can then be removed under prolonged balloon tamponade with vascular surgical support. Manual compression alone is associated with poor outcomes—stroke, airway obstruction, pseudoaneurysm, and death.

3. Lack of ultrasound guidance, high body mass index (BMI), emergency procedures, and multiple attempts at gaining access have been cited as risk factors for inadvertent arterial access.

4. Massive pleural effusion occurs rapidly.

5. Complications include pseudoaneurysm and arteriovenous fistula formation, arterial embolus and stroke, mediastinal hematoma, and airway compromise.

Pearls

- Consequences of inadvertent arterial placement of a central venous catheter can be severe and cause stroke or death.
- Ultrasound-guided access is recommended for all central line placements. Nevertheless, arterial puncture can still occur.
- A high BMI, multiple passes and attempts at line placement, previous surgery of and radiotherapy to the site, and coagulopathy are predictors of complications.
- Simple removal of the catheter carries high risk of hemorrhagic complications. Open surgical or endovascular-assisted retrieval is recommended.

Suggested Reading

Guilbert M-C, Elkouri S, Bracco D, et al. Arterial trauma during central venous catheter insertion: case series, review and proposed algorithm. *J Vasc Surg.* 2008;48(4):918-925; discussion 925.

54-year-old man who is status post coronary artery stent presents with sudden onset of right leg claudication

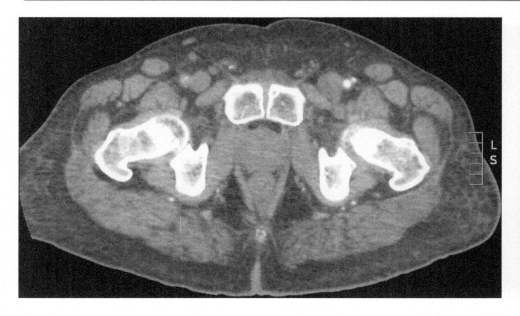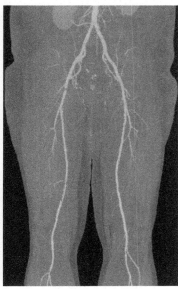

1. Review the image—where are the abnormalities?

2. What is the cause of the patient's symptoms?

3. Arterial closure devices are better than manual compression—true or false?

4. List some advantages of closure devices.

5. List some disadvantages of closure devices.

Case ranking/difficulty: **Category:** Arterial system

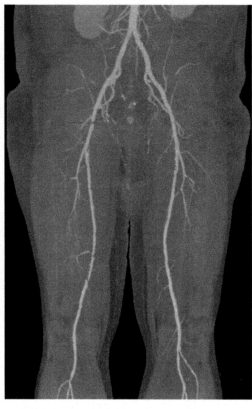

Maximum intensity projection (MIP) image.

3. Meta-analyses have found no significant statistical difference in reduction of complications. There is also no robust data to suggest discharge is improved. Data is indeterminate for patients on anticoagulation, obese patients, and for antegrade punctures.

4. Faster patient turnover. Faster patient recovery. Obviates need for manual compression.

5. Failure of closure still require manual compression. There are severe complications directly associated with the closure device such as vascular occlusion. Some devices stipulate that the arterial cannot be reaccessed immediately.

Pearls

- Closure devices can lead to major complications such as vessel occlusion, vessel dissection, and pseudoaneurysm formation. There are several commercially available closure devices, and appropriate operator experience is required for their use.
- There is no convincing data that arterial closure devices are safer, or in fact lead to earlier discharge.

Answers

1. The common femoral artery appears occluded and there is right superficial femoral artery (SFA) disease.

2. It is likely that the closure device has caused occlusion of the common femoral artery leading to the acute onset of claudication. The SFA disease is longstanding.

Suggested Readings

Das R, Ahmed K, Athanasiou T, Morgan RA, Belli AM. Arterial closure devices versus manual compression for femoral hemostasis in interventional radiological procedures: a systematic review and meta-analysis. *Cardiovasc Intervent Radiol.* 2011;34(4):723-738.

Reekers JA, Müller-Hülsbeck S, Libicher M, et al. CIRSE vascular closure device registry. *Cardiovasc Intervent Radiol.* 2011;34(1):50-53.

55-year-old-man with refractory hypertension presents for renal sympathetic denervation

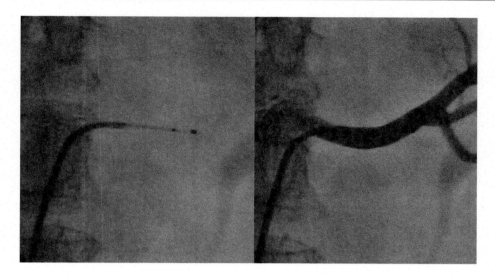

1. What is the definition of refractory hypertension?

2. Which arteries should be treated?

3. Which medications are needed for the procedure?

4. When does hypertension respond?

5. What are potential complications?

Case ranking/difficulty: **Category:** Arterial system

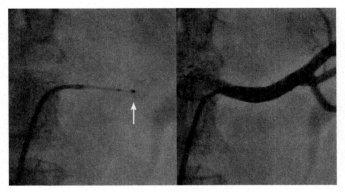

Fluoroscopy and contrast puff showing catheter tip position.

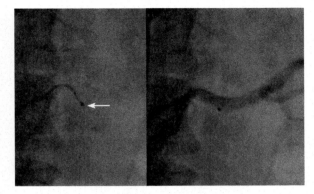

Fluoroscopy and contrast puff showing deflected catheter tip position.

Answers

1. Refractory hypertension occurs where the blood pressure (BP) is above 160/90 despite 3 oral medications and where secondary causes of hypertension have been excluded.

2. Both renal arteries need to be treated and possibly also large accessory renal arteries. Guidelines recommend that the renal artery should be 2 cm in length. These recommendations are in place to ensure that adequate ablation occurs to keep a high treatment response rate at around 85%-90%.

3. Nitrates are recommended to avoid renal artery spasm. Sedoanalgesia is recommended, as the ablation can cause some discomfort. Atropine is required should there be a bradycardic reaction.

4. There is a gradual decrease in blood pressure that is seen to occur over weeks and months, and the patient should have regular follow-up with an appropriate physician with an interest in hypertension.

5. Renal artery dissection is rare, but operators should be competent at managing this complication with renal stent placement. Hypotension can occur in 1%. Groin access complications are probably the most significant, highlighting the low-risk nature of this procedure.

Pearls

- Renal sympathetic denervation is a new alternative for treating refractory hypertension.
- Denervation catheters are placed into the renal arteries. Low-power radiofrequency ablations pass through the arterial wall and ablate the sympathetic nerves. Four to 6 ablations (each of 2-minute duration) are applied in sites that are longitudinally and rotationally separated.
- This appears to cause a decrease in blood pressure of 30/10 mmHg in patients with refractory hypertension that is sustained at 2 years. Long-term data are awaited.

Suggested Reading

Sapoval M, Azizi M, Bobrie G, Cholley B, Pagny JY, Plouin PF. Endovascular renal artery denervation: why, when, and how? *Cardiovasc Intervent Radiol.* 2012;35(3):463-471.

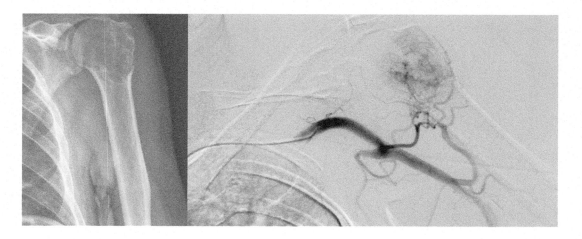

1. What sites may benefit from preoperative embolization?

2. Which tumors can cause hypervascular bone metastases?

3. What embolic agent would you use?

4. What are the advantages of pre-operative embolization?

5. What are disadvantages of pre-operative embolization?

Case ranking/difficulty: Category: Arterial system

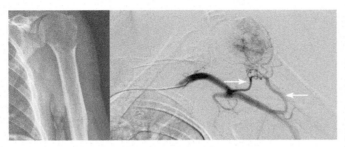

Plain radiograph and nonselective angiogram.

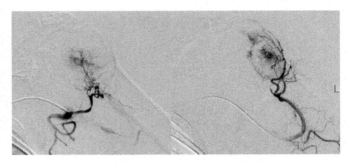

Selective angiograms of the feeding branches.

Answers

1. Surgery to lesions affecting the spine, long bones, and pelvis may particularly benefit from preoperative embolization.

2. Metastases from the above primary malignancies have been reported to have been embolized.

3. Gelfoam or medium-to-large particles would be the agent of choice. These would cause occlusion of the feeding vessels. Recanalization seen with gelatin sponge (Gelfoam) would not be an issue as the procedure would generally be performed in the (immediate) preoperative period. Smaller particles may increase the risk of nontarget embolization due to the presence of arteriovenous (AV) shunts. Trisacryl gelatin microspheres have been reported to be superior to polyvinyl alcohol (PVA) particles in one study. Coils have been reported to be ineffective as collateral channels can open within hours.

4. It can help by reducing vascularity in the operative field, it may be cost-effective, and it may reduce transfusion requirement.

5. It can be painful, and complications of angiography and embolization such as non-target embolization, pain, infection, and post-embolization syndrome can occur. Ideally, pre-operative embolization procedures are well co-ordinated with the timing of the surgical procedure.

Pearls

- Preoperative embolization of hypervascular bone metastases can facilitate challenging surgery improving clarity in the operating field. It may result in less intraoperative blood loss and is embolization associated with less intraoperative blood transfusions.
- Gelfoam or PVA particles may be used as the embolic agent. Medium-to-large particles in the order of 500 μm may be favorable, as there may be significant AV shunting through the tumor.
- The procedure should be coordinated with surgery, as the embolization itself can cause some pain. Complications include those related to arterial access, nontarget embolization, postembolization syndrome, abscess formation, and neurologic injury.

Suggested Readings

Chatziioannou AN, Johnson ME, Pneumaticos SG, Lawrence DD, Carrasco CH. Preoperative embolization of bone metastases from renal cell carcinoma. *Eur Radiol.* 2000;10(4):593-596.

Kickuth R, Waldherr C, Hoppe H, et al. Interventional management of hypervascular osseous metastasis: role of embolotherapy before orthopedic tumor resection and bone stabilization. *AJR Am J Roentgenol.* 2008;191(6):W240-W247.

Kwon JH, Shin JH, et al. Preoperative transcatheter arterial embolization of hypervascular metastatic tumors of long bones. *Acta Radiol.* 2010;51(4):396-401.

53-year-old man presenting for transarterial chemoembolization (TACE) for hepatocellular carcinoma (HCC), planning computed tomographic angiography (CTA) is performed

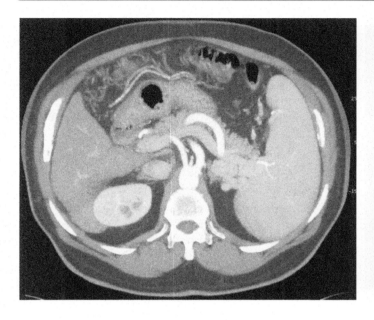
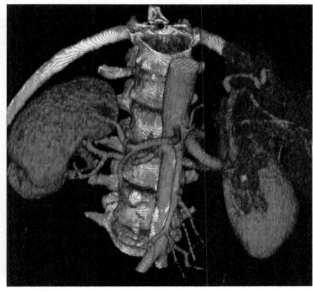

1. Review the 2 images, what do you notice?

2. Do you know any classifications of hepatic arterial anatomy?

3. Consider the advantages of knowing the vascular anatomy prior to an intervention such as TACE.

4. What other vessels might supply a hepatic lesion?

5. How could you go about studying the variations of hepatic arterial supply?

Case ranking/difficulty: **Category:** Arterial system

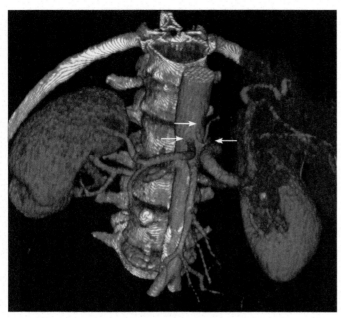

Volume-rendered reconstruction.

Answers

1. There are separate aortic origins of the left gastric artery, common hepatic artery, splenic artery, and the superior mesenteric artery (SMA).

2. Below is Michel's classification, derived from a series of 200 autopsies. This information has been largely replicated by large series that have reviewed transplant operations, angiograms, and CT scans. (1) Normal, 55%. (2) Replaced left hepatic artery (LHA) from left gastric artery (LGA), 10%. (3) Replaced right hepatic artery (RHA) from SMA, 11%. (4) Replaced LHA from LGA and replaced RHA from SMA, 1%. (5) Accessory LHA from LGA, 8%. (6) Accessory RHA from SMA, 7%. (7) Accessory LHA and accessory RHA, 1%. (8) Accessory LHA and replaced RHA, or accessory RHA and LHA, 2%. (9) Common hepatic artery (CHA) from SMA, 4.5%. (10) CHA from LGA, 0.5%.

3. Use of contrast medium can be reduced, as flush aortography may not be required because vessels can be selected directly. Knowledge of the angles and take-offs of vessels can aid catheter selection. Knowing angles

and take-offs can also aid planning tube angulation and projection of angiograms, which can reduce dose. Reviewing for the presence of significant atherosclerotic disease, iliac tortuosity, and aneurysmal disease can also facilitate a smoother TACE with the use of a long sheath that would improve catheter control. Understanding the variations and supply to the lesion increases the technical success of the procedure, reduces complications, reduces equipment cost, saves time, contrast dose, and radiation dose.

4. The cystic artery, the inferior phrenics, and intercostals, can be recruited to supply hepatic tumors. These vessels can also be reviewed on a pretreatment CTA.

5. Cadaveric studies/dissection, details at transplant and surgery, angiograms, and CTAs have been reviewed in large numbers and reported in the literature.

Pearls

- Any cross-sectional study must be reviewed prior to intervention. This process facilitates catheter selection, choice of tube angulation and projections and saves contrast medium, saves time, and reduces potential complications.
- The Michel's classification is commonly cited but is not comprehensive. This can be simplified conceptually (think: "50 normal, 40 replaced/accessory, 10 other"). About 50% of people have typical textbook hepatic artery anatomy. LHAs can arise from the LGA, and the RHAs can arise from the SMA (and these can be accessory or replaced)—these variations may account for up to 40%. Then the other variations, such as a replaced CHA, direct aortic, and other celiac variations can account for another 10%.

Suggested Readings

Michels NA. Newer anatomy of the liver and its variant blood supply and collateral circulation. *Am J Surg.* 1966;112(3):337-347.

Yi S-Q, Terayama H, Naito M, et al. Absence of the celiac trunk: case report and review of the literature. *Clin Anat.* 2008;21(4):283-286.

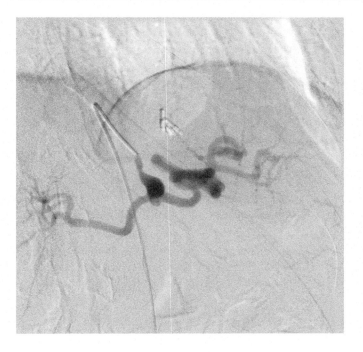
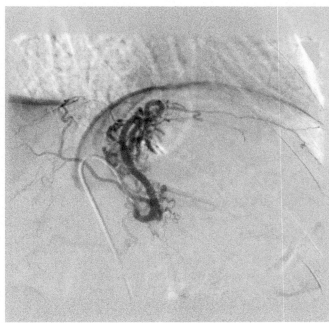

1. Describe the findings in the angiograms.

2. These lesions only occur in the stomach—true or false?

3. Describe the arterial supply to the stomach.

4. List some techniques for reforming a reverse curve catheter.

5. How would you go about selectively catheterizing the left gastric artery?

Case ranking/difficulty: **Category:** Arterial system

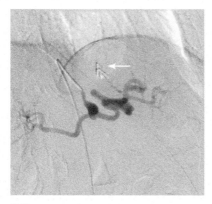

Celiac angiogram.

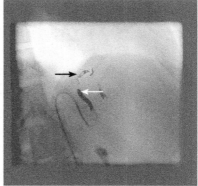

Postembolization image demonstrating stasis in the vascular arcade.

Answers

1. There is a selective celiac angiogram demonstrating a normal splenic artery. The origin of the left gastric artery is not seen. The selective left gastric angiogram demonstrates a tortuous and ectatic appearance of the left gastric artery. There is no evidence of active extravasation. There is no evidence of early venous filling. Endoscopic clips are also noted.

2. False, they can occur anywhere in the gastrointestinal (GI) tract.

3. The arteries that run in the lesser curve are the left and right gastric arteries (LGA and RGA). The LGA most commonly arises from the celiac trunk. Although the origin of the RGA is variable, it most commonly arises from the common hepatic artery. The arteries, which course along the greater curve, are the gastroepiploic (GE) arteries. The right GE artery is a branch of the gastroduodenal artery, whereas the left GE and short gastric arteries are branches of the splenic artery.

4. The reverse curve catheters can be reformed in several ways—reflected off the aortic valve, turned in the descending thoracic aorta against the arch, or reformed over the aortic bifurcation or using a renal artery (where the natural 90-degree bends facilitate reforming the catheter).

5. Any available preprocedural imaging should be reviewed. A computed tomographic (CT) angiogram should be carefully reviewed to look for the origins and orientation of the vessels. An aortogram, or lateral aortogram, can be useful to demonstrate the origins. Selective celiac trunk angiogram can be performed. Some operators prefer reverse curve catheters (eg, Simmonds). However, a Cobra or glide Cobra can be used in conjunction with a hydrophilic glidewire, particularly if there is a somewhat vertical origin of the left gastric from the celiac trunk. A microcatheter

can also facilitate selecting the LGA. In this case, the Simmonds catheter was used as the host catheter, and a microcatheter was used to select the LGA.

Pearls

- Dieulafoy lesions are a rare cause of bleeding and are potentially life threatening. The classic clinical presentation is with recurrent, massive GI bleeding.
- Hemorrhage occurs from an abnormally enlarged and eroded submucosal artery, most commonly located in the proximal stomach.
- Endoscopy is the mainstay of diagnosis and treatment.
- Angiographic findings include tortuous ectatic arteries without early venous return. (Angiographic finding of abnormal arteries with early venous filling of normal veins would indicate angiodysplasia.) The abnormal vessels can arise from the LGA or splenic artery.
- There is no consensus regarding embolization technique. We elected to coil the proximal and distal end of this arcade, and there has been no recurrence of the bleeding. Success with Gelfoam, particles, and coils has been reported.

Suggested Readings

Alshumrani G, Almuaikeel M. Angiographic findings and endovascular embolization in Dieulafoy disease: a case report and literature review. *Diagn Interv Radiol.* 2006;12(3):151-154.

Ashour MA, Millward SF, Hadziomerovic A. Embolotherapy of a Dieulafoy lesion in the cecum: case report and review of the literature. *J Vasc Interv Radiol.* 2000;11(8):1059-1062.

Baxter M, Aly EH. Dieulafoy's lesion: current trends in diagnosis and management. *Ann R Coll Surg Engl.* 2010;92(7):548-554.

42-year-old man with a history of cirrhosis undergoes paracentesis at the bedside. He rapidly becomes hypotensive

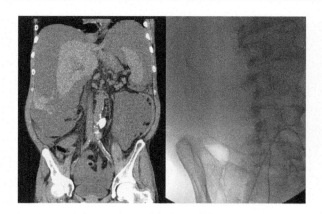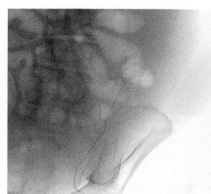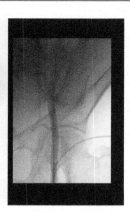

1. List some possible causes of inferior epigastric artery (IEA) injury.

2. Why might injury to this artery be more serious after paracentesis?

3. The inferior epigastric artery arises from the common femoral artery—true or false?

4. Which artery is referred to in this case—superficial or deep inferior epigastric artery?

5. What are the cardinal features and management of rectus sheath hematomas?

Case ranking/difficulty: 🏵🏵🏵

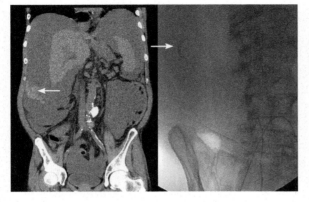

Right selective inferior epigastric artery angiogram from a contralateral "up and over" approach. Prior computed tomographic scan helped to localize the abnormality.

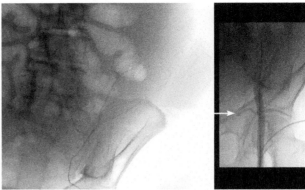

Left selective inferior epigastric angiogram from an ipsilateral access.

Answers

1. IEA injury can occur as a result of surgery, laparoscopic port insertion, percutaneous drain placement, or paracentesis. Blunt trauma is another cause. Bleeding can occur spontaneously in patients on Coumadin.

2. Hemorrhage occurring into ascites can accumulate rapidly, as there is no tamponade effect that might happen in the retroperitoneum or within the rectus sheath, all of which are sites for development of a hematoma after IEA injury.

3. False, the IEA arises from the external iliac artery. It takes a characteristic curved course as it passes the medial aspect of the inguinal ring, before piercing the transversalis fascia and entering the rectus sheath. It anastomoses with the lower intercostals and the superior epigastric branch of the internal thoracic artery.

4. This case refers to the deep IEA. There is also a superficial IEA that is a direct cutaneous branch of the common femoral artery. Knowledge of these arteries is important for radiologists involved in planning flap reconstructions such as the deep inferior epigastric perforator (DIEP) flap.

5. It can be an underrecognized cause of abdominal pain and usually occurs spontaneously in anticoagulated patients as is usually due to a muscle tear rather than a vascular injury. Intervention is rarely required.

Pearls

• IEA injury is rare. It can be life threatening, particularly in patients with coagulopathy and ascites, where there is no tamponade effect. Injury can occur after paracentesis, laparoscopic port placement, and percutaneous drain placement. Blunt trauma is another cause.

Suggested Readings

Park SW, Ko SY, et al. Transcatheter arterial embolization for hemoperitoneum: unusual manifestation of iatrogenic injury to abdominal muscular arteries. *Abdom Imaging.* 2011;36(1):74-78.

Sobkin PR, Bloom AI, Wilson MW, et al. Massive abdominal wall hemorrhage from injury to the inferior epigastric artery: a retrospective review. *J Vasc Interv Radiol.* 2008;19(3):327-332.

Yalamanchili S, Harvey SM, Friedman A, Shams JN, Silberzweig JE. Transarterial embolization for inferior epigastric artery injury. *Vasc Endovascular Surg.* 2008;42(5):489-493.

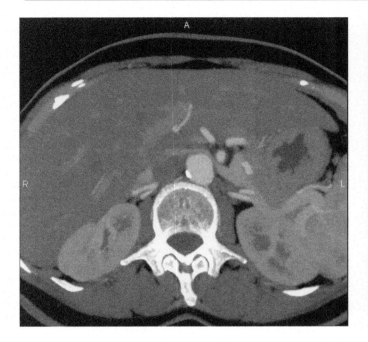
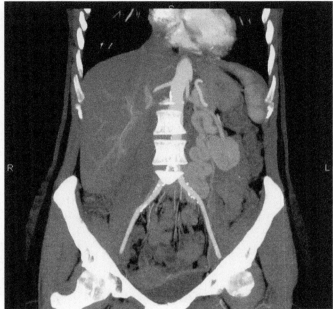

1. What is the condition?

2. This condition is due to what?

3. What features are seen in its clinical presentation?

4. What are treatment options?

5. What is traditionally the gold standard for diagnosis?

Case ranking/difficulty: 🌰 🌰 🌰

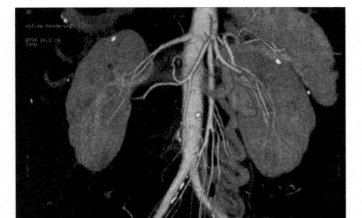

Volume-rendered image.

Answers

1. This is nutcracker syndrome.

2. Nutcracker syndrome is commonly due to compression of the left renal vein between the superior mesenteric artery (SMA) and aorta.

3. Hematuria, left flank pain, nausea, and vomiting are seen.

4. Conservative, stenting, renal vein reimplantation, and gonadal vein embolization have been performed.

5. Venogram is traditionally "gold standard."

Pearls

- The nutcracker syndrome is a clinical manifestation of the nutcracker phenomenon, where there is compression of the left renal vein, most commonly between the abdominal aorta and SMA.
- This is not to be confused with superior mesenteric artery (SMA) syndrome, which is where there is compression of the third part of the duodenum by the SMA and abdominal aorta.

Suggested Reading

Poyraz AK, Firdolas F, Onur MR, Kocakoc E. Evaluation of left renal vein entrapment using multidetector computed tomography. *Acta Radiol.* 2013;54(2):144-148.

53-year-old woman with a history of orthotopic liver transplant presents with swollen legs bilaterally

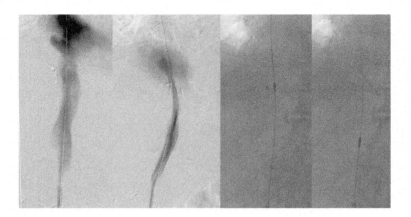

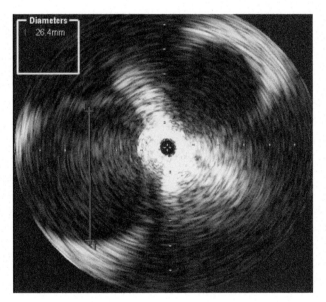

1. Review the cavagrams—is there a significant inferior vena cava (IVC) stenosis?

2. What are indications for intravascular ultrasound (IVUS)?

3. What is a typical IVUS probe frequency?

4. List some advantages of IVUS over angiography.

5. List some disadvantages of IVUS.

Case ranking/difficulty:

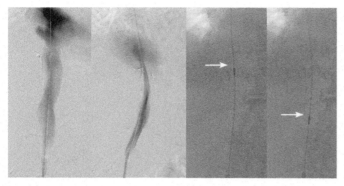

Cavagram in 2 projections and spot fluoroscopy demonstrating different positions of the probe as the cava is examined with IVUS.

Answers

1. The anteroposterior and oblique projections suggest that there may be a stenosis, but there are no significant collaterals. Pressure measurements did not demonstrate a significant pressure gradient across the narrowing. IVUS also did not demonstrate significant fixed caval stenosis.

2. There is a growing list of indications for IVUS. IVUS can aid the selection of appropriate angioplasty balloons and stents by facilitating accurate measurement. It can be used to assist percutaneous fenestration of dissection flaps, to guide filter placement, and to characterize the sites of chronic pulmonary emboli. It can be used to guide IVC filter placement, in critically ill patients at the bedside to avoid the risks of transfer, to reduce dose particularly in bariatric patients, and to avoid the use of contrast medium in selected patient groups. Cardiologic applications include the characterization of coronary atherosclerotic plaques.

3. 20 to 40 MHz.

4. Plaque and vessel wall can be imaged, and this can be done dynamically in real time.

5. Equipment and catheter cost. Increases procedural time. May require larger access than otherwise needed.

Pearls

- IVUS has many developing applications in interventional radiology and also interventional cardiology. IVUS-guided filter placement and IVUS assessment of the cava and pulmonary arteries in the setting of chronic pulmonary embolism (PE) are some indications. One particularly useful application may be the placement of IVC filters in critically ill patients at the bedside, which obviates the need for patient transfer to an intervention radiology (IR) suite or operating room (OR). IVUS probes come in a range of sizes and different arrays.

Suggested Readings

Killingsworth CD, Taylor SM, Patterson MA, et al. Prospective implementation of an algorithm for bedside intravascular ultrasound-guided filter placement in critically ill patients. *J Vasc Surg.* 2010;51(5):1215-1221.

Raju S, Hollis K, Neglen P. Obstructive lesions of the inferior vena cava: clinical features and endovenous treatment. *J Vasc Surg.* 2006;44(4):820-827.

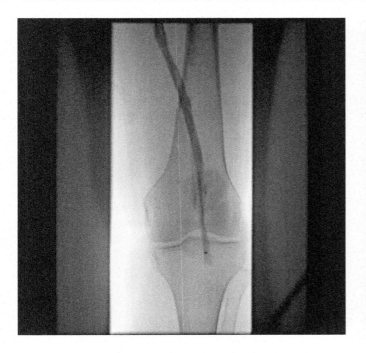
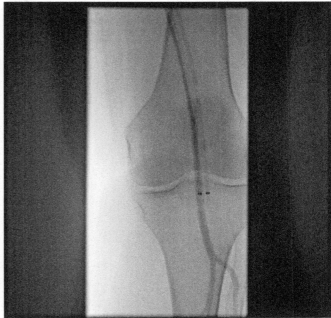

1. Where have these sheaths been placed?

2. Why?

3. What conditions are usually treated in this way?

4. What are the potential benefits of this treatment?

5. What are the complications?

Case ranking/difficulty:

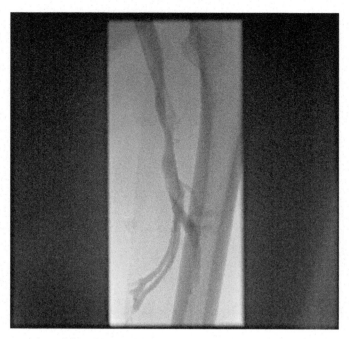

Venous collaterals and valves.

3. Melanoma and soft-tissue sarcoma.

4. Complete response and limb salvage.

5. Any complication related to arterial/venous punctures and angiography/venography can occur. Valves can potentially be damaged. Limb edema and erythema are usually self-limiting.

Pearls

- Isolated limb infusion/perfusion techniques allow the regional administration of chemotherapy. After sheath placement, patients are placed under general anesthesia and made mildly hyperthermic. This technique is used for treatment of melanoma and soft-tissue sarcoma.

Suggested Reading

Kroon HM, Moncrieff M, Kam PCA, Thompson JF. Outcomes following isolated limb infusion for melanoma. A 14-year experience. *Ann Surg Oncol.* 2008;15(11):3003-3013.

Answers

1. Popliteal artery and vein. Passing a catheter against the venous flow can be time consuming, as the guidewire does not easily cross valves and regularly finds collateral channels.

2. Isolated limb infusion allows regional chemotherapy to be administered. Cytotoxics such as melphalan or actinomycin-D as well as anti–tumor necrosis factor (TNF)-alpha can be infused.

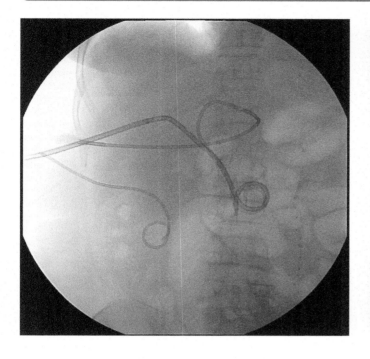
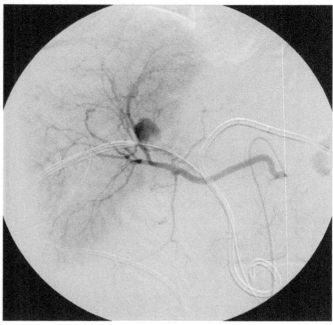

1. What are hemorrhagic complications after PTHC drain insertion?

2. How can bleeding through the biliary drain be managed?

3. What is the main disadvantage of CT in investigating post-PTHC bleeding?

4. What is the commonest cause of a hepatic artery pseudoaneurysm?

5. What is more common, splenic pseudoaneurysms or splenic aneurysms?

Case ranking/difficulty:

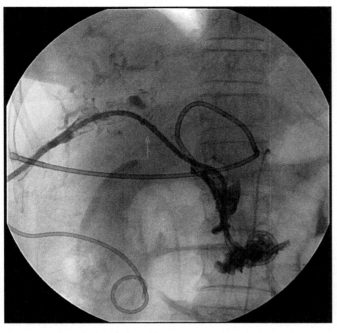

Post-coil embolization and replacement of drains.

biliary drain can be upsized. Coagulopathy should be correction. Angioembolization can be considered.

3. CT angiography can miss small pseudoaneurysm. The drain can have a tamponade effect, and so angiography may need to be performed with drains removed over access wires.

4. Hepatic artery pseudoaneurysms can occur after transplantation and they tend to be extrahepatic.

5. Pseudoaneurysms of the splenic artery are rare compared to true aneurysms. Large pseudoaneurysms tend to occur in the mid splenic artery over the body of the pancreas and are commonly associated with pancreatitis.

Pearls

• Bleeding complications occur in 2% to 3% of biliary drainage procedures. These range from subcapsular hematoma through to shock with hemobilia and resultant melena due to a hepatic artery pseudoaneurysm.

Answers

1. Subcapsular hematoma, arterioportal fistula, or hepatic artery pseudoaneurysms can occur.

2. The drain can be capped, which can lead to tamponading. Similarly, the existing internal-external

Suggested Reading

Saad WE, Dasgupta N, Lippert AJ, et al. Extrahepatic pseudoaneurysms and ruptures of the hepatic artery in liver transplant recipients: endovascular management and a new iatrogenic etiology. *Cardiovasc Intervent Radiol.* 2013;36(1):118-127.

44-year-old woman on hemodialysis with multiple failed fistulas and exhausted upper body central venous access due to multiple dialysis catheter placements presents for further line placement

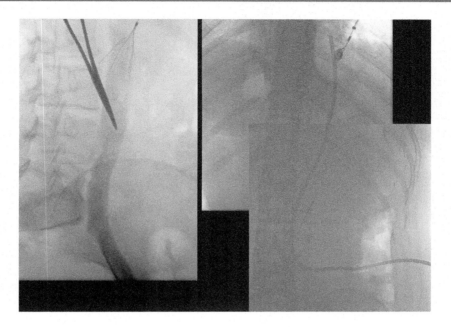

1. What is the rate of infection of dialysis catheters?

2. What is a fibrin sheath?

3. When would you recommend placement of a translumbar catheter?

4. What accesses are possible if the translumbar catheter fails?

5. What is the 1-year patency of a translumbar catheter?

Case ranking/difficulty:

Category: Venous system

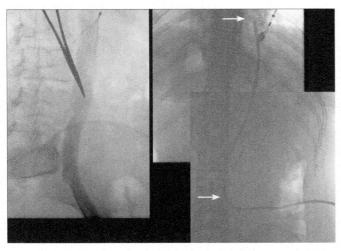

Unsubtracted venogram demonstrating the cava and bony landmarks used to facilitate percutaneous caval access. Postprocedure spot fluoroscopic images of the prone patient demonstrate the catheter in place, with its tip in the right atrium.

Answers

1. Catheter-related bloodstream infections (CRBSIs) are major causes of morbidity and mortality. Infection rates are quoted in events per 1000 catheter days. Tunneled dialysis catheters have an infection rate of 4.2 per 1000 catheter days.

2. A fibrin sheath can form around the tip of a dialysis catheter and result in malfunction. Simple catheter exchange over a guidewire does not necessarily deal with this problem. If a venogram demonstrates a fibrin sheath, after catheter removal, the fibrin sheath should be split with a standard angioplasty balloon before a new catheter is inserted.

3. Translumbar catheters are a useful and durable long-term dialysis option when traditional accesses have failed. Fistula and arteriovenous graft options as well as upper body and transfemoral central venous catheters should have been used prior to considering a translumbar catheter.

4. Transrenal and transhepatic venous accesses can also be established percutaneously.

5. One series of 26 translumbar catheters found a 1-year patency rate of 73% with a systemic bacteremia rate of 0.8 per 1000 days.

Pearls

- Translumbar venous access is resorted to when upper body and femoral access routes have been exhausted. Transrenal and transhepatic accesses can also be performed, as access to the cava itself becomes progressively lost.

Suggested Reading

Power A, Singh S, Ashby D, et al. Translumbar central venous catheters for long-term haemodialysis. *Nephrol Dial Transplant.* 2010;25(5):1588-1595.

35-year-old woman who is status post orthotopic liver transplant presents with bilateral swollen legs

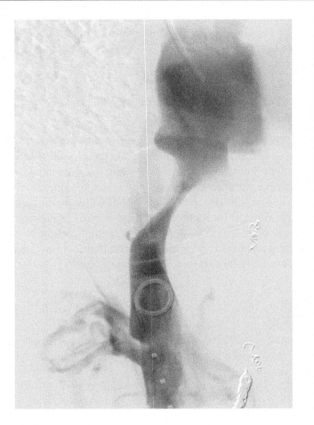 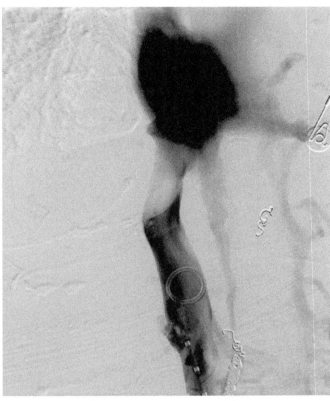

1. How can you be sure that a stenosis is genuine?

2. What is your management plan?

3. List 5 potential complications.

4. What pressure gradient indicates a stenosis?

5. What would you be concerned with, in your stent selection?

Case ranking/difficulty: **Category:** Venous system

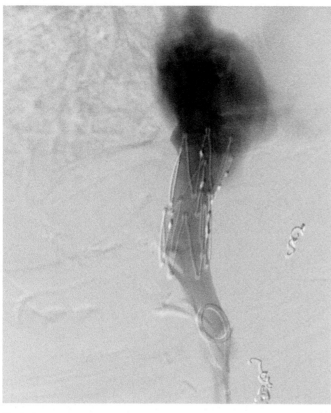

Post stent cavagram.

Answers

1. Multiple projections demonstrating a stenosis, filling of collaterals, and an elevated pressure gradient across the lesion would be indications of a true stenosis. Stenoses can be further characterized with intravascular ultrasonography.

2. A Gianturco Z stent was used in this case. Palmaz stents, Wallstents, and balloon angioplasty can also be used. Angioplasty is less favorable than stenting, as elastic recoil is commonly encountered. The inferior vena cava (IVC) has inherent elasticity; chronic stenosis may be due to fibrosis, and there may be some compressive element that requires stents to keep the lesion open. Stents are at risk of migration and may increase the risk of hepatic vein thrombosis and complicate the need for any further intervention and retransplantation.

3. Complications of IVC stenting include rupture of the anastomosis, hemopericardium, retroperitoneal hemorrhage, stent thrombosis, stent migration, and recurrent stenosis.

4. A gradient of 7 to 10 mmHg across the lesion is indicative of a significant stenosis. Posttreatment, the gradient is expected to reduce to <2 mmHg.

5. Care must be taken to choose an appropriate stent size and to avoid undersizing. The "watermelon-seed" effect describes the situation where the stent slips during placement—the analogy is that of squeezing a watermelon seed between finger and thumb, mimicking the effect of radial force within a stenosis. Z stents may be more stable than the Wallstent. Percutaneous stent retrieval is possible, but open thoracotomy may ultimately be required.

Pearls

- Stenosis of the IVC is a rare complication of liver transplantation, reported to occur in less than 3% of cases.
- Caval stenosis can be an early or late complication.
- Because of outflow obstruction, renal dysfunction, ascites, and lower limb edema can also occur. Mismatch of donor to recipient caval size, kinking, and repeat transplantation are risk factors. Stent placement may be favorable to angioplasty, if the stenosis is functional due to kinking or tortuosity.

Suggested Readings

Borsa JJ, Daly CP, Fontaine AB, et al. Treatment of inferior vena cava anastomotic stenoses with the Wallstent endoprosthesis after orthotopic liver transplantation. *J Vasc Interv Radiol.* 1999;10(1):17-22.

Guimarães M, Uflacker R, Schönholz C, Hannegan C, Selby JB. Stent migration complicating treatment of inferior vena cava stenosis after orthotopic liver transplantation. *J Vasc Interv Radiol.* 2005;16(9):1247-1252.

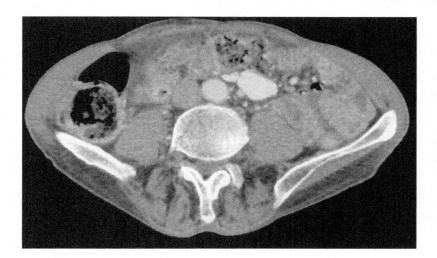

1. What is the diagnosis?

2. What is the incidence?

3. What conditions are associated with mesenteric venous thrombosis?

4. Name branches of the superior mesenteric vein.

5. Where is the commonest site of peripheral venous aneurysms?

Case ranking/difficulty:

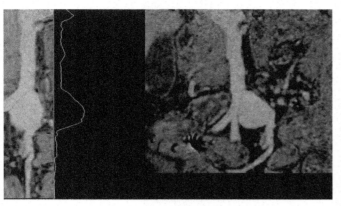

Centerline analysis and curvilinear reformatted image.

Answers

1. There is a superior mesenteric venous aneurysm.

2. It is very rare, with a number of case reports.

3. Thrombophilia, pancreatitis, inflammatory bowel disease, and malignancy are associations. Intra-abdominal sepsis is the commonest cause.

4. The superior mesenteric vein is formed by the jejunal, ileal, ileocolic, right colic, and middle colic veins, which drain the small intestine, cecum, ascending colon, and transverse colon. The right gastroepiploic vein and inferior pancreaticoduodenal vein are also SMV branches.

5. The popliteal vein is the most frequent site.

Pearls

- Venous aneurysms are rare and occur most commonly in the peripheral circulation.
- Mesenteric venous aneurysms are mostly asymptomatic, but have been reported to be a cause of abdominal pain that may be due to localized mass effect. They can rarely rupture or thrombose. There is some association with portal hypertension and cirrhosis.

Suggested Reading

Sfyroeras GS, Antoniou GA, Drakou AA, Karathanos C, Giannoukas AD. Visceral venous aneurysms: clinical presentation, natural history and their management: a systematic review. *Eur J Vasc Endovasc Surg.* 2009;38(4):498-505.

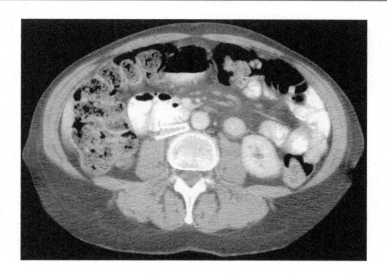

1. Review computed tomographic (CT) image, what surgery was performed and why?

2. What other equivalent surgical techniques were used? What is the modern alternative?

3. When was the first inferior vena cava (IVC) filter used?

4. How large a sheath was required for the early Greenfield filter?

5. When was the first percutaneous device used?

Case ranking/difficulty: **Category:** Venous system

Axial computed tomography.

Answers

1. The patient underwent surgical caval plication for pulmonary embolism (PE) protection.

2. Ligation, suture plication, and then clip applications were developed before the introduction of IVC filters.

3. The Mobin-Uddin filter was first developed in 1967 but was associated with high rates of IVC occlusion. This was replaced by the stainless steel Kimray-Greenfield filter in 1973.

4. The stainless steel Kimray-Greenfield filter in 1973, which was required to be placed via a 24-Fr sheath.

5. The first Greenfield filter was placed percutaneously in 1984, previously being placed via femoral or jugular cut-downs.

Pearls

• Surgery for PE prophylaxis started with interruption of the femoral vein, which was performed by Homans in 1934. Next, IVC ligation, and then partial caval interruption such as suture plication or clip application, was performed before the introduction of IVC filters such as the Mobin-Uddin umbrella and the Kim-Ray Greenfield filter. These were often performed in conjunction with open pulmonary embolectomy.

• Surgical caval interruptions carry significant risk of limb swelling while patients still developed fatal PE.

Suggested Readings

Greenfield LJ, McCurdy JR, Brown PP, Elkins RC. A new intracaval filter permitting continued flow and resolution of emboli. *Surgery.* 1973;73(4):599-606.

Mansour M, Chang AE, Sindelar WF. Interruption of the inferior vena cava for the prevention of recurrent pulmonary embolism. *Am Surg.* 1985;51(7):375-380.

Tadavarthy SM, Castaneda-Zuniga W, Salomonowitz E, et al. Kimray-Greenfield vena cava filter: percutaneous introduction. *Radiology.* 1984;151(2):525-526.

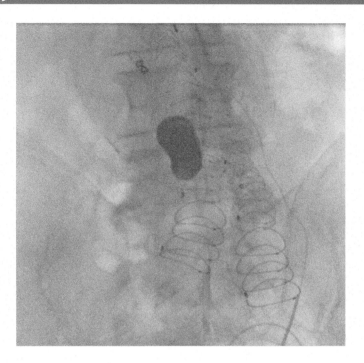

1. Review the image—which embolic agent has been used here?

2. What components make up this agent?

3. What are its advantages?

4. What are its disadvantages?

5. What are its main uses?

Case ranking/difficulty:

Category: Arterial system

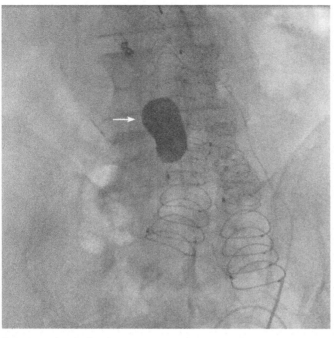

Status postembolization.

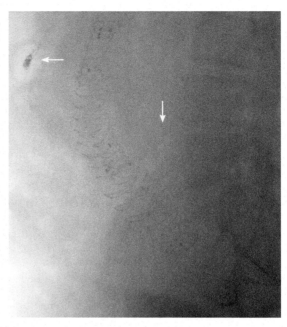

Preembolization—note the coils at the IMA origin anterior to the sac (arrow), and the radiopaque tip of the microcatheter that has been passed up an iliolumbar trunk and is seen at the back of the aortic sac (arrow).

Answers

1. Onyx has been used to embolize the aneurysm sac.

2. Onyx is composed of the ethylene vinyl alcohol (EVOH) polymer, a dimethyl sulfoxide (DMSO) solution, and tantalum particles for radio-opacity.

3. It can be handled with normal saline unlike glue and does not stick to catheters.

4. It requires mixing, and is expensive. Solidification can take a long time, particularly if large volumes are used. It must also be used with DMSO-compatible catheters. The DMSO can leave a garlicky smell that can linger around the patient for up to 48 hours.

5. Use in neurointerventions and aortic sac embolization is well reported, but other peripheral applications are growing.

Pearls

- Type 2 endoleaks can be considered as complex vascular lesions with inflow and outflow.
- It is becoming clear that there is poor outcome with microcatheter coil embolization, and better results may be obtained through the use of liquid embolic agents that fill the sac/nidus.
- Liquid embolic agents are well used by interventional neuroradiologists but have growing peripheral/body applications.
- In this case, Onyx was used, with a satisfactory clinical result with sac stability.
- Onyx is a nonadhesive liquid polymer composed of EVOH dissolved in DMSO and micronized tantalum powder. Onyx has lava-like properties, being a liquid that solidifies from outside to inside.

Suggested Reading

Guimaraes M, Wooster M. Onyx (ethylene-vinyl alcohol copolymer) in peripheral applications. *Semin Intervent Radiol.* 2011;28(3):350-356.

54-year-old man with hypertension and a computed tomographic scan revealing a left adrenal nodule

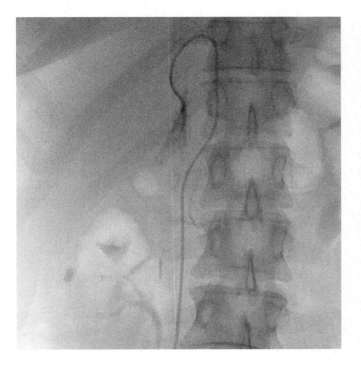 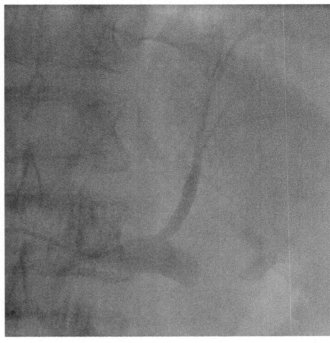

1. List some indications for adrenal vein sampling.

2. What is the commonest cause of primary aldosteronism?

3. What vein can be confused with the right adrenal vein?

4. What can you do if you have selected the vein, but cannot aspirate a sample?

5. Name some catheters that can be used to select the right adrenal vein.

Case ranking/difficulty:

Category: Genitourinary system

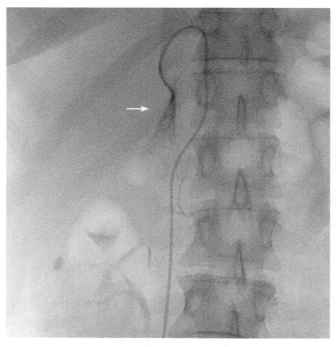

Right adrenal vein.

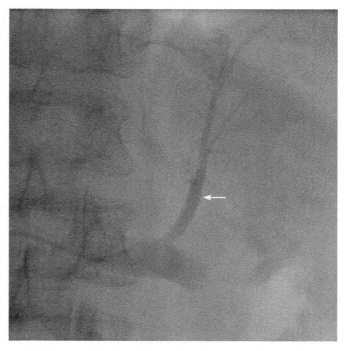

Left adrenal vein.

Answers

1. Adrenal vein sampling is performed to determine whether autonomous hormone production is unilateral or bilateral. It is most commonly performed for primary hyperaldosteronism but can also be used to sample in the setting of phaeochromocytoma, Cushing disease, and androgen excess.

2. Bilateral cortical hyperplasia is more common than unilateral nodular disease and unilateral hyperplasia.

3. The caudate lobe hepatic vein can be confused with the right adrenal vein.

4. If a sample cannot be obtained using a small syringe, drops can be collected directly from the back end of the catheter. A microwire and Tuohy-Borst valve can be used—a microwire used through the 0.035" catheter can push the catheter away from the vessel wall enough to get a sample.

5. One reported strategy is to use a C2, then C1, then reverse curve catheters like a Simmons 1 and Mikaelsson. Other operators use a heat source to reshape catheters.

Pearls

- Adrenal vein sampling (AVS) has a reputation as a difficult procedure. It is performed to assess whether autonomous hormone production is unilateral or bilateral. AVS is most commonly performed in primary hyperaldosteronism.
- Cannulating the right adrenal vein is difficult because of inconsistent origin. A variety of catheter shapes may be required to select the right adrenal vein.
- Samples are taken from both adrenal veins, as well as representative samples from other parts of the venous system such as from the suprarenal and infrarenal cava, as well as a peripheral sample should be obtained. Aldosterone and cortisol measurements can be taken. The sampling can occur in conjunction with hormonal stimulation.

Suggested Reading

Daunt N. Adrenal vein sampling: how to make it quick, easy, and successful. *Radiographics.* 2005;25(Suppl 1): S143-S158.

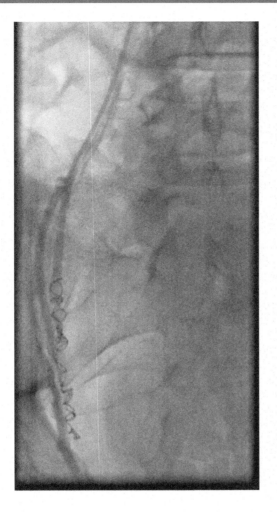
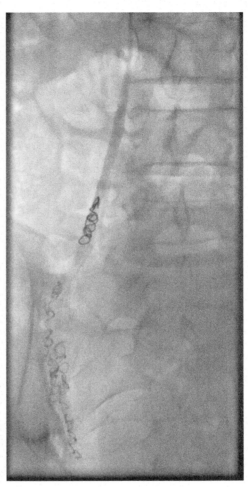

1. What is a varicocele?

2. How common are varicoceles?

3. List indications for treatment.

4. The right gonadal vein is best catheterized from a jugular approach—true or false?

5. How often does the right gonadal vein drain into the inferior vena cava (IVC)?

Case ranking/difficulty:

Answers

1. A varicocele is a dilatation of the pampiniform venous plexus and the internal spermatic vein.

2. They occur in 10%–15% of males, and are seen in up to 40% of infertile males.

3. Pain and infertility. The military often also require varicoceles to be treated.

4. False. Some operators prefer a jugular approach, others a femoral approach.

5. 95% of the time. In 5% of cases, it drains into the right renal vein.

Pearls

- Right-sided varicoceles are less common.
- The right gonadal vein normally arises from the anterolateral aspect of the IVC at the level of L3.

Suggested Reading

Bigot JM, Utzmann O. Right varicocele: contribution of spermatic phlebography. Results on 250 cases (article in French). *J Urol (Paris)*. 1983;89(2):121-131.

77-year-old man who is status post endovascular aneurysm repair (EVAR) presents for follow-up computed tomographic (CT) angiography

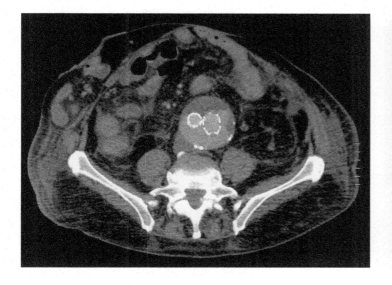 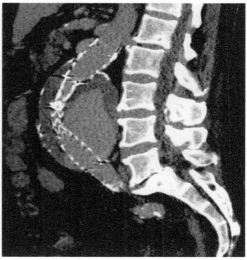

1. What is the most likely diagnosis based on CT angiography?

2. How would you classify the abnormality?

3. How urgent is the management?

4. What factors might predict this complication?

5. As well as leaks, what other factors should be sought for on EVAR follow-up imaging?

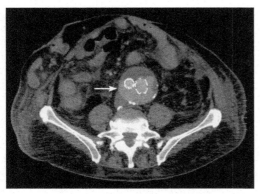

CT angiogram with EVAR in situ. Large region of contrast enhancement seen in the sac.

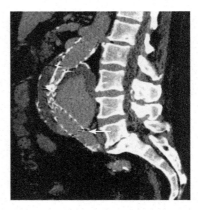

Sagittal reformats show the distal limb lies within the sac with retrograde flow into the sac.

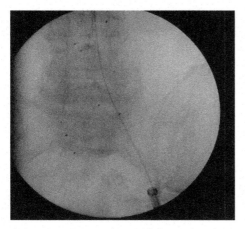

Fluoroscopic image pre-procedure with large sheath in the left iliac system.

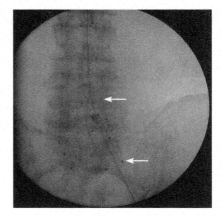

Fluoroscopic image post-procedure with stent extension in situ.

Answers

1. There is contrast seen in the sac. The large region involved suggests that the leak is probably more significant than a type 2 endoleak, and the limb is retracted in the sac and so this is in fact a distal type 1 endoleak.

2. 1a occurs at the neck, 1b at a distal limb, and 1c where there is failed iliac occlusion in the setting of an aorto-uni-iliac graft.

3. High-flow leaks should be managed on a relatively urgent basis.

4. Distal leaks can occur where there is sac growth and a reason for graft to move, and may be more likely to occur where the iliacs are native, and also if the initial stent was "short" and not flush to the iliac bifurcation.

5. Endoleaks, stent migration, kinking, fracture, sac enlargement, and non-vascular incidental findings should be reviewed on all post EVAR CT scans.

Pearls

- CT angiograms (CTAs) must be carefully reviewed to look for leaks, sac expansion, and graft migration.
- Graft migration can occur over time, particularly is the sac morphology changes due to enlargement. One series reported sac progression in 40% of cases, with a delayed rupture rate of 3%, presumably because of an unrecognized leak.
- High-pressure leaks require urgent management.
- Distal type 1 endoleaks can be treated with simple stent graft extension.

Suggested Reading

Stavropoulos SW, Charagundla SR. Imaging techniques for detection and management of endoleaks after endovascular aortic aneurysm repair. *Radiology*. 2007;243(3):641-655.

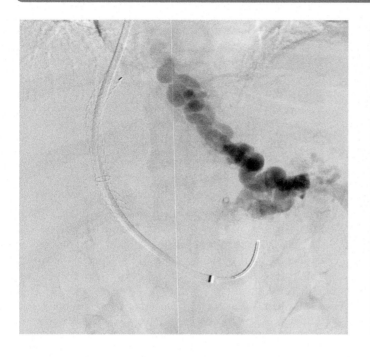 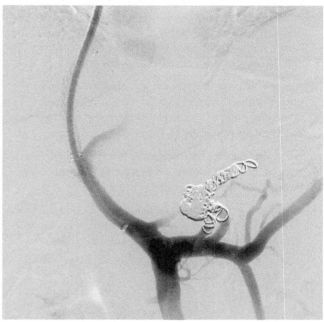

1. What are the afferent and draining veins involved in esophageal varices?

2. What is sinistral portal hypertension?

3. Are gastric varices more likely to bleed than esophageal varices?

4. What is BRTO?

5. Name some surgical shunts performed for portal hypertension.

Case ranking/difficulty:

Answers

1. Esophageal varices are extremely dilated submucosal veins in the lower third of the esophagus. They are most often a consequence of portal hypertension, commonly due to cirrhosis. The left gastric vein is the afferent vein, and the varices drain into the azygous vein.

2. Sinistral portal hypertension is a clinical syndrome of gastric variceal hemorrhage in the setting of splenic vein thrombosis due to a primary pancreatic pathology such as chronic pancreatitis.

3. No, esophageal varices are more likely to bleed. Gastric varices, however, can be very large and may be more likely to result in massive hemorrhage.

4. BRTO refers to a technique known as balloon-occluded retrograde transvenous obliteration, which is used to treat gastric varices through a gastrorenal shunt.

5. Portocaval, mesocaval, and splenorenal shunts can be created surgically.

Pearls

• Transjugular intrahepatic portosystemic shunt (TIPS) procedure can reduce the portoatrial gradient effectively to stop variceal hemorrhage. However, significant filling of the left gastric vein may be persistent despite adequate TIPS decompression because of the presence of a large competing collateral such as a splenorenal shunt. Embolization of the varices may be necessary after successful creation of a TIPS.

Suggested Readings

Chen T-W, Yang Z-G, Wang Q-L, et al. Evaluation of gastric fundic and oesophageal varices by 64-row multidetector computed tomography before and after transjugular intrahepatic portosystemic shunt with concurrent left gastric vein embolization. *Eur J Gastroenterol Hepatol.* 2010;22(3):289-295.

Ford JM, Shah H, Stecker MS, Namyslowski J. Embolization of large gastric varices using vena cava filter and coils. *Cardiovasc Intervent Radiol.* ;27(4):366-369.

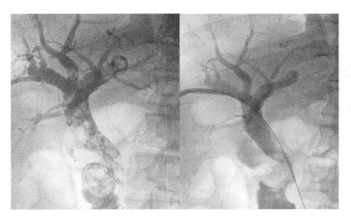 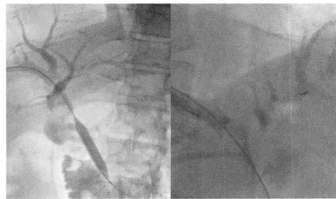

1. Review the first image—what is the abnormality and what has been done?

2. Review the second image—what 2 techniques are shown?

3. Define the terms *primary* and *secondary* bile duct stones.

4. What are the complications of endoscopic sphincterotomy?

5. What special techniques and agents can be used to perform percutaneous bile duct stone removal?

Case ranking/difficulty: **Category:** Gastrointestinal system

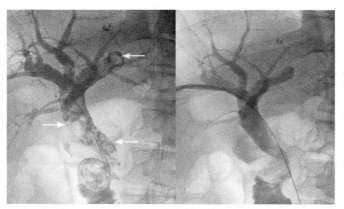

Cholangiograms, before and after the procedure.

Answers

1. There are multiple filling defects within the common bile duct and intrahepatic ducts consistent with stones. The stones have been removed from the biliary system.

2. Balloon sphincteroplasty and a Dormia basket are demonstrated. Both are techniques for biliary stone retrieval/removal. Percutaneous transhepatic balloon sphincteroplasty with transpapillary elimination of the stones can be performed at initial biliary access. Multistep procedure may still be required. Percutaneous retrieval with Dormia baskets require a larger and mature tract, at least 12 Fr, and so treatment is often performed over several stages.

3. Primary bile duct stones form in situ, and this is due to biliary stasis or bactibilia. Sphincter of Oddi dysfunction, sclerosing cholangitis, choledochal cysts, and benign biliary strictures are common causes of bile duct stasis. Secondary bile duct stones refer to the passage of gallstones via the cystic duct.

4. Endoscopic retrograde cholangiopancreatography (ERCP) and sphincterotomy is the first line for the management of common bile duct (CBD) stones and is frequently successful. It can be complicated by perforation, pancreatitis, and hemorrhage.

5. Glucagon should be administered to relax the sphincter of Oddi. Octreotide does reduce pancreatic secretions but is associated with sphincter of Oddi spasm. Somatostatin has a preferential pharmacologic profile, causing relaxation of the sphincter and reduced pancreatic secretions. A compliant occlusion balloon should be used to push the stones across the sphincter. Complications include pancreatitis (though this is less frequent than in ERCP sphincterotomy), cholangitis, and papillary stenosis. Hemobilia and sphincter of Oddi spasm may lead to the procedure needing to be abandoned, and stone retrieval can be reattempted at another sitting. The Dormia basket requires a larger percutaneous access. Eight- to 14-mm balloon angioplasty is common, but the size of the balloon should be tailored to the stone size and can be greater than 20 mm.

Pearls

- Bile duct stones can be primary (due to bile duct stasis or bactibilia) or secondary, migrating from the gallbladder. ERCP and sphincterotomy is the mainstay of management. Percutaneous bile duct stone procedures can be performed if there are contraindications to ERCP.

Suggested Readings

García-Vila JH, Redondo-Ibáñez M, Díaz-Ramón C. Balloon sphincteroplasty and transpapillary elimination of bile duct stones: 10 years' experience. *AJR Am J Roentgenol.* 2004;182(6):1451-1458.

Park YS, Kim JH, Choi YW, et al. Percutaneous treatment of extrahepatic bile duct stones assisted by balloon sphincteroplasty and occlusion balloon. *Korean J Radiol.* 2007;6(4):235-240.

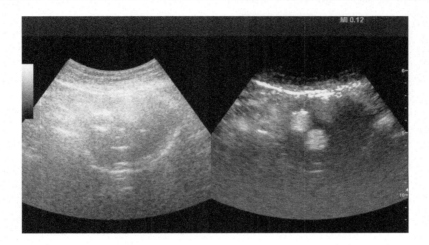

1. For which applications is contrast-enhanced ultrasonography (CEUS) useful?

2. How is CEUS performed?

3. What are the properties and pharmokinetics of microbubble preparations?

4. What are advantages of microbubble ultrasound?

5. What is a type 5 endoleak?

Case ranking/difficulty:

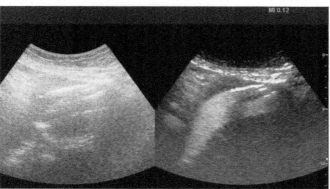

Longitudinal view, CEUS.

Answers

1. CEUS is useful in detecting occult endoleaks. It also can be a very useful tool to aid with characterizing endoleaks as the direction of flow can be seen. Similarly, as it is a time-resolving technique, the true and false lumen of a dissection can be seen. Inflammatory changes in the aortic wall are also highlighted with CEUS.

2. Venous access is required (eg, butterfly or intravenous cannula). The contrast agent is injected and then flushed through with saline.

3. SonoVue is made of SF6 gas contained within a phospholipid monolayer shell. At low–mechanical index (MI) imaging, ultrasonography causes the gas bubble to oscillate. High-MI images causes the bubble to burst, which otherwise, are eliminated via the lungs.

4. There are several advantages that can be utilized through contrast-enhanced microbubble ultrasonography.

5. Type 5 endoleaks have been attributed to "endotension," where pulsation of the graft wall can lead to growth of the perigraft space. It may be the case that type 5 endoleaks could be occult, undiagnosed small endoleaks from sources 1 through 3.

Pearls

- Ultrasonography contrast agents are composed of gas (eg, SF6) with a lipophilic shell. They are given intravenously and remain in the intravascular space and are excreted through the lungs.
- Its primary use has been the characterization of liver lesions. However, CEUS can help to differentiate between different types of endoleaks, eg, type 1 or type 2 as direction of the endoleak can be visualized. It may also be more sensitive than conventional modalities in characterizing endoleaks of otherwise unknown etiology.

Suggested Reading

Clevert DA, Minaifar N, Kopp R, et al. Imaging of endoleaks after endovascular aneurysm repair (EVAR) with contrast-enhanced ultrasound (CEUS). A pictorial comparison with CTA. *Clin Hemorrheal Microcirc.* 2009;41(3):151-168.

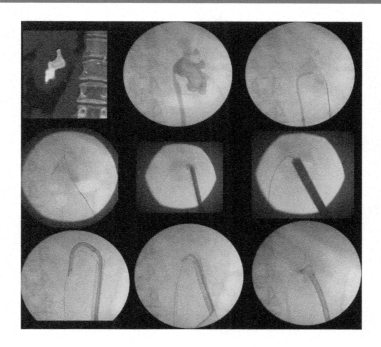

1. What are indications for percutaneous nephrolithotomy?

2. How many accesses are required to treat a staghorn calculus?

3. What techniques are available to dilate the access tract?

4. What is the role of the Malecot catheter?

5. What is the risk of stone recurrence at 10 years?

Case ranking/difficulty:

Category: Genitourinary system

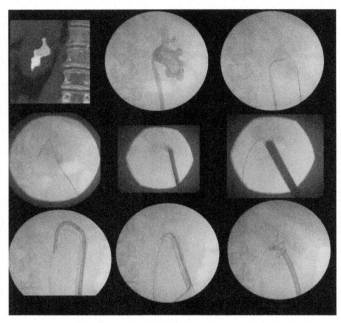

Multiple images pre- and post-PCNL.

Answers

1. Staghorn calculi, large stones, or stones behind stenosed infundibulae can be treated with PCNL. Small pelvic and ureteric stones can be treated with retrograde techniques or extracorporeal shock-wave lithotripsy.

2. Each access should be tailored to the anatomy of the kidney and the stone burden.

3. There is a variety of different equipment available to dilate the tract—serial plastic dilators, serial metallic dilator sets, and also a balloon inflation device. Fascial incising needle can also aid tract dilatation. A well-planned access with a well-placed stiff wire will facilitate tract dilatation.

4. The Malecot catheter is a large drainage tube that facilitates drainage of the collecting system and can also tamponade the access tract.

5. Large series have reported recurrence rates ranging from 25% to 50% and even 40% to 70%. Recurrent stone disease is a significant cause of ultimately needing renal replacement therapy.

Pearls

- Stones can be treated with extracorporeal shock wave lithotripsy, retrograde ureteroscopy, or PCNL.
- PCNL is indicated for staghorn calculi, stones >1.5 cm, stones present behind a stenosed infundibulum or in a kidney with pelviureteric junction obstruction.
- PCNL may require multiple percutaneous accesses, and there are multiple techniques, from fluoroscopic guidance, ultrasound guidance in interventional radiology, to combined techniques with retrograde ureteroscopy, and retrograde filling of the renal pelvis with contrast medium or methylene blue dye.

Suggested Reading

Dyer RB, Regan JD, Kavanagh PV, Khatod EG, Chen MY, Zagoria RJ. Percutaneous nephrostomy with extensions of the technique: step by step. *Radiographics.* 2002;22(3):503-525.

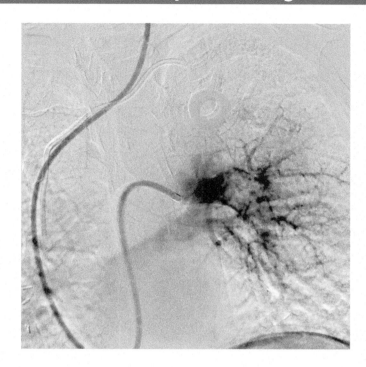

1. Define the term "thrombus."

2. Which tumors are associated with intravascular tumor thrombus?

3. Which signs distinguish acute versus chronic pulmonary embolisms (PEs)?

4. Intraluminal tumor emboli progress and lead to pulmonary metastases—true or false?

5. What treatments are useful?

Case ranking/difficulty:

Category: Arterial system

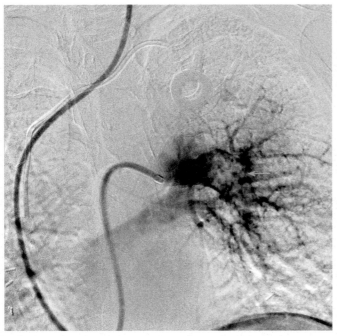

Pulmonary angiogram shows a filling defect. This was biopsied endovascularly using pinch biopsy forceps through the vascular sheath and the diagnosis of tumor thrombus was made.

Answers

1. A thrombus is usually defined as the presence or formation of a clot within the circulation. If the thrombus moves to a distant part of the circulation, then the term *thromboembolism* is used. However, thrombus can also refer to foreign bodies, which may include talc, tumor, or even bullets.

2. Renal cell carcinoma, hepatocellular carcinoma, and uterine leiomyosarcomas are the most common malignancies that are associated with intravascular tumor thrombus.

3. Signs of chronic pulmonary embolism include vessel tapering, intimal and laminar abnormalities, poststenotic dilatation, bands, and webs.

4. Tumor thrombi have not been reported to progress and directly cause lung metastases.

5. Surgical pulmonary embolectomy can be performed if tumor thrombi obstruct central pulmonary arteries.

Pearls

- A thrombus can be defined as an object present within the circulation. Though typically, it implies bland thrombus, thrombus can apply to other pathologies such as tumor thrombus.
- Tumors that enter the vasculature commonly include renal cell carcinoma (renal vein to inferior vena cava to right atrium) or hepatocellular carcinoma (into the portal vein).
- A biopsy was required to make a definitive diagnosis, and an endovascular biopsy was performed with pinch forceps placed through a vascular sheath.

Suggested Readings

Grosse C, Grosse A. CT findings in diseases associated with pulmonary hypertension: a current review. *Radiographics.* 2010;30(7):1753-1777.

Wittram C, Kalra MK, Maher MM, Greenfield A, McLoud TC, Shepard JA. Acute and chronic pulmonary emboli: angiography-CT correlation. *AJR Am J Roentgenol.* 2006;186(6 Suppl 2):S421-S429.

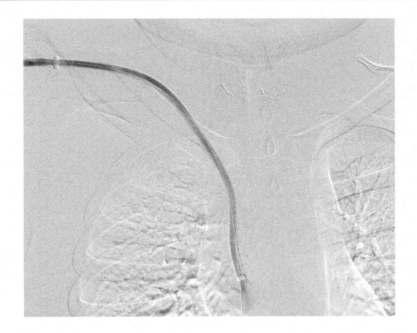

1. Review the image—what is the implant?

2. When can it be used?

3. What is the 6-month primary and secondary patency?

4. What management options are available if it becomes thrombosed?

5. What is the approval process for new medical devices in your country?

Case ranking/difficulty:

Category: Venous system

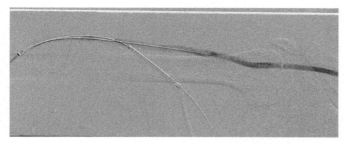

Note the corrugated appearance of the proximal graft component. There are 2 accesses to facilitate declot—antegrade for aspiration thrombectomy and retrograde to pull the arterial plug.

Answers

1. This is the HeRO device.

2. All options for native arteriovenous fistulas and grafts are considered before the HeRO device, which may be a better alternative to the use of lines.

3. The 6-month primary and secondary patency rates are reported to be 80 and 95%, respectively, based on a multicenter registry of over 150 implantations.

4. Rotational mechanical devices are contraindicated here due to the risk of damage to the venous outflow limb and the connector.

5. There are different regulations for medical devices in different countries, but you should be familiar with the approval processes and safety standards in your region. Device faults should be reported to the manufacturer and logged into any relevant national databases.

Pearls

- The HeRO vascular access device (Hemodialysis Reliable Outflow) is an option for long-term dialysis access. It is an option when other options have failed and where a patient is catheter dependent.
- It is surgically implanted. The venous outflow component is inserted using endovascular techniques and its distal radiopaque marker is sited at the right atrium. The arterial graft component is then surgically anastomosed to the native artery. The venous outflow component has an internal diameter (ID) of 5 mm. The arterial graft has an ID of 6 mm.

Suggested Reading

Gage SM, Katzman HE, Ross JR, et al. Multi-center experience of 164 consecutive Hemodialysis Reliable Outflow [HeRO] graft implants for hemodialysis treatment. *Eur J Vasc Endovasc Surg.* 2012;44(1):93-99.

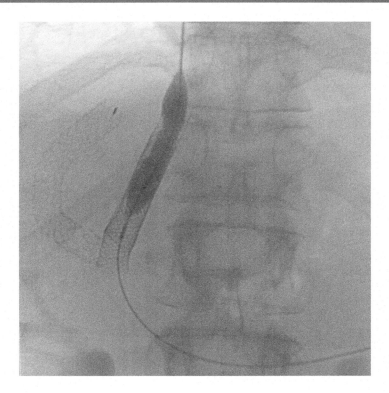

1. How can TIPS be monitored?

2. What is the 6-month patency of a covered stent?

3. What is the 6-month patency of an uncovered stent?

4. What can be done if the patient develops encephalopathy?

5. What is a parallel TIPS?

Category: Gastrointestinal system

Answers

1. TIPS can be monitored with ultrasonography. Further evaluation can be performed by transjugular access and direct portal pressure measurement. Portograms can be used to assess TIPS shunt narrowing and the presence of portosystemic collaterals.

2. Primary patency at 6 months is 62%; secondary patency is greater than 90%.

3. Primary patency is 48%, secondary patency is 60%.

4. Encephalopathy can be managed medically. TIPS may not cause encephalopathy—encephalopathy may occur because of progression of underlying disease. However, in the setting of encephalopathy, the TIPS can be reduced or occluded.

5. A parallel TIPS is a second TIPS stent. If the first TIPS was placed from the right hepatic vein to the right portal vein, a second TIPS can be created from the middle hepatic vein to the left portal vein, or from the left hepatic vein to the left portal vein.

Pearls

- TIPS can stenose, thrombose, and occlude. Therefore, routine surveillance after TIPS procedure is necessary. TIPS can be revised, with angioplasty and stenting.
- Ultrasonography is a noninvasive method that can be used to check TIPS patency, but transjugular portography and pressure gradient measurement is both definitive diagnostic procedure and treatment can be performed at the same sitting.
- Parallel TIPS can be performed to treat portal hypertension that does not respond to a primary well-functioning TIPS.

Suggested Reading

Jung HS, Kalva SP, Greenfield AJ, et al. TIPS: comparison of shunt patency and clinical outcomes between bare stents and expanded polytetrafluoroethylene stent-grafts. *J Vasc Interv Radiol.* 2009;20(2):180-185.

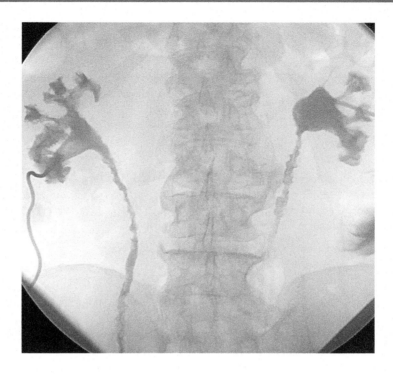

1. Review the image—what is the diagnosis?

2. What blood marker is associated with this condition?

3. What is the pathological mechanism here?

4. What are possible treatments?

5. Describe the anatomy of the ureter.

Case ranking/difficulty:

Category: Genitourinary system

Answers

1. There is ureteric inflammation and the underlying cause here is due to Wegener granulomatosis (WG).

2. A raised c-ANCA can help to establish the diagnosis of WG.

3. There is vasculitis causing inflammation in the ureteric wall.

4. Medical therapy involves cyclophosphamide and prednisolone. Decompression and stenting can manage the ureteric obstruction. However, nephrectomy and transplantation may ultimately be required.

5. The ureter is normally 25 to 30 cm in length and passes anterior to the iliac vessels (though a retroiliac ureter can occur). It has a transitional epithelium.

Pearls

• Ureteritis can be caused by xanthogranomatous or emphysematous inflammation. Ureteritis cystica, TB, or local inflammation (eg, due to pelvic inflammatory disease or Crohn diease) may give similar appearances.

Suggested Reading

Davenport A, Downey SE, Goel S, Maciver AG. Wegener's granulomatosis involving the urogenital tract. *Br J Urol.* 1996;78(3):354-357.

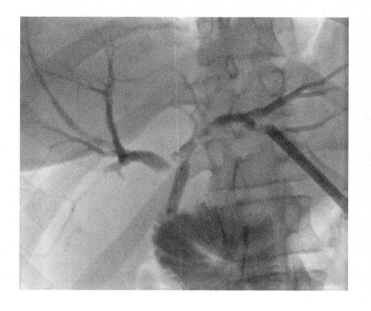 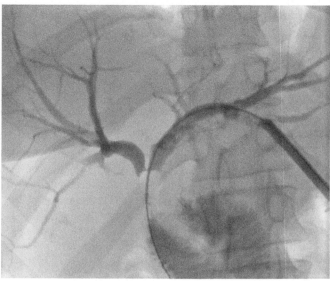

1. How does the bile drain in this antegrade cholangiogram?

2. List some reasons why hepaticojejunostomy might be performed.

3. How can strictures of the hepaticojejunostomy anastomosis be treated?

4. What is the rate of posttransplant biliary-enteric anastomotic stenosis?

5. What is a cutting balloon?

Answers

1. The left and right hepatic ducts drain into a jejunal loop. This patient underwent hepaticojejunostomy because of prior common bile duct (CBD) transection.

2. Hepaticojejunostomy is commonly performed for a variety of extrahepatic ductal disease such as iatrogenic bile injury, resection of benign or malignant lesions, and orthotopic liver transplantation.

3. Surgical revision, balloon dilatation (including cutting balloon dilatation), and stent placement are options.

4. This is reported to occur in up to 10% of cases.

5. A cutting balloon is a noncompliant balloon with a number of longitudinal atherotomes. Balloon expansion results in a number of longitudinal cuts being delivered to the host lumen. These balloons have been shown to have favorable results in certain situations such as in coronary angioplasty, fistuloplasty, and relevant to this case, the dilatation of biliary-enteric stenoses.

Pearls

- Biliary-enteric anastomotic strictures are difficult to treat surgically and are often inaccessible by endoscopy. A choledochojejunostomy or hepaticojejunostomy are commonly encountered as both native and posttransplant anastomoses.
- Posttransplant strictures may occur in up to 10% of transplant recipients. Native anastomoses may occur after CBD resection due to bile duct injury, benign strictures, choledochal cysts, or resection for malignancy.
- Percutaneous treatment involves repeated balloon dilatation of the anastomosis and serial upsizing of the drain until adequate patency is achieved. Cutting balloon dilatation can be useful in resistant strictures.

Suggested Readings

Ko G-Y, Sung K-B, Yoon H-K, Kim KR, Gwon DI, Lee SG. Percutaneous transhepatic treatment of hepaticojejunal anastomotic biliary strictures after living donor liver transplantation. *Liver Transpl.* 2008;14(9):1323-1332.

Saad WEA. Percutaneous management of postoperative anastomotic biliary strictures. *Tech Vasc Interv Radiol.* 2008;11(2):143-153.

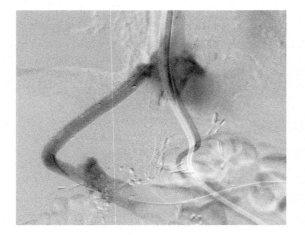
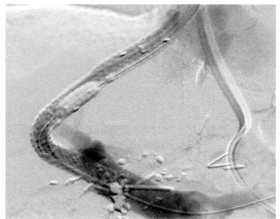
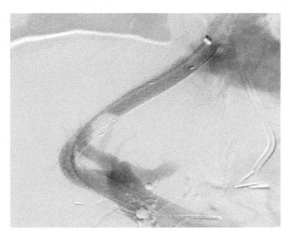

1. What is the incidence of encephalopathy after TIPS?

2. What causes encephalopathy?

3. What is appropriate medical management?

4. Shunt occlusion is free of complications—true or false?

5. How can shunts be reduced?

Case ranking/difficulty:

Answers

1. Increased encephalopathy is reported to be within 5% and 35%. The majority can be managed medically, with only around 5% requiring intervention.

2. Constipation, high dietary protein, GI bleeds, hypokalemia, and narcotic analgesics can cause hepatic encephalopathy.

3. Low-protein diet, lactulose, and neomycin aim to reduce the nitrogenous load and toxins from the gut. Zinc supplements and branched-chain amino acids can also be used.

4. Shunt occlusion can be life threatening, as portal hypertension recurs along with the risk of variceal hemorrhage.

5. Many methods exist—popular approaches include the use of a constrained covered stent (coaxially through a balloon-mounted stent to provide the "waisting"), or in parallel (eg, shotgun barrels).

Pearls

- About 3% to 7% of hepatic encephalopathy after TIPS procedure require intervention treatment.
- Treatment may include shunt occlusion or shunt reduction, which can be performed in a variety of ways. In this case, 2 accesses are obtained into the TIPS—in one, a new covered stent is deployed to reline the TIPS, and in the other, a balloon-mounted stent is used to titrate the portosystemic gradient.

Suggested Reading

Madoff DC, Wallace MJ, Ahrar K, Saxon RR. TIPS-related hepatic encephalopathy: management options with novel endovascular techniques. *Radiographics.* 2004;24(1):21-36; discussion 36-37.

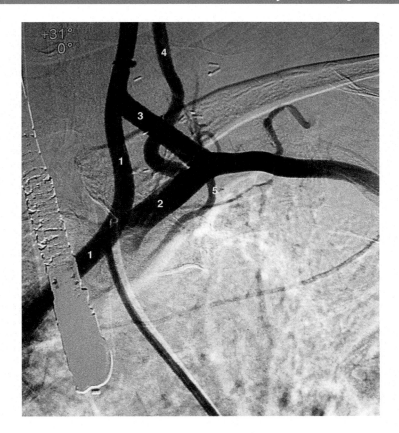

1. Review the image and name the structures 1 to 5.

2. What are the options when left subclavian
   artery overstenting is required?

3. What are the complications of left subclavian
   artery overstenting in TEVAR?

4. What vascular territories contribute to cord
   supply and should be considered when
   planning TEVAR?

5. Which aortic landing zone requires LSA
   coverage?

Category: Arterial system

Answers

1. (1) Left common carotid artery, (2) left subclavian artery, (3) carotid–subclavian bypass, (4) left vertebral artery, (5) left internal mammary artery.

2. The left subclavian can be sacrificed, or carotid subclavian by-pass can be performed in conjunction with coiling or plugging of the proximal LSA. Subclavian transposition may be favored by some surgeons, but there is a risk of massive stump hemorrhage and thoracic duct injury. The LSA can be ignored in more elderly patients who may tolerate a 50 mmHg BP drop in the left arm.

3. Complications include vertebrobasilar ischemia, arm ischemia, type 2 endoleak, and increased risk of cord ischemia.

4. Left subclavian, intercostals, lumbar, and internal iliac arteries contribute to cord supply. Intrathecal drains can help reduce the risk of cord ischemia.

5. Zone 0 is the ascending aorta with the brachiocephalic trunk, and zone 1 would include coverage of the left carotid and subclavian arteries. Landing in zone 2 would cover the left subclavian artery. Zone 3 is distal to, but does not cover, the left subclavian artery. Zone 4 is the descending thoracic aorta.

Pearls

- Evaluation for the need for left subclavian artery revascularization is required prior to thoracic endovascular aortic repair.
- Covering the left subclavian arteries increases the number of patients for whom TEVAR would be suitable as the landing zone is increased.
- Left carotid subclavian bypass can be performed to allow overstenting of the left subclavian artery. The proximal LSA is then occluded with coils or plugs to prevent a type 2 endoleak.

Suggested Reading

Reece TB, Gazoni LM, Cherry KJ, et al. Reevaluating the need for left subclavian artery revascularization with thoracic endovascular aortic repair. *Ann Thorac Surg.* 2007;84(4):1201-1205; discussion 1205.

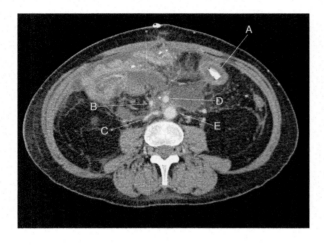 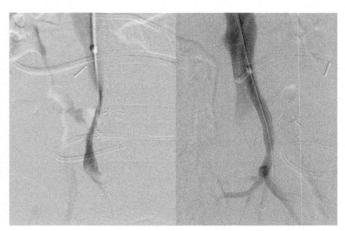

1. Name structures A to E.

2. Why is there an increased risk of complication with intestinal transplantation over solid visceral transplants?

3. What factors have improved results of intestinal transplantation over the past few decades?

4. What is the 1-year patient survival and 1-year graft survival?

5. What are the complications of intestinal transplantation?

Case ranking/difficulty:

Category: Venous system

Answers

1. A shows mucosal edema in the small bowel transplant. B is the donor superior mesenteric vein (SMV), C is the recipient inferior vena cava (IVC), D is the donor superior mesenteric artery, and E is the aorta. Systemic venous drainage is used if the access to the portal vein is difficult, or if its patency is compromised. No survival advantage has, as yet, been demonstrated for splanchnic over systemic venous return.

2. With intestinal transplants, there is a large number of immunocompetent donor lymphocytes in the gut-associated lymphoid tissue and mesenteric nodes. There is also increased risk of bacterial contamination. Both of these factors increase the risk of rejection.

3. Improved surgical technique, immunosuppressant regimes, antimicrobial treatment of opportunistic infections, as well as better critical care and interventional radiology services have improved outcomes.

4. One-year patient survival is 81% and 1-year graft survival is currently around 63%.

5. Vascular complications include dissection, thrombosis, occlusion, stenosis, and pseudoaneurysm formation. Knowledge of vascular anatomy is key—is there an aortic conduit, a caval stump, and so on? In this case, there is a venous stenosis that is simply stented from a jugular approach with resultant graft salvage.

Pearls

- Familiarity with surgical anatomy is key when diagnosing and treating complex transplant complications. Where are the gastrointestinal anastomoses? End-to-end? End-to-side? Where are the arteriovenous anastomoses? Is there an aortic, iliac, or carotid conduit?
- There are different patterns of small bowel transplantation—ranging from isolated small bowel transplant through to multivisceral transplantation.

Suggested Reading

Towbin AJ, Towbin RB, Di Lorenzo C, Grifka RG. Interventional radiology in the treatment of the complications of organ transplant in the pediatric population—part 1: the kidneys, heart, lungs, and intestines. *Semin Intervent Radiol.* 2004;21(4):309-320.

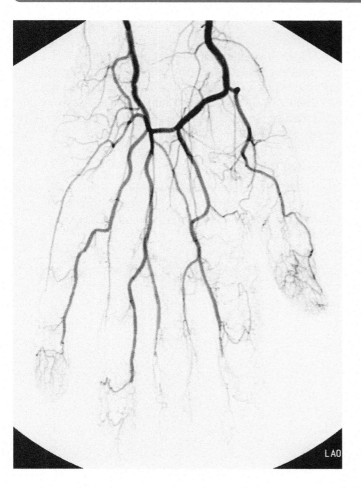
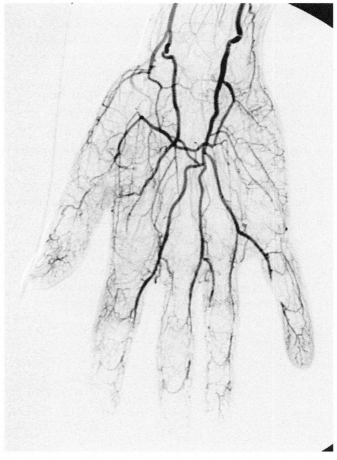

1. Give a differential diagnosis.

2. What features are seen in systemic sclerosis?

3. What is the reported rate of digital ulceration in systemic sclerosis?

4. What is Raynaud's phenomenon?

5. How can this be managed?

Case ranking/difficulty: **Category:** Arterial system

Answers

1. Digital arterial embolic occlusion can occur in thromboembolic disease, connective tissue diseases, hypothenar hammer syndrome, and, as in this case, scleroderma.

2. Systemic sclerosis can result digital artery ischemia, but not aneurysm formation. All the other digital complications are due to ischemia.

3. Digital ulcers are seen in more than half of the patients with scleroderma.

4. Raynaud phenomenon is an almost universal manifestation, affecting 95% of scleroderma patients.

5. Management often relies on nonpharmacologic measures, with lifestyle modifications as smoking cessation, avoidance of cold exposure, appropriate clothing, and if possible, avoiding psychological stress that can trigger attacks. Pharmacologic treatment is offered, with calcium channel blockers or other vasodilators used.

Pearls

- Occlusive digital artery disease with Raynaud phenomenon is not specific for scleroderma. Raynaud phenomenon should lead to a search for a systemic disease, and scleroderma is the most common associated condition.

Suggested Reading

Maiman MH, Bookstein JJ, Bernstein EF. Digital ischemia: angiographic differentiation of embolism from primary arterial disease. *AJR Am J Roentgenol.* 1981;137(6): 1183-1187.

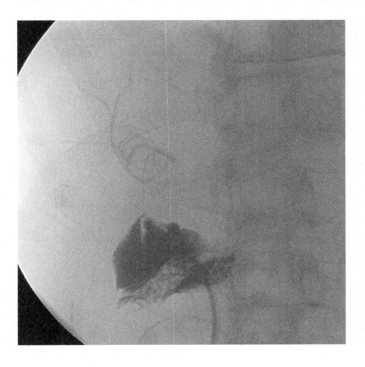 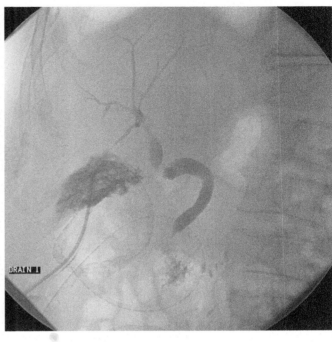

1. Review the images, how were they obtained and what do they show?

2. What causes bile leak after laparoscopic cholecystectomy?

3. Which duct is most commonly the source of a bile leak?

4. How are bile duct injuries managed?

5. What are risk factors for bile duct injury?

Case ranking/difficulty:

Answers

1. A drainogram has been performed and contrast medium has refluxed from the collection up into the biliary tree. Hepatobiliary 99mTc-iminodiacetic acid (HIDA), endoscopic retrograde cholangiopancreatography (ERCP), or percutaneous transhepatic cholangiography (PTHC) may ultimately be required in the diagnosis of bile duct leaks.

2. Common bile duct laceration or thermal injury, non-closure of the cystic duct, and cystic duct stump necrosis can result in bile leak. Clipping the CBD will cause biliary obstruction. Opening of the ducts of Luschka can also be a source of leak.

3. Cystic duct is reported to be the source of bile leak in 78%, subvesical ducts 26%, and major ducts in 9% of cases.

4. Small leaks can resolve spontaneously. Collections should be drained. Internal stenting is required in larger leaks, which is usually performed via ERCP. Sphincterotomy may also be required. PTHC is reserved when ERCP fails or is contraindicated. Laparotomy, lavage, and direct closure of the ducts of Luschka may be required. Surgical ligation or repair of ducts is definitive.

5. Technical factors and the underlying pathology can influence the risk of bile duct injury. For example, operator experience, dense scarring, and inflammation increase the risk of injury.

Pearls

- Major bile duct injury after laparoscopic cholecystectomy is around 0.5%. This can occur if the common duct is mistaken for the cystic duct and is clipped and divided, or if a segment of an aberrant right hepatic duct (taken between the cystic duct and the common hepatic duct) is mistaken as the cystic duct.
- The bile ducts of Luschka are also called subvesical ducts and are small ducts that originate from the right hepatic lobe, course along the gallbladder fossa, and usually drain into the extrahepatic bile ducts. Injuries to these ducts are a frequent cause of post cholecystectomy bile leaks.
- HIDA scans can demonstrate active bile leak and aid to localize the general anatomic site, but ERCP or PTHC may be required.
- Bile duct injuries have been classified into low-grade or high-grade leaks. Drainage, stenting, sphincterotomy, or surgery may be required.

Suggested Readings

Rulli F, Grasso E. Biliary peritonitis for duct of Luschka bile leak after laparoscopic cholecystectomy performed with a 10-mm harmonic scalpel. *Langenbecks Arch Surg.* 2007;392(1):111-112; author reply 113.

Spanos CP, Syrakos T. Bile leaks from the duct of Luschka (subvesical duct): a review. *Langenbecks Arch Surg.* 2006;391(5):441-447.

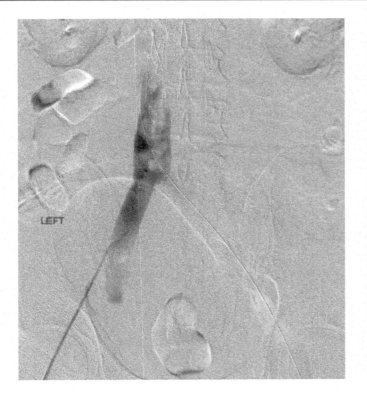

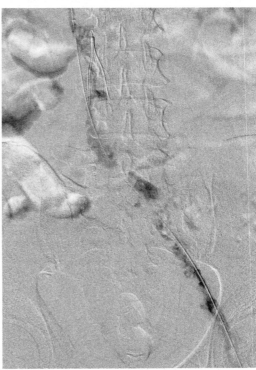

1. What is the natural history of thrombus in an IVC filter?

2. When is thrombolysis indicated?

3. What factors influence the risk of caval occlusion?

4. When does transplant renal vein thrombosis occur and how can it be managed?

5. What size of thrombus present in a filter is considered "safe" to remove?

Case ranking/difficulty:

Answers

1. Symptomatic IVC filter thrombosis is rare. Thrombosis can progress to caval occlusion. Anticoagulation is recommended when possible.

2. Most filter thrombus resolves spontaneously. In symptomatic acute/subacute thrombosis with caval or renal vein occlusion or a large clot burden, the patient must be referred for catheter-directed thrombolysis. When there is associated iliocaval stenosis or occlusion, angioplasty and stenting can be performed. Chronic filter-related IVC occlusion can similarly be treated safely with stenting and displacement of the obstructed filter.

3. The risk of filter thrombosis may also be influenced by the study population, underlying hypercoagulable states, use of anticoagulation, and the specific method used to assess for thrombosis. The data show higher IVC filter thrombosis rates associated with a double-basket or double-trap filter design.

4. Transplant renal vein thrombosis tends to be an early complication occurring in the first week. The venous anastomosis typically is with an external iliac vein. Thrombectomy can salvage the graft, which is at risk for rupture from the high venous pressure. The role of intervention radiology is not well defined, but there are several reports of successful graft salvage.

5. All current retrievable IVC filters are approved by the Food and Drug Administration as permanent filters. About 10% IVC filters cannot be removed due to tilt or attachment to the caval wall. There have been many reports describing successful removal of permanent IVC filters. Thrombus less than 2×1 cm is considered safe to remove.

Pearls

- New formation of thrombus within an IVC filter cannot be differentiated from captured thrombus that has migrated from a distal source. Thrombus can also propagate and extend up to, and beyond, a filter.
- Anticoagulation following filter placement has been associated with an approximately 50% reduction in the incidence of IVC filter thrombosis. Similarly, thrombus seen in a filter can regress spontaneously.
- Thrombectomy and thrombolysis are indicated with symptomatic patients. There are a number of different devices available that aid aspiration and mechanical or infusional thrombolysis.

Suggested Reading

Habito CR, Kalva SP. Inferior vena cava filter thrombosis: a review of current concepts, evidence, and approach to management. *Hosp Pract (Minneap).* 2011;39(3):79-86.

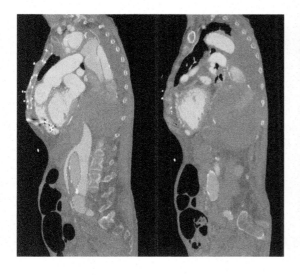
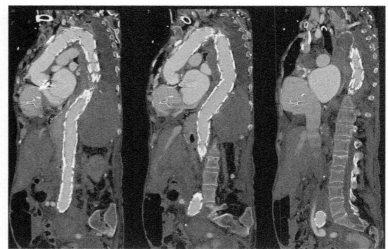

1. Review the sagittal computed tomographic (CT) images—what is the diagnosis?

2. What are indications to intervene in the descending thoracic aorta?

3. What is an elephant trunk procedure?

4. How is the diagnosis of Marfan syndrome made?

5. What is Loeys-Dietz syndrome?

Case ranking/difficulty:

Answers

1. There is a large saccular aneurysm seen related to the descending thoracic aorta and associated dissection. Such advanced disease is seen with patients with Marfan syndrome.

2. Large aneurysms, pseudoaneurysms, or complicated dissections are indications for stent grafting.

3. This is a 2-stage aortic repair, where the ascending aorta and arch are repaired first and an excess length of graft is left in the true lumen of the descending aorta.

4. The Ghent criteria use familial, genetic information as well as the presence of skeletal and cardiovascular manifestations.

5. Loeys-Dietz syndrome has been likened to a severe form of a combination of Marfan and Ehlers-Danlos syndromes.

Pearls

- Thoracoabdominal grafting and reconstruction of all visceral branches is an option preferred by some centers, as it can be definitive and avoids the need for multiple or future aortic operations.
- Marfan syndrome is caused by a mutation in *FBN-1* gene on chromosome 15.
- Loeys Dietz syndrome is caused by transforming growth factor–beta receptor abnormalities and manifests with severe aortic, aneurysmal, and dissecting disease.

Suggested Reading

Omura A, Tanaka A, Miyahara S, et al. Early and late results of graft replacement for dissecting aneurysm of thoracoabdominal aorta in patients with Marfan syndrome. *Ann Thorac Surg.* 2012;94(3):759-765.

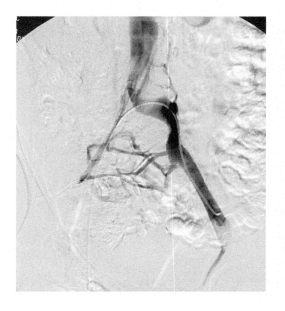
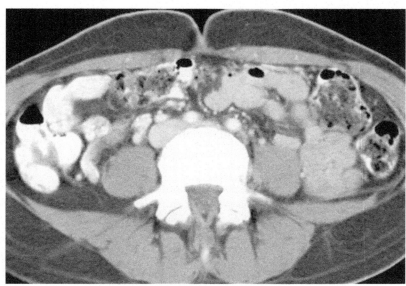

1. What is the diagnosis?

2. What are its other names and what is the usual
   underlying cause?

3. What physical lesions are described?

4. What are diagnostic signs?

5. How is this condition managed?

Case ranking/difficulty: **Category:** Venous system

Answers

1. This is May-Thurner syndrome.

2. Other names are iliac vein compression syndrome or Cockett syndrome. Pulsatile compression induces tissue changes that lead to deep vein thrombosis or venous hypertension in the left lower extremity. The majority of cases are due to compression of the left common iliac vein between the right common iliac artery and vertebral body.

3. May and Thurner described 3 variations of "spurs": a lateral spur where the lesion protrudes from the lateral wall of the vessel, a central spur that divides the lumen in an anteroposterior fashion, and a membranous spur that obstructs the lumen diffusely.

4. The characteristic May-Thurner lesion is diagnosed with contrast venography showing a left common iliac stenosis with a demonstrable pressure gradient.

5. Venoplasty has a poor outcome. Venous stenting has gained popularity as a minimally invasive technique, but long-term behavior of stents is undefined. Excision of intraluminal adhesions has provided significant symptomatic relief to patients with high patency rates. Anticoagulation or antiplatelet medication is recommended to keep the stents open.

Pearls

- May-Thurner syndrome occurs as a result of compression of the left common iliac vein between the right common iliac artery and the vertebral column, commonly affects females, and is associated with deep vein thrombosis. It can also occur on the right.
- Venography, intravascular ultrasonography, computed tomographic angiogram, and magnetic resonance venography all can demonstrate this abnormality with high sensitivity.
- Iliac vein stenting is accepted practice. Thrombolysis can be required in the acute setting.

Suggested Reading

O'Sullivan GJ, Semba CP, Bittner CA, et al. Endovascular management of iliac vein compression (May-Thurner) syndrome. *J Vasc Interv Radiol.* 2003;11(7):823-836.

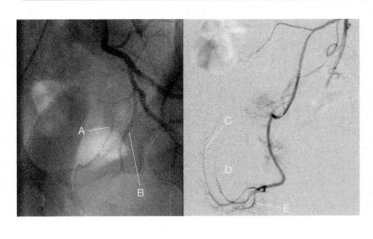
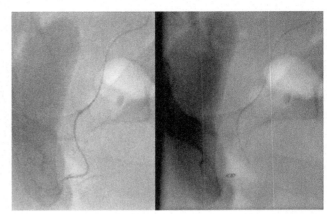

1. Name the arteries A to E.

2. How can priapism be classified?

3. What are the clinical features of low-flow priapism?

4. What are the clinical features of high-flow priapism?

5. What is the management of high-flow priapism?

Answers

1. A is the internal pudendal artery, B is the obturator artery, C is the dorsal artery of the penis, D is a cavernosal artery, and E is the scrotal artery.

2. It can be classified into high-flow and low-flow states.

3. It is due to venous stasis and is a urological emergency with risk of fibrosis, scarring, and erectile dysfunction. Sickle cell patients are particularly at risk. Measurement of oxygenation from a cavernosal blood sample is diagnostic. Low-flow priapism is treated by aspiration. Flushing, phenylephrine, or shunting may be required.

4. High-flow priapism typically occurs secondary to trauma and is due to underlying AV shunting. It is rarely painful and rarely leads to erectile dysfunction. It can be treated with embolization.

5. Doppler tumescent ultrasound can confirm the diagnosis prior to treatment. Unilateral internal pudendal artery embolization is performed. Gelfoam embolization reduces the risk of erectile dysfunction but increases the risk of recurrence compared to coiling. Cavernosal arterial ligation is needed if embolization fails. It can also be managed conservatively.

Pearls

- Internal iliac artery anatomy is variable. The internal pudendal artery arises from the anterior division of the internal iliac artery, and divides into the dorsal artery of the penis and the cavernosal artery.
- Priapism is divided into low-flow and high-flow states, and embolization is a treatment for high-flow lesions.

Suggested Reading

O'Sullivan P, Browne R, McEniff N, Lee MJ. Treatment of "high-flow" priapism with superselective transcatheter embolization: a useful alternative to surgery. *Cardiovasc Intervent Radiol.* 2006;29(2):198-201.

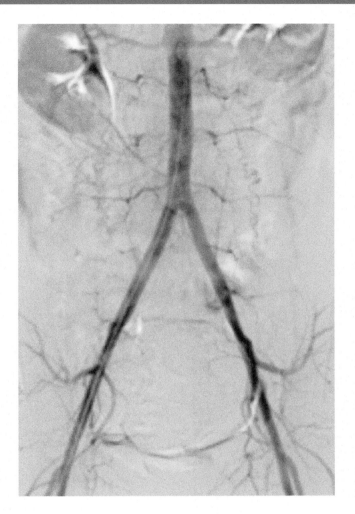

1. Patient presents for fibroid embolization—where is the vessel of interest on image 1?

2. How common is it to see these arteries using flush aortograms in this clinical setting?

3. What are the risk factors for ovarian artery supply of a fibroid?

4. When should ovarian arteries be looked for and what is the effect of embolization?

5. What are the potential origins of the ovarian artery?

Case ranking/difficulty: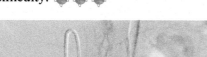

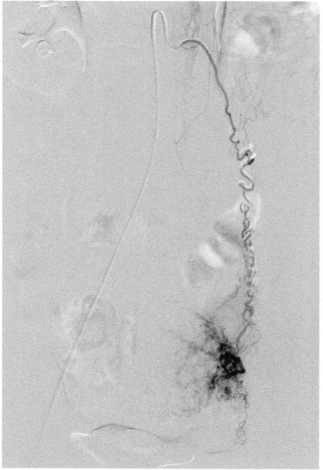

Selective left ovarian artery angiogram shows supply to the fibroid uterus.

Answers

1. Flush aortogram at the level of the renal arteries shows bilateral ovarian arteries.

2. One series of 300 patients identified 16 bilateral and 43 unilateral cases of visible ovarian arteries. The artery is usually more than 1 mm in size when identified on an aortogram, and in some cases can be hypertrophied and very large.

3. Previous pathology, surgery, and the presence of large fundal fibroids are risk factors.

4. Unilateral ovarian artery embolization increases clinical success in fibroid embolization, but does not cause early menopause and should be looked for if the uterine arteries are not hypertrophied or do not supply all of the uterus.

5. Aortic, renal, lumbar, phrenic, adrenal, and iliac sources have been described.

Pearls

- Ovarian arteries contribute to the pathologic blood supply in fibroids—this can be seen in around 1 in 20 of cases. They normally arise from the anterolateral aspect of the aorta between the renal arteries and the IMA.

Suggested Reading

Pelage JP, Walker WJ, Le Dref O, Rymer R. Ovarian artery: angiographic appearance, embolization and relevance to uterine fibroid embolization. *Cardiovasc Intervent Radiol.* 2003;26(3):227-233.

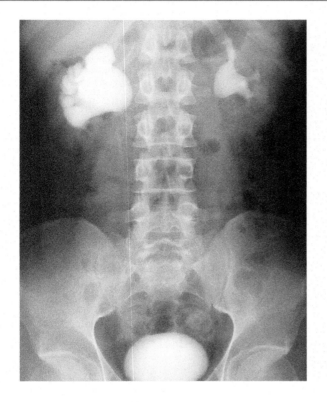
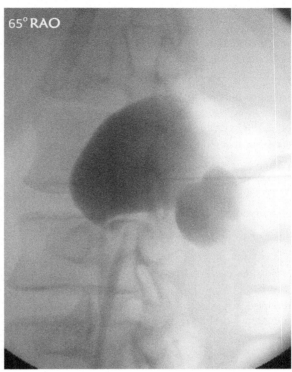

1. What is the most common etiology of ureteropelvic junction (UPJ) obstruction?

2. What contributes to primary UPJ obstruction?

3. What sign on antegrade pyelography is indicative of the crossing vessel phenomenon?

4. What are the causes of secondary UPJ obstruction?

5. What is the management of UPJ obstruction?

Case ranking/difficulty:

Answers

1. Most common cause of UPJ obstruction is primary (congenital) and is attributed to ureteral bud development. It is associated with excessive collagen tissue in the affected segment of the ureter.

2. Arrange of the muscle layers, excessive collagen deposition, ischaemia, and abnormal intercellular conduction have all been implicated as the underlying cause of primary UPJ obstruction.

3. An acute anterior indentation seen in the upper ureter 2 to 3 cm below the UPJ is a unique sign. Crossing can be anterior, posterior, or both, and both artery and vein can be involved.

4. Causes of secondary UPJ obstruction include infection, stones, surgery, ischemia, and iatrogenic injury.

5. Endopyelotomy is contraindicated because of potential risk of vascular injury. Surgical vascular reimplantation is required. An infected obstructed system requires percutaneous drainage as well as antibiotics.

Pearls

• A crossing vessel is one of the uncommon causes of UPJ or pelviureteric junction obstruction. There is a unique of sign of anterior crossing vessel that can be seen on a lateral projection, with an acute anterior indentation on the upper ureter 2 to 3 cm below the UPJ or a "tucked back" configuration. Endopyelotomy is contraindicated in this entity, and reimplantation of the crossing vessel is required.

Suggested Readings

Kletscher BA, Segura JW, LeRoy AJ, Patterson DE. Percutaneous antegrade endopyelotomy: review of 50 consecutive cases. *Urology* 1995;153(3 pt 1):701-703.

Wang W, LeRoy AJ, McKusick MA, Segura JW, Patterson DE. Detection of crossing vessels as the cause of ureteropelvic junction obstruction: the role of antegrade pyelography prior to endopyelotomy. *J Vasc Interv Radiol.* 2004;15(12):1435-1441.

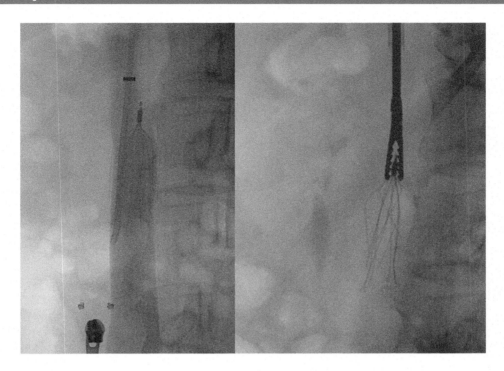

1. What is a valid reason to leave a filter in situ rather than retrieve it?

2. List some advanced techniques that can be used for filter retrieval.

3. What is the most serious potential complication that could be encountered during a difficult retrieval?

4. When should a filter be considered "unretrievable"?

5. What are the potential long-term risks of leaving a filter in situ permanently?

Case ranking/difficulty: 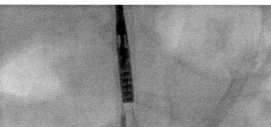   **Category:** Venous system

3. Detachment and subsequent loss of control of the filter could potentially result in its migration into the right heart with risk of arrhythmia, pericardial tamponade, and death.

4. In many cases, filters can be removed if the benefit-to-risk ratio remains in the patient's favor. However, loss of appropriate central access probably makes a filter irretrievable—for example, if there is superior vena cava occlusion.

5. These complications include fracture, migration, caval penetration, caval occlusion, and breakthrough pulmonary embolization.

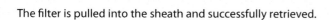

The filter is pulled into the sheath and successfully retrieved.

Pearls

- Up to 10% of retrievable IVC filters may not be able to be removed with conventional retrieval techniques. Filter tilt and endothelial overgrowth resulting in incorporation into the caval wall are 2 major causes of failure of filter retrieval.
- The use of self-made wire loop snares, balloon, and laser-assisted retrieval techniques are reported.
- Forceps-assisted filter retrieval may itself cause severe deformity and fracture of the filter components.

Answers

1. Large thrombus caught in IVC will eventually resolve. Therefore, the filter still can be removed after anticoagulation and appropriate follow-up.

2. Use of any equipment different to manufacturer guidance such as snare or dedicated retrieval sets may be seen as "advanced" techniques. The use of rigid bronchoscopy forceps and laser-assisted sheath techniques is also reported.

Suggested Readings

Kuo WT, Cupp JS, Louie JD, et al. Complex retrieval of embedded IVC filters: alternative techniques and histologic tissue analysis. *Cardiovasc Intervent Radiol.* 2012;35(3):588-597.

White SB, Stavropoulos SW. Retrieval of a wall-embedded recovery inferior vena cava filter using rigid bronchoscopy forceps. *Semin Intervent Radiol.* 2007;24(1):15-19.

Subject Index

Difficulty Level Index

Easy Cases

153, 2432, 154, 2425, 189, 2478, 237, 155, 157, 240, 177, 241, 1629, 450, 384, 196, 159, 161, 576, 206, 364, 2409, 2243, 2051, 2043, 2408, 288, 302, 2070, 207, 300, 289, 2013, 1671, 295, 274, 451, 301, 1603, 2004, 277, 296, 418, 243, 7, 332, 2503, 657, 247, 329, 294, 1751, 333, 385, 281, 179, 284, 2405, 2002, 2509, 2003, 2404, 2466, 2486, 2546, 2583, 2434, 2433, 2431, 656, 2586, 2620, 2417, 2413, 2472, 2410, 2076, 2584, 2005, 2491

Moderately Difficult Cases

2530, 2423, 2723, 238, 2421, 2467, 158, 156, 166, 2406, 2226, 1587, 1, 235, 577, 1586, 1998, 236, 267, 1696, 1748, 2045, 1747, 2078, 1613, 2044, 251, 2237, 383, 2637, 2033, 1750, 297, 287, 2481, 337, 330, 244, 245, 2426, 270, 298, 1791, 252, 1658, 362, 180, 2075, 2428, 282, 1855, 248, 2724, 249, 325, 327, 1752, 2427, 2403, 2412, 2411, 2254, 2456, 2526, 2505, 2424, 2485, 2479, 2475, 2494, 2402, 2469

Most Difficult Cases

1767, 2223, 2558, 2074, 2430, 2731, 1604, 2733, 338, 2001, 2071, 261, 250, 266, 268, 1697, 272, 409, 2077, 275, 271, 2416, 366, 2429, 331, 455, 2407, 328, 278, 2415, 1999, 181, 2585, 326, 2457, 283, 2079, 2531, 2730, 2495, 2414, 2621, 2640, 2660, 2729, 2588, 2484, 2587

Author Index

Acknowledgement Index